"HER BALICIOUS"

The Smile Enthusiast's Book of Bountiful Botanicals

THE SMILE ENTHUSIAST
Author of #FUTURECENTURIONLIFE, My Longevity Lifestyle

FOREWORD BY JENNY DIEHL, BCHN
BOARD-CERTIFIED HOLISTIC NUTRITIONIST

"HERBALICIOUS"
The Smile Enthusiast's Book of Bountiful Botanicals

"HERBALICIOUS"
Copyright © 2024 by The Smile Enthusiast

All rights reserved. No part of this publication may be reproduced, distributed, or transmitted in any form or by any means, including photocopying, recording, or other electronic or mechanical methods, without the prior written permission of the author, except in the case of brief quotations embodied in critical reviews and certain other non-commercial uses permitted by copyright law.

For permissions, inquiries, or for bulk sales, email: itsherbalicious@gmail.com

This textbook is for educational purposes only. The publisher and the author disclaim liability for any medical outcomes as a result of using any of the information which is outlined in this book.

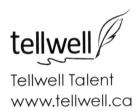

Tellwell Talent
www.tellwell.ca

ISBN
978-1-77941-012-2 (Paperback)

This book is dedicated to all the beautiful souls—

…Who are seeking to explore the vast realm of herbal medicine. I extend my warmest embrace to you.

I have been captivated by the enchanting world of herbalism since 2014, delving deep into the secrets of medicinal herbs. This journey has been more than a personal quest; it has been a relentless pursuit to unlock the wonders that the Divine forces have bestowed upon us. Today, as I stand at the crossroads of this profound exploration, I realize that keeping this treasure chest of herbal wisdom to myself would be a disservice to the world.

So, with a heart brimming with passion, I present this book to you. It is a labor of love, meticulously crafted to share the insights and knowledge gained along my odyssey of herbal discovery. This book is more than a collection of data; it is a testament to the remarkable potential that plants hold to enrich our existence and help us attain our best and longest lives.

Through these pages, I invite you to explore the power and possibilities of over 200 medicinal herbs from my herbal collection. Each page within this book is a celebration of Mother Nature and her bounty, carefully curated from years of study and unwavering dedication to herbalism. My purpose is simple yet profound: to ignite your curiosity, foster a deeper understanding, and empower you on your own path to well-being.

With love and gratitude,

Smile

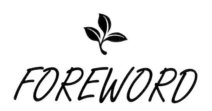

FOREWORD

I am absolutely honored and thrilled to have the opportunity to write the foreword for The Smile Enthusiast's incredible book, "HERBALICIOUS." As a board-certified holistic nutritionist, I have witnessed firsthand the transformative power of embracing Mother Nature's abundant offerings as a form of medicine. While traditional approaches and processed supplements have their place, there is something truly special about the healing properties of whole medicinal herbs and making our own fresh medicine with them.

Let's take a moment to celebrate Smile's incredible journey. For nearly a decade, she has been captivated by the world of medicinal herbs, fueled by her insatiable thirst for self-healing. What's truly remarkable is that she is entirely self-taught, accumulating a treasure chest of herbal wisdom over the years, which she has now lovingly translated into "HERBALICIOUS."

This remarkable soul overcame her own health challenges, including spending five years of her healing journey on an unsustainable supplement-heavy healing protocol (which didn't translate into the results that she hoped for). *This* was the catalyst that inspired her to use the tools and techniques her ancestors practiced—using weeds, roots, berries, twigs, bark, blossoms, roots, spices, and extracting these in water to make herbal infusions and decoctions (homemade herbal medicine).

Propelled by her own journey, Smile poured her heart into creating "HERBALICIOUS"—a book that shines a light on the wonders of Mother Nature's bounty. Smile opens up her vault of knowledge and wisdom about medicinal herbs and blesses us with this gift from the depths of her caring soul. Smile's passion shines through every page, and her dedication to helping others reclaim their health and extend their proverbial "shelf life" is truly uplifting.

Get ready to have your mind blown with "HERBALICIOUS!" This book is a true labor of love, meticulously crafted to shine a light on a collection of over 200 medicinal herbs and spices. What makes it truly unique is that it serves not only as a personal herbal pantry of a woman passionately striving to become a Guinness World Record holder in longevity, but it's also designed as a comprehensive reference guide. This book takes you on an educational journey, alphabetically listing each herb in The Smile Enthusiast's herbal pantry and delving into its origin, history, and not just a few but ten exceptional health benefits. But that's not all! Smile's attention to detail extends to the final paragraph for each herb, highlighting important contradictions that may arise. Think of it as having a wise and knowledgeable herbalist-friend by your side, educating you along your journey. With *"HERBALICIOUS,"* you've hit the mother lode—a single book that provides you with an extensive and exhaustive list of herbs and their capacity to provide value to human health in the name of longevity. My friends, this is a book brimming with a wealth of herbal education. Smile has gone above and beyond, delving deep into the world of active compounds: antioxidants, alkaloids, flavonoids, polyphenols, tannins, terpenoids, and so many other phytochemical wonders that make each herb truly remarkable.

In this impressively formulated herbal textbook, Smile has packed it with knowledge yet made it incredibly approachable and easy to understand. Whether you're new to the world of herbs or already have some herbal knowledge under your belt, this book is the perfect herbal reference tool. It's like embarking on a herbal odyssey through the realm of plant medicine. You will dive deep into these pages and emerge with a profound understanding of why these herbs hold such incredible value for human health and longevity. It will come as no surprise why these herbs are in The Smile Enthusiast's herbal pantry.

Now, I must confess my own admiration for Smile's work. As a board-certified holistic nutritionist, I can wholeheartedly endorse the information presented in *"HERBALICIOUS."* The level of detail and authenticity is amazing! Smile's ability to navigate through the sea of misinformation and present the most valuable information is a testament to her expertise. I am honored to be a part of *"HERBALICIOUS"* and lend my support to her extraordinary work.

"HERBALICIOUS" is not just a companion textbook to her longevity textbook, *"#FUTURECENTURIONLIFE;"* it's a gateway to a world of vibrant health, vitality, and longevity, shining a spotlight on plant medicine. *"HERBALICIOUS"* is a tool to mentor you in the field of medicinal herbs. It will positively accompany you on your own healing journey and quest to live your best, longest life.

So, my dear readers, I invite you to dive into the pages of *"HERBALICIOUS"* with an open heart, an open mind, and a sense of excitement. Let Smile's wisdom and passion for holistic healing and medicinal herbs inspire you as you uncover the secrets of herbal medicine and journey toward wellness, longevity, and a life well-lived.

Jenny Diehl, BCHN

TABLE OF CONTENTS

AÇAI BERRY (POWDER) 1
ALFALFA LEAF 3
ALLSPICE 7
ALOE VERA 9
AMLA BERRY (POWDER) 11
ANGELICA ROOT 13
ANISE SEED 17
ANISE, STAR (WHOLE) 19
ARNICA FLOWERS 21
ARONIA BERRY (POWDER) 23
ARTICHOKE LEAF 25
ASHWAGANDHA 27
ASTRAGALUS ROOT 29
BARBERRY BARK 31
BARBERRY FRUIT 33
BARLEY GRASS 35
BAY LEAF 37
BEETROOT POWDER 39
BILBERRIES 41
BILBERRY LEAF 43
BLACK COHOSH 47
BLACK PEPPERCORN 49
BLACK WALNUT 51
BLACKBERRY LEAF 53
BLADDERWRACK 55
BLESSED THISTLE 57
BLUE VERVAIN 59
BOLDO LEAF 61
BONESET 63
BORAGE 65
BOSWELLIA 69
BRAHMI LEAF (BACOPA) 71
BURDOCK ROOT 75
BUTTERBUR ROOT 77
CALENDULA FLOWERS 79

CALIFORNIA POPPY	83
CAMU CAMU BERRY (POWDER)	85
CARDAMOM	87
CINNAMON	91
CAT'S CLAW	95
CAYENNE PEPPER	99
CELERY SEED	101
CHAGA MUSHROOM	103
CHAMOMILE	107
CHAPARRAL LEAF	109
CHASTEBERRY (VITEX)	111
CHICORY ROOT	115
CHIPOTLE POWDER	117
CHRYSANTHEMUM FLOWERS	119
CLEAVERS	123
CLOVES	125
COMFREY LEAF	127
COMFREY ROOT	129
CORDYCEPS MUSHROOM	131
CORIANDER SEED	135
CORNFLOWERS	137
CORYDALIS ROOT	139
CURRY POWDER	141
DAMIANA	143
DANDELION LEAF	145
DANDELION ROOT	147
DEVIL'S CLAW	149
DILL WEED	151
DONG QUAI ROOT	153
DULSE FLAKES	155
ECHINACEA ANGUSTIFOLIA LEAF	157
ECHINACEA ANGUSTIFOLIA ROOT	159
ECHINACEA PURPUREA LEAF	161
ECHINACEA PURPUREA ROOT	165
ELDERFLOWER	167
ELDERBERRIES	169
ELECAMPANE ROOT	171
ELEUTHERO (SIBERIAN GINSENG)	173

ESSIAC TEA BLEND	175
EUCALYPTUS LEAF	177
EYEBRIGHT	179
FENNEL SEED	181
FENUGREEK LEAF	183
FENUGREEK SEED	187
FEVERFEW	191
FO-TI ROOT	193
GINGER ROOT	195
GINKGO	197
GINSENG, AMERICAN	201
GINSENG, KOREAN RED	205
GOAT'S RUE	207
GOJI BERRY (POWDER)	209
GOLDENSEAL	213
GOTU KOLA	217
GRAPEFRUIT PEEL	219
GREEK MOUNTAIN TEA	223
GUDUCHI	225
GYNOSTEMMA	227
HAWTHORN	231
HIBISCUS	235
HOLY BASIL (KRISHNA TULSI)	237
HOLY BASIL (RAMA TULSI)	239
HOLY BASIL (VANA TULSI)	243
HONEYSUCKLE	247
HOPS	251
HORSETAIL	253
HYSSOP	257
INDIAN SARSAPARILLA	261
JAMAICAN DOGWOOD	265
JAMAICAN SARSAPARILLA	269
JUJUBE SEED	273
JUNIPER BERRIES	275
KAVA KAVA	277
KELP	279
KNOTTED WRACK	281
KOMBU	283

KELPWEED	285
LAVENDER	287
LEMON BALM	289
LEMON PEEL	293
LEMON VERBENA	295
LEMONGRASS	299
LICORICE ROOT	303
LINDEN LEAF AND FLOWER	307
LION'S MANE MUSHROOM	309
LOBELIA	313
LOMATIUM ROOT	317
MANGOSTEEN PEEL (POWDER)	321
MAQUI BERRY (POWDER)	325
MARJORAM	329
MARSHMALLOW ROOT	331
MEADOWSWEET	335
MILK THISTLE SEED	339
MIMOSA ROOT	343
MISTLETOE (EUROPEAN)	347
MORINGA	351
MOTHERWORT	353
MUGWORT	357
MULLEIN LEAF	361
MUSTARD SEED	365
MYRRH GUM	367
NEEM LEAF	371
NETTLE LEAF	375
OATSTRAW	379
ORANGE PEEL	383
OLIVE LEAF	385
OREGANO LEAF	389
OREGON GRAPE ROOT	393
ORRIS ROOT	397
OSHA ROOT	401
PAPAYA SEED	405
PAPRIKA	409
PASSIONFLOWER	411
PAU D'ARCO	415

PEPPERMINT LEAF	419
PERIWINKLE	423
PERSIMMON LEAF	427
PINE NEEDLES	431
PLANTAIN LEAF	435
PSYLLIUM SEED	439
RED CLOVER	443
RED DRAGON FRUIT (POWDER)	447
RED RASPBERRY LEAF	451
REDROOT	455
REISHI MUSHROOM	459
RHODIOLA ROOT	463
ROSE BUD AND PETALS	467
ROSEHIPS	471
ROSEMARY	475
SAGE	479
SASSAFRAS ROOT	483
SAW PALMETTO BERRIES	487
SCHISANDRA BERRIES	491
SEA BUCKTHORN (POWDER)	495
SEA LETTUCE	499
SHANKHPUSHPI	503
SHATAVARI	507
SHEEP SORREL	511
SHEPHERD'S PURSE	515
SKULLCAP (AMERICAN)	519
SLIPPERY ELM BARK	523
SOLOMON'S SEAL	527
SPEARMINT LEAF	531
ST. JOHN'S WORT	535
SUMAC BERRIES	539
SWEETGUM BALLS	543
SWEET WOODRUFF	547
TANSY	551
THUJA	555
THYME	559
TURKEY TAIL MUSHROOM	563
TURMERIC	567

UVA URSI	571
VALERIAN ROOT	575
WAKAME	579
WHITE OAK BARK	583
WHITE PINE BARK	587
WHITE WILLOW BARK	591
WILD CHERRY BARK	595
WILD YAM	599
WINTERGREEN LEAF	603
WITCH HAZEL BARK	607
WOOD BETONY	611
WORMWOOD	615
YARROW	619
YELLOW DOCK	623

Mother Nature's Bounty: Exploring the World of Medicinal Herbs

Welcome to the world of medicinal herbs, a realm where nature's gifts intertwine with our journey toward wellness and longevity. As you embark on this exploration, it is essential to approach these herbs with love and the utmost respect, for they are treasures bestowed upon us by Mother Nature herself.

Within these pages reside a wealth of wisdom, held within each herb, unique fruit, and spice. Their profound essence stems from a harmonious blend of compounds and constituents, offering the potential to nourish, heal, and uplift. Cultivated by the Earth, nurtured by the sun, and caressed by the breeze, they embody the fruits of countless seasons and cycles, patiently awaiting to share their bountiful gifts with those who seek their solace.

As you delve into the world of plant medicine, I invite you to embrace these pages with an open heart and an open mind. Approach these botanical tools as allies on your journey toward optimal well-being and longevity. Honor their ancient lineage and the wisdom they have carried through generations. Let them be a source of inspiration, reminding us of our deep connection to the natural world.

As you embark on this enlightening journey, exploring the inherent value that each medicinal herb holds, may you not only discover a profound sense of inner balance and connection to Mother Earth but also appreciate the remarkable gifts from Mother Nature that provide our bodies with the tools to heal, thrive and survive in the the twenty-first century and beyond. These botanical wonders hold the potential to enrich our lives and support our well-being, empowering us to adopt a path of holistic vitality. Cherish the rituals and practices that honor their presence, for it is in these moments of deep respect and purpose that their innate healing abilities come alive. Let the wisdom of these herbs be a guiding light, illuminating the path toward holistic well-being and a harmonious connection with the natural world around you.

May you cultivate a loving relationship with these botanical gems and allow their energy to infuse your being, awakening a sense of gratitude and wonder for the intricate tapestry of life.

I warmly welcome you to this journey through the world of medicinal herbs. May the wisdom and healing power of Mother Nature's bounty guide you on a path of great health and longevity.

AÇAI BERRY (POWDER)

Açaí berries, scientifically known as Euterpe oleracea, is a small, purple fruit that grows on açaí palm trees native to the Amazon rainforest in Brazil. For centuries, the indigenous people of the Amazon have revered this fruit for its remarkable health benefits and ability to support longevity. Açaí berries have gained popularity around the world in recent years due to their high antioxidant content and various nutritional properties. Açaí berry powder is derived from the freeze-dried pulp of the fruit, which helps preserve its nutrient content.

Now, let's explore ten extensive health and longevity benefits associated with açaí berries:

1. **Antioxidant Powerhouse:** Açaí berries are packed with antioxidants, including anthocyanins, proanthocyanidins, and vitamin C. These antioxidants help combat free radicals, protect cells from oxidative damage, and support overall cellular health.
2. **Cardiovascular Health:** Açaí berries contain heart-healthy compounds like omega-3 fatty acids, phytosterols, and polyphenols, including resveratrol. These nutrients support cardiovascular health by reducing inflammation, improving blood circulation, and promoting healthy cholesterol levels.
3. **Brain Health:** Açaí berries are rich in polyphenols, such as catechins and quercetin, which have been linked to improved cognitive function, memory, and neuroprotective effects. They also contain essential fatty acids that support brain health.
4. **Anti-inflammatory Effects:** Açaí berries contain several anti-inflammatory compounds, including anthocyanins, quercetin, and omega-3 fatty acids. These compounds help reduce inflammation throughout the body, supporting joint health and potentially reducing the risk of chronic diseases.
5. **Immune System Support**: Açaí berries' high vitamin C content, along with other antioxidants like beta-carotene, helps strengthen the immune system and protect against infections and diseases.
6. **Eye Health:** Açaí berries contain nutrients like vitamin C, vitamin E, and anthocyanins, which contribute to healthy vision and may help protect against age-related macular degeneration and other eye disorders.
7. **Antimicrobial Effects:** Açaí berries contain antimicrobial compounds, such as ellagic acid and quercetin, that may help fight against certain pathogens, including bacteria and viruses, supporting overall immune health.

8. **Digestive Health:** Açaí berries are loaded with polyphenols and flavonoids; these berries possess potential prebiotic effects that foster a thriving gut microbiome. Beyond this, açaí berries also contain compounds like anthocyanins, which exhibit antioxidant and anti-inflammatory properties. These attributes contribute to a balanced gut environment by potentially deterring harmful pathogens, aiding in the maintenance of regular bowel movements, and supporting overall digestive harmony.
9. **Skin Health:** Açaí berries' abundance of antioxidants, particularly anthocyanins and vitamin C, may help protect the skin from oxidative stress and promote a youthful appearance. They also provide essential fatty acids that nourish the skin and support its elasticity.
10. **Detoxification:** Açaí berries contain antioxidants and phytochemicals that assist in the body's natural detoxification processes by neutralizing toxins and supporting liver function.

While açaí berries are generally considered safe to consume, there are a few warnings and contradictions to be aware of. Açaí berry supplements should be used with caution if you are taking specific medications, such as anticoagulants (e.g., warfarin) or antiplatelet drugs (e.g., aspirin), as they may interact with these medications and increase the risk of bleeding. Additionally, individuals with pollen allergies may be sensitive to açaí berries. Açaí berries in culinary amounts are generally considered safe for those who are pregnant or lactating. Consult with your herbalist/practitioner prior to using these berries in large therapeutic doses.

ALFALFA LEAF

Alfalfa leaf, scientifically known as Medicago sativa, holds a captivating history that stretches back centuries, spanning diverse cultures and lands. Originating in Central Asia, this perennial flowering plant quickly garnered attention for its exceptional adaptability, becoming a cherished forage crop across various climates and soils. But alfalfa's tale goes beyond agriculture; it ventured into the realms of traditional medicine, capturing the imaginations of ancient healing practices like Ayurveda and Chinese medicine. Celebrated for its unique qualities, alfalfa earned the evocative moniker "father of all foods," signifying its rich nutritional value and versatile applications. Its journey from humble beginnings to a revered herb showcases a captivating narrative of resilience, nourishment, and cultural significance, making it an enchanting botanical ally worth exploring.

Now, let's explore ten extensive health and longevity benefits associated with alfalfa leaf:

1. **Nutrient-Dense:** Alfalfa leaf is a powerhouse of essential nutrients, including vitamins A, C, E, and K, as well as minerals like calcium, magnesium, potassium, and iron. These nutrients play vital roles in supporting overall health and proper bodily functions.
2. **Antioxidant Powerhouse:** Alfalfa leaf is abundant in antioxidants such as flavonoids, phenolic compounds, carotenoids, and various saponins. These antioxidants help neutralize harmful free radicals, protect cells from oxidative stress, and contribute to graceful aging and longevity.
3. **Digestive Health:** The high fiber content in alfalfa leaf promotes healthy digestion by aiding in regular bowel movements and preventing constipation. It can also support the growth of beneficial gut bacteria, contributing to a balanced gut microbiome.
4. **Detoxification:** Alfalfa leaf contains chlorophyll, a natural pigment that has been shown to aid in detoxification processes in the body. Chlorophyll helps eliminate toxins and heavy metals, supporting liver health and overall detoxification.
5. **Immune System Support:** Alfalfa leaf possesses immune-enhancing properties attributed to its high vitamin C content and the presence of immune-modulating compounds, including L-canavanine—an amino acid found in alfalfa. L-canavanine is known for its immunomodulatory effects, contributing to the regulation of immune responses.

6. **Cardiovascular Health:** The presence of bioactive compounds like saponins and flavonoids in alfalfa leaf has been linked to improved cardiovascular health. These compounds help reduce cholesterol levels, lower blood pressure, and prevent the formation of blood clots.
7. **Hormonal Balance:** Alfalfa leaf contains plant compounds called phytoestrogens, such as coumestrol and isoflavones, which have estrogen-like effects in the body and may help balance hormone levels (they have a similar structure to human estrogen). These phytoestrogens may help balance hormone levels, particularly in menopausal women, reducing symptoms like hot flashes and mood swings.
8. **Bone Health:** Alfalfa leaf is a good source of calcium, magnesium, and vitamin K, all of which are essential for maintaining strong and healthy bones. Regular intake may help reduce the risk of osteoporosis and improve bone density.
9. **Menstrual Support:** The phytoestrogens present in alfalfa leaf can provide relief from menstrual discomfort and symptoms such as bloating, cramps, and mood swings. Its anti-inflammatory properties may also help reduce pain and inflammation associated with menstruation.
10. **Skin Health:** The antioxidants and anti-inflammatory compounds in alfalfa leaf contribute to healthy, glowing skin. Regular consumption or topical use of alfalfa leaf extract may help reduce signs of aging, improve skin tone, and promote a youthful appearance.

While alfalfa leaf is generally considered safe to consume for most individuals, there are a few medical contradictions and precautions to be aware of. It is important to note that alfalfa leaf may interact with blood-thinning medications, such as warfarin or heparin, potentially increasing the risk of bleeding. If you are taking these medications, it is essential to consult with your healthcare professional before incorporating alfalfa leaf into your routine. Individuals with known allergies to plants in the Fabaceae/Leguminosae family, such as peanuts, soybeans, or lentils, may also experience allergic reactions to alfalfa leaf. It is crucial to exercise caution or consult a healthcare professional if you have specific medical conditions or are taking medications that may interact with the herb. Regarding safety during pregnancy and lactation, it is advisable to consult with your herbalist/practitioner before consuming alfalfa leaf to ensure it is safe for you and your baby.

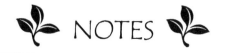

NOTES

ALLSPICE

Allspice, scientifically known as Pimenta dioica, is a fragrant spice with a fascinating origin and a wide array of health benefits. Native to the Caribbean and Central America, allspice gets its name from its unique flavor, which resembles a combination of cloves, cinnamon, and nutmeg. The spice is derived from the dried, unripe berries of the allspice tree, which is an evergreen tree belonging to the Myrtle family. Allspice has been used for centuries as a culinary ingredient, as well as in traditional medicine, due to its aromatic properties and potential health-promoting effects.

Now, let's explore ten extensive health and longevity benefits associated with allspice:

1. **Antioxidant Powerhouse:** Allspice contains a rich concentration of antioxidants, including phenolic compounds like eugenol, which help neutralize free radicals and protect cells from oxidative damage.
2. **Digestive Health:** Allspice provides digestive support by offering carminative properties that aid in digestion, alleviate indigestion, bloating, and flatulence, and promote a healthy gut function. Additionally, it has a traditional use as a natural remedy for digestive discomfort, including nausea and diarrhea.
3. **Anti-inflammatory Effects:** The active compounds in allspice, such as eugenol and caryophyllene, have been found to possess anti-inflammatory properties, potentially reducing inflammation throughout the body and alleviating symptoms of inflammatory conditions.
4. **Pain Relief:** Allspice has traditionally been used for its analgesic properties. The eugenol compound found in allspice may have mild pain-relieving effects and can be used topically to relieve muscle aches and joint pain.
5. **Respiratory Health:** Allspice contains compounds that have expectorant properties, which may help alleviate congestion and promote respiratory health by loosening phlegm and mucus.
6. **Blood Pressure Regulation:** Preliminary studies suggest that allspice may have hypotensive effects, potentially aiding in the regulation of blood pressure levels and reducing the risk of hypertension.
7. **Oral Health:** The antibacterial properties of allspice may help combat oral bacteria, potentially preventing gum disease, cavities, and bad breath.

8. **Antimicrobial Effects:** Allspice possesses antimicrobial properties, making it a potential natural remedy for certain infections. The active compound responsible for its antimicrobial activity is eugenol, which exhibits strong antibacterial and antifungal properties.
9. **Immune System Support:** Allspice contains essential vitamins and minerals, such as vitamin C, vitamin A, and iron, which can support a healthy immune system and enhance the body's ability to fight infections and diseases.
10. **Mood Support:** Allspice has been used traditionally for its uplifting aroma and potential mood-enhancing effects. Its fragrance is believed to have a calming influence, potentially reducing stress and promoting relaxation.

> While allspice is generally considered safe to consume, it is important to be aware of potential contradictions and interactions, especially if you are taking certain medications or have underlying health conditions. Allspice may interact with specific medications, including anticoagulants like warfarin, as it contains eugenol, a compound that may increase the risk of bleeding. It is advisable to consult with a healthcare professional if you are taking anticoagulant medications or have a bleeding disorder before using allspice as a herbal supplement. It is important to note that individuals with allergies to spices, particularly those in the Myrtle family, such as cloves or eucalyptus, may also be allergic to allspice due to potential cross-reactivity. Regarding pregnancy and lactation, allspice is generally considered safe when used in culinary amounts.

ALOE VERA

Aloe vera, scientifically known as Aloe barbadensis miller, boasts a history that spans centuries, interwoven with tales of discovery, healing, and cultural significance. Originating from the Arabian Peninsula, this succulent plant's legacy is dotted with fascinating anecdotes from ancient civilizations like the Egyptians, who revered it as the "plant of immortality." Renowned for its resilience and ability to thrive in arid environments, aloe vera's widespread cultivation gradually spread across the globe, transcending geographical boundaries. Its gel-like sap, extracted from its fleshy leaves, has found multifaceted applications throughout history, serving not only as a natural remedy for various ailments but also as a valuable ingredient in beauty and skincare rituals.

Now, let's explore ten extensive health and longevity benefits associated with aloe vera gel:

1. **Skin Health:** Aloe vera gel is renowned for its soothing and moisturizing properties. It contains vitamins such as vitamin E and vitamin C, which help nourish and protect the skin. Additionally, antioxidants like polyphenols and flavonoids in aloe vera gel can support healthy skin aging and combat oxidative stress.
2. **Wound Healing:** Aloe vera gel contains compounds like polysaccharides and glycoproteins that contribute to its wound-healing properties. These compounds aid in reducing inflammation, promoting cell growth, and increasing collagen synthesis, thus accelerating the healing process.
3. **Digestive Health:** Aloe vera gel contains enzymes such as amylase and lipase, which aid in the digestion of carbohydrates and fats. It also contains polysaccharides, including acemannan, that support gut health by promoting a healthy balance of gut flora and enhancing nutrient absorption.
4. **Immune System Support:** Aloe vera gel contains various antioxidants, including vitamins A, C, and E, as well as polyphenols. These antioxidants help neutralize free radicals and support a strong immune system, reducing the risk of chronic diseases and promoting longevity.
5. **Anti-inflammatory Effects:** Aloe vera gel contains several anti-inflammatory compounds, such as bradykinase and salicylic acid. These compounds help reduce inflammation and alleviate associated discomfort, supporting the health of various organs and body systems.

6. **Cardiovascular Health:** The antioxidant properties of aloe vera gel, attributed to compounds like vitamins C and E, help protect against oxidative stress and inflammation, both of which are risk factors for cardiovascular diseases. Aloe vera gel may also support healthy cholesterol levels, promoting heart health.
7. **Detoxification:** Aloe vera gel contains compounds like polysaccharides and antioxidants, including glutathione and superoxide dismutase (SOD), which help support the body's natural detoxification processes. These compounds aid in eliminating toxins, reducing oxidative stress, and supporting overall health and longevity.
8. **Oral Health:** Aloe vera gel possesses antimicrobial properties attributed to compounds like anthraquinones, which help combat harmful bacteria in the oral cavity. It can be used as a natural mouthwash to promote healthy gums and reduce the risk of oral infections.
9. **Joint Health:** Aloe vera gel contains anti-inflammatory compounds, such as bradykinase and salicylic acid, which may help alleviate joint pain and stiffness. Additionally, the vitamins and minerals in aloe vera gel support the health of bones and joints.
10. **Antimicrobial Effects:** Aloe vera gel contains compounds like anthraquinones, which possess antimicrobial properties against various pathogens, including bacteria and fungi. These properties may help fight against harmful microorganisms and support overall health.

> While aloe vera gel, derived from the inner part of the leaf, is generally considered safe for consumption, the green outer leaf should be avoided. It's important to carefully process and extract the gel to ensure minimal contamination with the latex containing aloin. Consuming aloe leaf, specifically the green outer portion, is generally not recommended as it contains a compound called aloin (also known as anthraquinone glycosides), which can have laxative effects and potentially cause adverse gastrointestinal symptoms if consumed in large quantities. Aloin is found in the latex layer located just beneath the skin of the aloe leaf. It is important to note that aloe vera gel and aloe leaf may interact with certain medications, including diuretics, steroids, and medications that affect blood sugar levels. Consult with a healthcare professional before using aloe vera gel in such cases to avoid potential interactions or adverse effects. Aloe vera gel is generally considered safe to consume during pregnancy and lactation.

AMLA BERRY (POWDER)

Amla berries, scientifically known as Emblica officinalis, has a rich history dating back thousands of years to ancient India and Southeast Asia. Revered as the "fruit of life" or "Indian gooseberry," amla holds deep cultural significance and diverse traditional uses. It comes from the deciduous tree Emblica officinalis, thriving in various climates across India and Southeast Asia. Ayurvedic medicine values amla as a potent rejuvenative tonic and elixir of life due to its abundant phytonutrients and antioxidants. The tangy fruit can be enjoyed fresh or as amla powder, obtained by sun drying and grinding the fruit.

Now, let's explore ten extensive health and longevity benefits associated with amla berries:

1. **Immune System Support:** Amla berries are rich in vitamin C, providing a significant boost to the immune system. Vitamin C helps stimulate the production of white blood cells, enhances immune response, and acts as an antioxidant to protect against free radicals.
2. **Antioxidant Powerhouse:** Amla berries contain potent antioxidants such as ellagic acid, gallic acid, and quercetin. These antioxidants help neutralize harmful free radicals, protecting cells from oxidative damage and reducing the risk of chronic diseases.
3. **Liver Health:** Amla berries contain phytochemicals like phyllanthin and gallic acid, which exhibit hepatoprotective properties, supporting liver health and detoxification processes.
4. **Cardiovascular Health:** The antioxidants in amla berries, including gallic acid and ellagic acid, help reduce oxidative stress and inflammation in the cardiovascular system, promoting heart health and reducing the risk of heart disease.
5. **Digestive Health:** Amla berries are rich in dietary polyphenols, including tannins and flavonoids, which possess anti-inflammatory and gastroprotective properties. These compounds help soothe the digestive tract, reduce inflammation, and support healthy digestion.
6. **Brain Health:** Amla berries contain antioxidants like quercetin and vitamin C, which may help protect against neurodegenerative diseases and support cognitive function. They also enhance the production of acetylcholine, a neurotransmitter important for memory and learning.

7. **Graceful-aging Effects:** Amla berries' high antioxidant content, including vitamin C and ellagic acid, helps combat oxidative stress, which contributes to the graceful aging process. These antioxidants support healthy skin, hair, and overall cellular health.
8. **Eye Health:** Amla berries are a rich source of vitamin C, which supports the health of blood vessels in the eyes and may help reduce the risk of age-related macular degeneration. The berries also contain carotenoids, such as zeaxanthin and lutein, which protect the eyes from oxidative damage.
9. **Anti-inflammatory Effects:** Amla berries contain quercetin, gallic acid, and ellagic acid, which possess anti-inflammatory properties. These compounds help reduce inflammation throughout the body, supporting joint health and reducing the risk of chronic diseases associated with inflammation.
10. **Antimicrobial Effects:** Amla berries exhibit antimicrobial properties due to the presence of compounds like ellagitannins and emblicanin. These properties help inhibit the growth of harmful bacteria, fungi, and viruses, supporting overall health and reducing the risk of infections.

> While amla berries are generally considered safe to consume, it is important to note a few warnings and contradictions. Individuals taking blood-thinning medications, such as warfarin, should exercise caution as amla berries may potentiate the effects of these medications. Additionally, individuals with hypoglycemia should monitor their blood sugar levels closely when consuming amla berries as it may lower blood sugar levels. It is also advised to consult a healthcare professional before using amla berries as a dietary supplement if you have any underlying health conditions or are taking medications. Amla berries are generally considered safe for consumption during pregnancy and lactation when consumed in moderate amounts as a food. Consult with your herbalist/practitioner prior to using amla berry supplements or extractions in large therapeutic doses during these times.

ANGELICA ROOT

Angelica root, scientifically known as Angelica archangelica, has a captivating and storied history that spans centuries. Originating in the northern regions of Europe, including Scandinavia, Iceland, and Russia, this herb has played a prominent role in various cultural practices and traditional remedies. Its name, "Angelica," is often associated with angelic symbolism, though its exact origin remains a subject of historical intrigue. Revered for its aromatic properties, angelica root has been used in culinary delights, such as flavoring liqueurs and confectionery treats. It also holds a deep significance in folklore and herbal folklore, with legends attributing its discovery to divine revelation, linking it to angels' protective powers. Throughout history, angelica root has been valued for its versatility, not only as a medicinal herb but also as a flavoring agent, aromatic stimulant, and even a talisman against evil spirits.

Now, let's explore ten extensive health and longevity benefits associated with angelica root:

1. **Digestive Health:** Angelica root contains essential oils like limonene and terpinen-4-ol, which have carminative properties. These compounds help relax and soothe the digestive tract, reducing bloating, gas, and indigestion. Additionally, the herb's coumarins and flavonoids may stimulate digestive enzyme secretion, promoting efficient nutrient absorption and overall digestive health.
2. **Immune System Support:** Angelica root's coumarins, such as osthol and bergapten, exhibit immunomodulatory effects, supporting the immune system's response to pathogens. These active constituents may enhance the activity of immune cells, aiding in the body's defense against infections.
3. **Respiratory Health:** The essential oils, including β-phellandrene and β-caryophyllene, found in angelica root possess expectorant and anti-inflammatory properties. These compounds help ease respiratory congestion, promote mucus clearance, and soothe inflamed airways, providing relief from respiratory discomforts.
4. **Hormonal Balance:** The phytoestrogens present in angelica root, such as coumarins and flavonoids, can interact with estrogen receptors and help regulate hormonal balance. This may be particularly beneficial for women experiencing hormonal fluctuations during menopause.

5. **Cardiovascular Health:** Angelica root's coumarins, such as umbelliferone and herniarin, possess vasodilatory properties that help relax blood vessels, potentially reducing blood pressure. This herb's antioxidant compounds may help prevent oxidative damage to blood vessels, supporting cardiovascular health.
6. **Anti-inflammatory Effects:** The active compounds in angelica root, such as ferulic acid and various flavonoids, inhibit pro-inflammatory pathways, reducing the production of inflammatory molecules. This may alleviate symptoms of inflammatory conditions and promote overall well-being.
7. **Liver Health:** Angelica root's essential oils, like a-pinene and limonene, have hepatoprotective properties that help protect the liver from damage and enhance its detoxification processes. These active constituents may also stimulate the production of liver-protective enzymes.
8. **Anxiety and Stress Relief:** The herb's coumarins and polysaccharides may modulate the release of neurotransmitters like serotonin and dopamine, contributing to a sense of calmness and reducing anxiety and stress levels.
9. **Antioxidant Powerhouse:** Angelica root's phenolic compounds, including ferulic acid and various flavonoids, act as potent antioxidants, neutralizing harmful free radicals in the body. This antioxidant defense may help prevent oxidative stress and cellular damage.
10. **Antimicrobial Effects:** Angelica root's essential oils, such as terpinen-4-ol and β-phellandrene, exhibit antimicrobial properties that can inhibit the growth of bacteria and fungi. These active constituents may support the body's natural defense against microbial infections.

While angelica root is generally considered safe to consume, there are certain medical contradictions and drug interactions that individuals should be aware of. This herb may interact with anticoagulant medications, increasing the risk of bleeding. It is not recommended for individuals with bleeding disorders or those preparing for surgery. Angelica root can also interact with certain medications metabolized by the liver's CYP3A4 enzyme, potentially altering their effectiveness. Allergy to angelica root is rare, but individuals with known allergies to plants in the Apiaceae family, such as celery, carrots, or dill, should exercise caution. Pregnant women should avoid using angelica root, as it may stimulate uterine contractions and affect hormone levels, potentially posing risks to the pregnancy. Those who are breastfeeding should consult with their herbalist/practitioner prior to using angelica root.

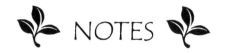

NOTES

ANISE SEED

Anise seed, scientifically known as Pimpinella anisum, is a flavorful and aromatic spice with a fascinating history and an array of health benefits. Native to the Mediterranean region and parts of Asia, anise seed has been cultivated and used for its medicinal properties for thousands of years. The seeds of the anise plant resemble small, brownish-green crescents and have a distinct licorice-like flavor and scent. Anise seed has a rich cultural heritage and has been a prominent ingredient in various culinary traditions, herbal remedies, and traditional medicine systems around the world.

Now, let's explore ten extensive health and longevity benefits associated with anise seed:

1. **Digestive Health:** Anise seeds contain anethole, a compound that has been shown to possess antispasmodic properties, helping to relax the muscles of the gastrointestinal tract and alleviate digestive issues such as bloating, gas, and indigestion.
2. **Respiratory Health:** Anise seeds have expectorant properties, which may help loosen and expel mucus from the respiratory system. This is beneficial for respiratory conditions like coughs, bronchitis, and asthma. The active compound responsible for this effect is called anethole.
3. **Anti-inflammatory Effects:** Anise seeds contain antioxidants like quercetin and kaempferol, which have anti-inflammatory properties. These compounds may help reduce inflammation in the body and support overall health.
4. **Liver Health:** Anise seeds contain essential oils, including anethole, which have been shown to have hepatoprotective properties, supporting liver health and detoxification processes.
5. **Antimicrobial Effects:** Anethole, present in anise seeds, exhibits antimicrobial activity against various bacteria and fungi. It may help inhibit the growth of pathogens, contributing to improved overall health.
6. **Detoxification:** Anethole and other compounds present in anise seeds have been found to support the detoxification processes of the liver, aiding in the elimination of toxins from the body and promoting a healthy digestive system.
7. **Antispasmodic Effects:** Anise seeds have been used traditionally to alleviate muscle spasms and cramps. This is attributed to the presence of anethole, which acts as a relaxant for smooth muscles.

8. **Hormonal Balance:** Anise seeds contain phytoestrogens, such as anethole, which have estrogenic effects and may help regulate hormonal imbalances. This can be beneficial for conditions related to hormonal fluctuations, such as menstrual discomfort and menopausal symptoms.
9. **Antioxidant Powerhouse:** Anise seeds are rich in antioxidants like quercetin, kaempferol, and coumarins, which help neutralize harmful free radicals and protect cells from oxidative stress, supporting longevity and overall health.
10. **Mood Support:** Anise seeds have been associated with potential mood-enhancing effects. Compounds like anethole and estragole may help alleviate symptoms of anxiety and promote a sense of calm and relaxation.

> While anise seed is generally considered safe to consume, there are a few important warnings and contradictions to consider. Individuals with estrogen-sensitive conditions, such as breast cancer, endometriosis, or uterine fibroids, should exercise caution as anise seed may have estrogenic effects. It is also recommended to avoid anise seed if you are taking anticoagulant medications, such as warfarin, as it may enhance the effects of these drugs and increase the risk of bleeding. Those who are pregnant or breastfeeding should consult with their herbalist/practitioner prior to using star anise seeds.

ANISE, STAR (WHOLE)

Star anise, scientifically known as Illicium verum, boasts a fascinating and diverse history dating back centuries. Originating in East Asia, particularly China and Vietnam, this star-shaped spice has been revered for its unique flavor and aromatic properties. Its botanical name, "Illicium verum," translates to "true anise," distinguishing it from the unrelated common anise (Pimpinella anisum). Star anise's striking appearance, resembling a star with eight points, is both visually captivating and a testament to its botanical wonder. Notably, this spice has been widely used in various cuisines worldwide, adding a distinct licorice-like flavor to both sweet and savory dishes. Beyond culinary use, star anise has played a vital role in traditional medicine and cultural practices, where it symbolizes luck, protection, and divine inspiration.

Now, let's explore ten extensive health and longevity benefits associated with star anise:

1. **Digestive Health:** Star anise contains anethole, a compound known for its carminative properties that can aid in relieving digestive issues such as bloating, indigestion, and gas.
2. **Anti-inflammatory Effects:** The antioxidants found in star anise, including quercetin, exhibit anti-inflammatory properties, helping to reduce inflammation and support overall health.
3. **Respiratory Health:** The essential oil in star anise contains compounds such as terpineol and shikimic acid, which have expectorant properties and may help alleviate respiratory conditions like coughs, colds, and bronchitis.
4. **Immune System Support:** Star anise is rich in vitamin C, known for its immune-boosting effects, helping to strengthen the immune system and protect against infections.
5. **Antioxidant Powerhouse:** Star anise is a potent source of antioxidants, including flavonoids like quercetin, which help combat oxidative stress and reduce the risk of chronic diseases.
6. **Cardiovascular Health:** Star anise contains minerals like potassium and magnesium, which contribute to maintaining a healthy cardiovascular system, including regulating blood pressure and supporting heart function.
7. **Anti-cancer Effects:** Star anise contains certain compounds, such as quercetin, that have been associated with potential anti-cancer effects, including inhibiting the growth of cancer cells and protecting against oxidative damage.

8. **Liver Health:** The compound anethole found in star anise has shown hepatoprotective properties, supporting liver health and aiding in detoxification processes.
9. **Antimicrobial Effects:** Star anise contains compounds such as anethole and eugenol, which have antimicrobial properties, potentially helping to combat harmful pathogens.
10. **Anti-viral Effects:** Star anise is a natural source of shikimic acid, which is used in the production of antiviral drugs, including those used to combat influenza viruses. Shikimic acid is an important compound in the synthesis of the antiviral medication oseltamivir (Tamiflu).

> While star anise is generally considered safe to consume, there are a few important warnings and contradictions to consider. Star anise contains a compound called anethole, which can have estrogenic effects and may interfere with certain medications, particularly hormone therapies or contraceptives. Individuals using medications such as tamoxifen or other selective estrogen receptor modulators should exercise caution when consuming star anise. Additionally, individuals with estrogen-sensitive conditions, such as breast cancer, should avoid star anise or consult with a healthcare professional before using it. Those who are pregnant or breastfeeding should consult with their herbalist/practitioner prior to using star anise.

ARNICA FLOWERS

Arnica flowers, scientifically known as Arnica montana, are vibrant yellow blooms with a rich history and a host of health benefits. Native to mountainous regions of Europe and Siberia, arnica flowers have been revered for centuries for their medicinal properties. These daisy-like flowers thrive in rocky, alpine environments and have been used in traditional medicine practices around the world. The flowers are carefully harvested and dried to preserve their therapeutic compounds, making them a valuable ingredient in herbal remedies and topical applications.
Now, let's explore ten extensive health and longevity benefits associated with arnica flowers:

1. **Anti-inflammatory Effects:** Arnica flowers contain flavonoids, such as quercetin and luteolin derivatives, as well as sesquiterpene lactones, which possess anti-inflammatory effects when used topically, potentially reducing inflammation and associated discomfort.
2. **Insect Bite and Sting Relief:** Arnica can be applied to insect bites and stings to reduce itching and discomfort.
3. **Wound Healing:** Arnica flowers contain flavonoids such as quercetin, along with thymol derivatives which possess antioxidant and anti-inflammatory properties that may aid in wound healing and tissue repair when applied topically. Arnica also contains various triterpenoid compounds that may enhance cell proliferation and collagen synthesis, which are essential processes for wound closure and tissue regeneration.
4. **Bruising Reduction Effects:** The flavonoid content in arnica flowers may help strengthen blood vessels and reduce leakage, potentially reducing bruising, when applied topically.
5. **Muscle Pain Relief:** Arnica's anti-inflammatory and analgesic properties may provide topical relief from muscle soreness and stiffness, aiding in post-exercise recovery.
6. **Skin Health:** Arnica flowers contain antioxidants, such as phenolic acids and flavonoids, which can protect the skin from oxidative stress and support skin health when used topically.
7. **Hair and Scalp Health:** The flavonoids and essential oils in arnica flowers may promote hair growth, improve scalp health, and reduce dandruff, when used topically.
8. **Swelling Reduction Effects:** Arnica may assist in reducing localized swelling, such as swelling associated with injuries.

9. **Antimicrobial Effects:** Some studies suggest that arnica extracts exhibit antimicrobial properties, which may help inhibit the growth of certain bacteria and fungi when used topically.
10. **Anti-edema Effects:** Arnica flowers have been traditionally used to reduce edema by potentially improving circulation and reducing fluid retention.

Arnica flowers are *not* generally considered safe to consume, as they can be toxic in high quantities and can lead to severe adverse effects. Arnica flowers are commonly used for topical applications and should be used with caution and under the guidance of your herbalist. Topical use of arnica may cause skin irritation or allergic reactions in some individuals, especially those with sensitive skin. It is essential to avoid using arnica on broken skin or open wounds. If you are taking any medications, especially blood thinners like warfarin, or have any underlying health conditions, it is crucial to consult with a healthcare professional before using arnica to avoid potential interactions or complications. Individuals with known allergies to plants in the Asteraceae family, such as ragweed or daisies, should exercise caution when using arnica. It is *not* recommended to use arnica flowers internally during pregnancy or lactation.

ARONIA BERRY (POWDER)

Aronia berries, scientifically known as Aronia melanocarpa, are small, dark berries with a fascinating history and an impressive range of health benefits. Native to North America, particularly the eastern regions of the United States and Canada, aronia berries have been cherished by Native American tribes for centuries due to their medicinal properties. Also known as chokeberries, these berries grow on shrubs that thrive in wetlands and forests. Aronia berries are rich in antioxidants and phytochemicals, making them a popular choice for both culinary and medicinal purposes. Aronia berry powder is derived by harvesting the aronia berries at peak ripeness, washing them to remove impurities, and then air drying or dehydrating them to reduce moisture content. High quality aronia berry powder is derived from the freeze-dried pulp of the fruit, which helps preserve its nutrient content.

Now, let's explore ten extensive health and longevity benefits associated with aronia berries:

1. **Antioxidant Powerhouse:** Aronia berries are packed with antioxidants, anthocyanins, and flavonoids such as quercetin and epicatechin. These compounds help neutralize harmful free radicals, which are known to contribute to aging and various age-related diseases. By reducing oxidative stress and cellular damage, antioxidants can support overall health and potentially extend lifespan.
2. **Cardiovascular Health:** The high levels of antioxidants and polyphenols in aronia berries contribute to heart health. They may help lower blood pressure, reduce inflammation in the arteries, improve blood circulation, and reduce the risk of cardiovascular diseases.
3. **Immune System Support:** Aronia berries contain immune-boosting compounds that help strengthen the immune system. They may enhance the body's natural defense mechanisms, reduce the risk of infections, and promote overall immune health.
4. **Anti-inflammatory Effects:** The phytochemicals present in aronia berries possess anti-inflammatory properties, which may help alleviate chronic inflammation in the body. They may be beneficial in reducing inflammation-related conditions such as arthritis and inflammatory bowel disease.

5. **Digestive Health:** Aronia berries are rich in polyphenols, which have been shown to support gut health by promoting the growth of beneficial gut bacteria and maintaining a balanced gut microbiome.
6. **Cognitive Function:** The antioxidant compounds in aronia berries have been linked to improved cognitive function and brain health. They may help protect against age-related cognitive decline, enhance memory, and support overall brain function.
7. **Skin Health:** Aronia berries' high antioxidant content can benefit the skin by protecting it against oxidative stress and promoting a youthful appearance. They may help reduce the signs of aging, improve skin elasticity, and support overall skin health.
8. **Antimicrobial Effects:** Aronia berries possess antimicrobial properties attributed to their polyphenols, which can inhibit the growth of certain bacteria and fungi, supporting overall health and aiding in pathogen defense.
9. **Eye Health:** The anthocyanins found in aronia berries are beneficial for eye health. They may help reduce the risk of age-related macular degeneration and protect the eyes from oxidative damage.
10. **Anti-cancer Effects:** Aronia berries have shown promising anti-cancer properties in various studies. The antioxidants and phytochemicals they contain may help inhibit the growth of cancer cells, reduce inflammation, and support overall cellular health.

While aronia berries are generally considered safe to consume, there are a few important warnings and contradictions to consider. Individuals taking anticoagulant medications, such as warfarin, should exercise caution, as aronia berry may interact with these medications and increase the risk of bleeding. Those with low blood pressure should also be cautious when consuming aronia berries, as it may further lower blood pressure levels. Additionally, individuals with known allergies to berries or similar fruits should avoid consumption of aronia berries. It is generally considered safe to consume culinary amounts of aronia berries during pregnancy and lactation. Seek the advice of your herbalist/practitioner before consuming large quantities of aronia berries during these periods.

ARTICHOKE LEAF

Artichoke leaf, scientifically known as Cynara cardunculus var. scolymus, has a captivating history that traces its origins back to ancient times. Native to the Mediterranean region, this herbaceous perennial plant has been cultivated for centuries for its delectable and nutritious edible buds. The ancient Greeks and Romans highly revered the artichoke, considering it a delicacy and a symbol of prosperity and fertility. In fact, the term "artichoke" is believed to have been derived from the Greek word "artikhokhion." As it traveled through different languages and cultures, the artichoke continued to hold cultural significance and symbolism. Beyond its culinary appeal, artichoke leaf has also been associated with various tales of love and romance in ancient folklore.

Now, let's explore ten extensive health and longevity benefits associated with artichoke leaf:

1. **Liver Health:** Artichoke leaf contains cynarin, silymarin, and caffeoylquinic acids, which support liver function, promote bile production, and help protect against liver damage.
2. **Antioxidant Powerhouse:** Artichoke leaf is rich in flavonoids (such as apigenin and luteolin), caffeic acid derivatives, and quercetin, providing potent antioxidant properties that help reduce oxidative stress and support cellular health.
3. **Digestive Health:** Artichoke leaf's active compounds, cynarin and cynaropicrin, stimulate the production of digestive enzymes, improving digestion and nutrient absorption while alleviating symptoms of indigestion.
4. **Cardiovascular Health:** Artichoke leaf contains flavones and luteolin, which support cardiovascular health by reducing cholesterol levels, maintaining healthy blood pressure, and protecting against oxidative stress.
5. **Blood Sugar Regulation:** The active compound chlorogenic acid in artichoke leaf may improve insulin sensitivity and help regulate blood sugar levels, reducing post-meal blood sugar spikes.
6. **Kidney Health:** Artichoke leaf's diuretic properties support kidney function by promoting urine production and aiding in the elimination of toxins and excess fluid.
7. **Immune System Support:** Artichoke leaf's antioxidants and flavonoids, such as apigenin and luteolin, support the immune system by protecting cells from oxidative stress and modulating immune responses.

8. **Anti-inflammatory Effects:** Artichoke leaf's luteolin and caffeic acid derivatives possess anti-inflammatory properties that help reduce inflammation throughout the body.
9. **Skin Health:** Artichoke leaf's antioxidants and flavonoids contribute to skin health by protecting against oxidative damage and promoting a youthful appearance.
10. **Detoxification:** Artichoke leaf stimulates liver function and bile production and contains cynarin and silymarin, which help protect the liver from toxins, aiding in the detoxification process.

> While artichoke leaf is generally considered safe to consume, there are a few important warnings and contradictions to consider. Individuals taking medication for gallstones, bile duct obstruction, or other liver conditions should consult their healthcare provider before using artichoke leaf. Additionally, individuals with known allergies to plants in the Asteraceae family, such as ragweed or daisies, may be at a higher risk of allergic reactions. It is recommended to avoid artichoke leaf supplementation during pregnancy or lactation unless advised by your herbalist/practitioner.

ASHWAGANDHA

Ashwagandha, scientifically known as Withania somnifera, is an ancient medicinal herb with a rich history and a wide array of health benefits. Originating from the dry regions of India, Northern Africa, and the Middle East, ashwagandha has been used for over 3,000 years in traditional Ayurvedic medicine. Also known as "Indian ginseng" or "winter cherry," this small shrub with yellow flowers has a reputation for its adaptogenic properties and ability to promote overall well-being. The root and leaves of the ashwagandha plant are utilized for their medicinal properties, making it a versatile herb with a significant impact on health and longevity.

Now, let's explore ten extensive health and longevity benefits associated with ashwagandha:

1. **Stress Relief:** Ashwagandha contains active compounds called withanolides, which have adaptogenic properties, helping the body adapt to stress. It supports healthy cortisol levels and reduces stress-related symptoms.
2. **Cognitive Support:** Withanolides in ashwagandha support brain health by enhancing neuroprotective activity, improving cognitive function, and supporting memory recall.
3. **Anti-inflammatory Effects:** Ashwagandha contains steroidal lactones, including withaferin A, which possess anti-inflammatory properties, helping to reduce inflammation and promote overall well-being.
4. **Immune System Support:** Ashwagandha contains antioxidants like withanolides, alkaloids, and flavonoids, which strengthen the immune system, protect against oxidative stress, and support healthy immune function.
5. **Cardiovascular Health:** Ashwagandha supports heart health by reducing cholesterol and triglyceride levels. It contains antioxidants like catalase and glutathione peroxidase that help protect against oxidative damage to the cardiovascular system.
6. **Thyroid Health:** Ashwagandha supports thyroid health by aiding in the conversion of the T4 hormone to the active T3 hormone. It contains compounds that help regulate thyroid function and support optimal hormone balance.
7. **Graceful-aging Effects:** Ashwagandha's antioxidant compounds, including withanolides, help protect against oxidative stress and cellular damage, which can contribute to aging and age-related diseases.

8. **Liver Health:** Ashwagandha supports liver detoxification processes by increasing antioxidant enzymes like superoxide dismutase (SOD) and glutathione, protecting the liver from toxins and promoting its overall health.
9. **Anxiety Relief:** Ashwagandha's active compound, withanolides, exhibits anxiolytic effects, reducing anxiety symptoms and promoting a sense of calm.
10. **Antimicrobial Effects:** Ashwagandha possesses antimicrobial and antiviral properties, thanks to compounds like withanolides, alkaloids, and flavonoids, which help combat pathogens and support a healthy immune response.

> While ashwagandha is generally considered safe to consume, there are several important medical contradictions and precautions to be aware of. Individuals taking immunosuppressant medications, such as corticosteroids or medications used in organ transplantation, should avoid ashwagandha as it may interfere with the effectiveness of these medications. Ashwagandha may also interact with medications for thyroid disorders, such as levothyroxine, as it can affect thyroid hormone levels. Allergy warnings include potential cross-reactivity with plants in the Solanaceae family, such as tomatoes, potatoes, and bell peppers. It is also advisable to avoid ashwagandha during pregnancy or lactation unless otherwise stipulated by your herbalist/practitioner.

ASTRAGALUS ROOT

Astragalus root, scientifically known as Astragalus membranaceus, is a medicinal herb with a long history of use in traditional Chinese medicine. Originating from the regions of China, Mongolia, and Korea, astragalus root has been revered for over 2,000 years for its health-promoting properties. This perennial plant, characterized by its distinct yellow flowers and the presence of a woody root, is highly regarded for its adaptogenic and immune-boosting qualities. The root of astragalus is harvested and used in various forms, such as teas, extracts, and supplements, to harness its extensive health benefits and contribute to longevity.

Now, let's explore ten extensive health and longevity benefits associated with astragalus root:

1. **Immune System Support:** Astragalus contains polysaccharides that have shown immunomodulatory effects, helping to enhance immune function and stimulate the production of immune cells, including T cells and natural killer (NK) cells.
2. **Antioxidant Powerhouse:** Astragalus is rich in flavonoids and saponins, which exhibit potent antioxidant properties. These antioxidants help neutralize harmful free radicals, protecting cells from oxidative damage and promoting longevity.
3. **Anti-inflammatory Effects:** Astragalus contains saponins, such as astragaloside IV, which possess anti-inflammatory properties. They may inhibit the production of pro-inflammatory cytokines, reducing inflammation and supporting various organ systems.
4. **Cardiovascular Health:** Astragalus has been linked to cardiovascular benefits due to its flavonoids and saponins. It may help regulate blood pressure, improve lipid profiles, and enhance cardiac function, promoting cardiovascular health. Astragaloside IV, a saponin in astragalus, is under research for potential cardioprotective effects.
5. **Liver Health:** Astragalus has been found to have hepatoprotective properties. Its active compounds, including astragalosides and flavonoids, may help protect liver cells from damage, support detoxification processes, and promote liver health.
6. **Respiratory Health:** Astragalus has been used to support respiratory health and may be beneficial in conditions such as asthma and chronic obstructive pulmonary disease (COPD). Its polysaccharides and flavonoids may have bronchodilatory and anti-inflammatory effects.

7. **Graceful-aging Effects:** Astragalus has been associated with graceful aging-supportive benefits. Its antioxidants, such as astragalosides and flavonoids, help combat oxidative stress, preserve cellular health, and support longevity.
8. **Kidney Health:** Astragalus has been used in traditional medicine for kidney-related conditions. Its compounds may protect against kidney damage, enhance renal function, and support urinary health.
9. **Diabetes Management:** Astragalus shows potential in managing diabetes by regulating blood sugar levels. Its active compounds may enhance insulin sensitivity, inhibit glucose absorption, and support pancreatic function.
10. **Antimicrobial Effects:** Astragalus exhibits antimicrobial activity against certain bacteria and viruses. Some studies suggest its polysaccharides and flavonoids may have antiviral effects, potentially inhibiting the replication of viruses.

> While astragalus is generally considered safe to consume, there are several important medical contradictions and precautions to be aware of. Astragalus may interact with immunosuppressant medications, such as corticosteroids or medications used in organ transplantation, as it can affect immune function. Individuals with hypotension or low blood pressure should use astragalus with caution, as it may further lower blood pressure levels. Allergy warnings include potential cross-reactivity with plants in the Fabaceae family, such as peanuts, lentils, and soybeans. Pregnant or lactating women should consult with their herbalist/practitioner before using astragalus root.

BARBERRY BARK

Barberry bark, derived from the barberry plant (Berberis vulgaris), has a rich history and a wide range of health benefits. This shrub is native to regions of Europe, Africa, and Asia and has been utilized for centuries in traditional medicine systems such as Ayurveda and Chinese medicine. The bark of the barberry plant is particularly prized for its medicinal properties and is known for its distinct yellow color and bitter taste. Barberry bark contains various bioactive compounds, including berberine, which contribute to its therapeutic potential.

Now, let's explore ten extensive health and longevity benefits associated with barberry bark:

1. **Liver Health:** Barberry bark contains berberine, a compound known for its hepatoprotective properties. Berberine helps support liver function and detoxification processes.
2. **Cardiovascular Health:** Berberine in barberry bark has been linked to cardiovascular benefits. It may help maintain healthy cholesterol levels and support optimal heart function.
3. **Anti-inflammatory Effects:** Barberry bark contains various antioxidants, including isoquinoline alkaloids such as berberine and berbamine. These compounds have shown anti-inflammatory properties, potentially benefiting various organs and body systems.
4. **Immune System Support:** The active compounds in barberry bark, including berberine, have antimicrobial and immunomodulatory properties. They may help support a healthy immune system and combat pathogens.
5. **Digestive Health:** Berberine in barberry bark has been found to have antibacterial properties against harmful bacteria, such as Helicobacter pylori, supporting digestive health.
6. **Antioxidant Powerhouse:** Barberry bark is rich in antioxidants, including berberine and phenolic compounds. These antioxidants help combat free radicals and oxidative stress, contributing to cellular health and overall longevity.
7. **Blood Sugar Regulation:** Research suggests that berberine in barberry bark may help regulate blood sugar levels by enhancing insulin sensitivity and reducing glucose production.
8. **Eye Health:** Barberry bark contains antioxidants like berberine, which may have protective effects against age-related eye conditions, supporting eye health.

9. **Anti-cancer Effects:** Some studies have shown that the active compounds in barberry bark, such as berberine, may have anti-cancer properties by inhibiting tumor growth and inducing apoptosis in cancer cells.
10. **Antimicrobial Effects:** Barberry bark's active compounds, particularly berberine, have been recognized for their broad-spectrum antimicrobial properties, making it useful against various pathogens, including bacteria, viruses, and fungi.

> While barberry bark is generally considered safe to consume, there are important medical contradictions to be aware of. Barberry bark should not be used without proper guidance if you are taking medications such as anticoagulants (e.g., warfarin) or antiplatelet drugs, as it may enhance their effects and increase the risk of bleeding. Individuals with diabetes should exercise caution, as barberry bark may lower blood sugar levels and require adjustments in medication dosages. Allergy warnings include potential cross-reactivity with plants in the same family, such as Oregon grape (Mahonia spp.) and goldenseal (Hydrastis canadensis). It is advisable to consult with a healthcare professional or herbalist before using barberry bark, especially if you have any specific health conditions or concerns. Barberry bark is not recommended during pregnancy or lactation unless otherwise stipulated by your herbalist/practitioner.

BARBERRY FRUIT

Barberry fruit, derived from the barberry plant (Berberis vulgaris), has a long history of use in traditional medicine and culinary practices. The barberry plant is native to regions of Europe, Africa, and Asia, and its vibrant red berries have been harvested for centuries for their medicinal properties and culinary uses. Barberry fruit is known for its tart and tangy flavor, which adds a unique taste to various dishes and beverages. Rich in beneficial compounds such as berberine and antioxidants, barberry fruit offers an array of health benefits that contribute to overall well-being and longevity.

Now, let's explore ten extensive health and longevity benefits associated with barberry fruit:

1. **Immune System Support:** Barberry fruit contains vitamin C, a potent antioxidant that supports the immune system by protecting cells from damage and promoting immune cell function.
2. **Cardiovascular Health:** The active compound berberine found in barberry fruit has been associated with various cardiovascular benefits, including maintaining healthy cholesterol levels and supporting heart function.
3. **Liver Health:** The berberine in barberry fruit has shown potential in supporting liver health by promoting healthy liver function and aiding in detoxification processes.
4. **Anti-inflammatory Effects:** Berberine may help reduce inflammation and support overall health.
5. **Antioxidant Powerhouse:** Barberry fruit is rich in antioxidants such as berberine and phenolic compounds, which may help neutralize harmful free radicals, protect against oxidative stress, and support longevity.
6. **Digestive Health:** Berberine has been studied for its potential to support digestive health by promoting a healthy microbial balance in the gut and aiding in the management of certain gastrointestinal conditions.
7. **Antimicrobial Effects:** The berberine in barberry fruit exhibits broad-spectrum antimicrobial effects, potentially inhibiting the growth of various bacteria, viruses, fungi, and parasites.
8. **Blood Sugar Regulation:** Berberine in barberry fruit has been studied for its potential to help regulate blood sugar levels by improving insulin sensitivity and reducing glucose production in the liver.

9. **Eye Health:** Barberry fruit contains antioxidants, such as vitamin C, zeaxanthin, and lutein, which are beneficial for eye health, helping to protect against age-related macular degeneration and supporting vision.
10. **Graceful-aging Effects:** Barberry fruit's high antioxidant content, including berberine and phenolic compounds, may help combat oxidative stress, a key contributor to aging processes in the body, supporting overall longevity and graceful aging.

> While barberry fruit (or barberries) are generally considered safe to consume, there are a few important contradictions and warnings to keep in mind. Individuals taking blood thinners, anticoagulants, or antiplatelet drugs should exercise caution, as barberries contain natural compounds that may enhance the effects of these medications, increasing the risk of bleeding. Allergy warnings should be noted, as some individuals may have allergies or sensitivities to barberries, particularly if they have known allergies to plants in the Berberidaceae family, such as Oregon grape or goldenseal. Cross-reactivity may occur. Regarding safety during pregnancy and lactation, while barberries are generally considered safe to consume, it is always recommended to consult with your herbalist/practitioner for personalized advice and to ensure safety during these periods.

BARLEY GRASS

Barley grass, scientifically known as Hordeum vulgare, has emerged as a nutrient-rich superfood renowned for its extensive health benefits. Originating in the Fertile Crescent of the Middle East, barley, one of the earliest cultivated grains, has served as a dietary staple for millennia. Barley grass is loaded with essential vitamins, minerals, antioxidants, and enzymes, making it a valuable source of crucial nutrients. However, to acquire the most of these nutrient benefits, consuming barley grass in the form of a fresh pressed juice extraction allows the natural integrity of the nutrients, antioxidants and enzymes to be retained. Moreover, fresh pressed barley grass juice is more readily absorbed by the body because it doesn't require digestion to break down the plant cell walls. A dried, processed powdered barley grass juice supplement risks the enzymes and some other valuable nutrients to be destroyed in the drying and powdering process. Importantly, it's worth noting that the young grass lacks gluten, and consequently, so does barley grass juice, making it suitable for those with gluten sensitivities.

Now, let's explore ten extensive health and longevity benefits associated with fresh barley grass and its juice:

1. **Immune System Support:** Barley grass juice is rich in vitamin C, which strengthens the immune system and supports the production of white blood cells, enhancing the body's ability to fight off infections.
2. **Antioxidant Powerhouse:** Barley grass juice contains potent antioxidants such as vitamin E, beta-carotene, and superoxide dismutase (SOD), which help protect cells from oxidative damage, reducing the risk of chronic diseases.
3. **Detoxification:** Barley grass juice is rich in chlorophyll, a powerful detoxifying compound that helps eliminate toxins, heavy metals, and harmful pollutants from the body, supporting liver health.
4. **Digestive Health:** Barley grass juice contains enzymes, including protease and amylase, which aid in digestion, ensuring efficient nutrient absorption and promoting a healthy gut.
5. **Cardiovascular Health:** Barley grass juice is a good source of heart-healthy nutrients like potassium, magnesium, and vitamin K, which help maintain normal blood pressure, support optimal circulation, and reduce the risk of cardiovascular diseases.
6. **Blood Sugar Regulation:** Barley grass juice contains chromium, a mineral that assists in regulating blood sugar levels, enhancing insulin sensitivity, and promoting stable energy levels.

7. **Anti-inflammatory Effects:** The abundance of antioxidants, including vitamin E and chlorophyll, in barley grass juice helps reduce inflammation in the body, protecting against chronic diseases and supporting overall well-being.
8. **Bone Health:** Barley grass juice provides essential minerals such as calcium, phosphorus, and manganese, which contribute to bone health, density, and the prevention of osteoporosis.
9. **Eye Health:** Barley grass juice contains lutein and zeaxanthin, antioxidants that accumulate in the retina, helping to protect against age-related macular degeneration and promoting optimal vision health.
10. **Energy Boost:** Barley grass juice supplies a range of B vitamins, iron, and magnesium, which are essential for energy production, reducing fatigue, and supporting overall vitality.

> Barley grass juice is generally considered safe to consume, however, there are a few important warnings and contradictions to consider. Individuals taking blood-thinning medications, such as warfarin, should be cautious, as barley grass juice may interact with these medications and increase the risk of bleeding. While barley grass itself is gluten-free, individuals with gluten sensitivity or celiac disease should exercise caution when consuming supplemental barley grass juice powder. Cross-contamination during processing or potential contamination in the supply chain can occur, so it is important to choose certified gluten-free products to avoid adverse reactions. It is also important to note that while barley grass juice during pregnancy or lactation is generally considered safe, the processed version (the powdered supplement) may contain impurities, so it is advisable to consult with your herbalist/practitioner before incorporating processed barley grass supplements into your routine, to ensure supplementation is right for you and your baby.

BAY LEAF

Bay leaves, known scientifically as Laurus nobilis, have a rich history and have been prized for their culinary and medicinal uses for centuries. Native to the Mediterranean region, bay leaves were highly regarded by the ancient Greeks and Romans, who considered them sacred and associated them with wisdom and protection. These aromatic leaves come from the bay laurel tree, an evergreen tree with glossy leaves. Bay leaves are widely used in various cuisines for their distinctive flavor and fragrance, but they also offer a host of health benefits that contribute to overall well-being and longevity.

Now, let's explore ten extensive health and longevity benefits associated with bay leaves:

1. **Anti-inflammatory Effects:** Bay leaves contain specific antioxidants such as quercetin and eugenol, which have demonstrated anti-inflammatory properties, helping to reduce inflammation in the body and potentially support various organs and systems.
2. **Digestive Health:** Bay leaves contain compounds like cineole and eugenol that may promote digestive health by stimulating the secretion of digestive enzymes, reducing gastrointestinal spasms, and aiding in nutrient absorption.
3. **Antioxidant Powerhouse:** Bay leaves are rich in antioxidants like rutin and lutein, which help neutralize harmful free radicals and protect cells from oxidative stress, supporting overall health and potentially slowing down the aging process.
4. **Cardiovascular Health:** The phytonutrients in bay leaves, including caffeic acid and rutin, have been associated with cardiovascular benefits, including supporting healthy cholesterol levels, reducing inflammation in blood vessels, and potentially lowering the risk of heart disease.
5. **Blood Sugar Regulation:** Certain compounds in bay leaves, such as flavonoids and polyphenols, have shown potential in helping regulate blood sugar levels and improve insulin sensitivity, making it beneficial for individuals with diabetes or prediabetes.
6. **Antimicrobial Effects:** Bay leaves contain antimicrobial compounds like eugenol and linalool, which have demonstrated inhibitory effects against various bacteria and fungi, potentially helping to combat certain pathogens and support the body's defense against infections.

7. **Respiratory Health:** Bay leaves contain volatile compounds like eucalyptol and cineole, which have expectorant properties and may help alleviate respiratory issues, such as coughs, congestion, and bronchitis.
8. **Liver Health:** The active compound caffeic acid present in bay leaves have been shown to support liver health by stimulating the production of detoxifying enzymes, aiding in the elimination of toxins from the body.
9. **Stress Relief:** The compounds in bay leaves, including linalool and eugenol, have been associated with calming effects and may contribute to stress relief, supporting mental well-being and indirectly impacting longevity.
10. **Anti-cancer Effects:** Some studies have suggested that the phytochemicals present in bay leaves, such as quercetin, may possess anti-cancer properties, potentially inhibiting the growth and spread of cancer cells.

> Bay leaves are generally considered safe to consume in moderate culinary preparations. However, there are a few important warnings and contradictions to consider. Individuals allergic to other plants in the Lauraceae family, such as cinnamon or camphor, may also be allergic to bay leaves and should exercise caution. Bay leaves may interact with certain medications, such as diabetes medications, by lowering blood sugar levels. Therefore, individuals taking medications for diabetes should monitor their blood sugar levels closely when using bay leaves as a culinary ingredient. Bay leaves are generally considered safe to use in moderate culinary preparations for those who are pregnant or lactating. Consult with your herbalist/practitioner before using bay leaves in large therapeutic quantities during these periods.

BEETROOT POWDER

Beetroot powder, derived from the root vegetable known as the beetroot (Beta vulgaris), has a rich history and is widely celebrated for its vibrant color and numerous health benefits. The beetroot is believed to have originated in the Mediterranean region and was highly regarded by ancient civilizations for its culinary and medicinal properties. Beetroot powder is typically created by freeze drying the beets and then grinding it into a fine powder, preserving its natural compounds and nutritional value. Packed with essential vitamins, minerals, antioxidants, and dietary fiber, beetroot powder has gained popularity as a superfood supplement with a wide range of health benefits that promote longevity and overall well-being. Now, let's explore ten extensive health and longevity benefits associated with beetroot powder:

1. **Cardiovascular Health:** Beetroot powder's high concentration of dietary nitrates, which are converted into nitric oxide in the body, helps improve blood flow and lower blood pressure. It also contains potassium, magnesium, and vitamin C, which promote heart health.
2. **Enhanced Exercise Performance:** The natural nitrates in beetroot powder improve oxygen utilization and increase stamina during exercise. It also contains betaine, which enhances muscle strength and performance.
3. **Anti-inflammatory Effects:** Beetroot powder contains betalains which possess potent anti-inflammatory properties, reducing inflammation in the body.
4. **Immune System Support:** Beetroot powder is rich in vitamin C and antioxidants like betalains, which strengthen the immune system and protect against infections.
5. **Digestive Health:** The fiber content in beetroot powder promotes healthy digestion and regular bowel movements. It also contains digestive enzymes that support proper nutrient absorption.
6. **Blood Sugar Regulation:** Beetroot powder's low glycemic index and fiber content help regulate blood sugar levels. It also contains alpha-lipoic acid, which enhances insulin sensitivity and glucose metabolism.
7. **Graceful-aging Effects:** Beetroot powder's antioxidants, including betalains, vitamin C, and manganese, combat free radicals and oxidative stress, protecting against cellular damage and contributing to graceful-aging.

8. **Anemia Support:** Beetroot's role in anemia support is notable due to its rich iron and folate content. Iron is a critical component of hemoglobin, the protein responsible for transporting oxygen in the blood. When the body lacks sufficient iron, it can lead to iron-deficiency anemia, characterized by fatigue, weakness, and pale skin. Beetroot provides a plant-based source of iron that can contribute to maintaining healthy iron levels, especially important for individuals with dietary restrictions or those who prefer non-meat sources. Furthermore, beetroot contains folate, a B-vitamin essential for the production of red blood cells and their proper functioning. Folate deficiency can also lead to anemia, making beetroot an excellent dietary choice to help prevent and address this condition.
9. **Detoxification:** Betalains, antioxidants, and fiber assist in liver detoxification and aid in the elimination of toxins from the body.
10. **Cognitive Function:** Beetroot powder's nitrates improve blood flow to the brain, supporting cognitive function. It also contains folate, vitamin C, and antioxidants, which contribute to brain health.

> While organic beetroot powder is generally considered safe to consume, there are a few important warnings and contradictions to consider. Individuals with low blood pressure or those taking blood pressure medications should exercise caution, as beetroot powder may lower blood pressure. It is advisable to monitor blood pressure levels regularly and consult with a healthcare professional if necessary. It is also important to note that while organic NON-GMO beets are generally considered safe to consume during pregnancy or lactation, the processed version (the powdered supplement) may contain impurities, so it is advisable to consult with your herbalist/practitioner before incorporating processed beetroot powder into your routine, to ensure purity, and to ensure that supplementation is right for you and your baby.

BILBERRIES

Bilberries, scientifically known as Vaccinium myrtillus, are small, dark purple berries that grow on shrubs native to Europe, North America, and certain parts of Asia. These delicious berries have a long history of use in traditional medicine and folklore. Bilberries are close relatives of blueberries and are often referred to as "European blueberries." They have been harvested for centuries and were consumed by ancient civilizations for their unique flavor and potential health benefits. Bilberries are known for their rich content of anthocyanins, powerful antioxidants that give them their deep purple color and contribute to their numerous health benefits.

Now, let's explore ten extensive health and longevity benefits associated with bilberries:

1. **Eye Health:** Bilberries contain anthocyanins, particularly cyanidin-3-glucoside, which support eye health by improving night vision, reducing eye fatigue, and protecting against age-related macular degeneration.
2. **Cardiovascular Health:** The flavonoids present in bilberries, including quercetin and resveratrol, have antioxidant and anti-inflammatory properties that support cardiovascular health, reducing the risk of heart disease and promoting healthy blood circulation.
3. **Cognitive Support:** Bilberries' high content of anthocyanins and proanthocyanidins may enhance cognitive function, memory, and learning abilities, as these compounds help protect brain cells from oxidative stress and improve blood flow to the brain.
4. **Anti-inflammatory Effects:** Bilberries contain various antioxidants, including vitamin C and quercetin, that help reduce inflammation in the body, potentially benefiting conditions such as arthritis and inflammatory bowel disease.
5. **Graceful-aging Effects:** The antioxidants in bilberries, such as vitamin C, supports healthy skin by protecting against oxidative stress, promoting collagen synthesis, and reducing the signs of aging. Resveratrol protects against cellular damage and environmental toxins, contributing to a youthful appearance and supporting longevity.
6. **Digestive Health:** Bilberries contain tannins and anthocyanins that have been associated with improved digestion, reduced inflammation in the gastrointestinal tract, and protection against stomach ulcers.

7. **Immune System Support:** The vitamin C and antioxidants in bilberries help strengthen the immune system, protecting against infections and supporting the body's defense mechanisms.
8. **Liver Health:** The antioxidants in bilberries, including anthocyanins, support liver health by protecting against oxidative stress and inflammation, promoting detoxification processes, and maintaining liver function.
9. **Urinary Tract Health:** The compounds in bilberries, such as proanthocyanidins, may prevent urinary tract infections by inhibiting the adhesion of bacteria to the urinary tract walls.
10. **Anti-cancer Effects:** Bilberries' diverse array of antioxidants, including anthocyanins and resveratrol, have been linked to potential anti-cancer effects, such as inhibiting the growth of cancer cells and reducing oxidative stress-induced DNA damage.

While bilberries are generally considered safe to consume, there are a few important warnings and contradictions to consider. Individuals taking anticoagulant medications, such as warfarin, should exercise caution as bilberries may enhance the effects of these medications, increasing the risk of bleeding. Bilberries may also interact with medications metabolized by the liver's cytochrome P450 enzyme system. Allergy warnings should be noted for individuals with known allergies to berries or other fruits from the Ericaceae family, such as blueberries or cranberries, as they may also be allergic to bilberries. It is advisable to consult with a healthcare professional if there are concerns regarding specific medications or allergies. Additionally, individuals with diabetes should monitor their blood sugar levels closely when consuming bilberries as they may lower blood sugar levels. Consuming bilberries during pregnancy or lactation is generally considered safe in mindful quantities. Consult with your herbalist/practitioner prior to consuming bilberries in large therapeutic quantities during these times.

BILBERRY LEAF

Bilberry leaf, derived from the bilberry plant (Vaccinium myrtillus), is a herbal remedy with a rich history and a wide array of potential health benefits. The bilberry plant, native to Europe, North America, and certain parts of Asia, is known for its small, dark purple berries, but its leaves also hold significant therapeutic value. Traditionally, bilberry leaves have been used in various herbal preparations and teas for their potential medicinal properties. The leaves contain a range of bioactive compounds, including antioxidants and plant polyphenols, which contribute to their extensive health benefits.

Now, let's explore ten extensive health and longevity benefits associated with bilberry leaf:

1. **Skin Health:** Bilberry leaf contains tannins, a type of polyphenol that possess astringent properties. When applied topically, tannins may help tighten the skin and reduce excessive oiliness. In the context of certain skin conditions like eczema and psoriasis, the astringent properties of tannins may help soothe and dry out weeping or oozing lesions, promoting the healing process. Tannins have been used in traditional medicine as topical treatments for various skin ailments due to their ability to provide a drying and soothing effect
2. **Cardiovascular Health:** The flavonoids present in bilberry leaf, including quercetin and catechins, have antioxidant properties that may help reduce inflammation and support cardiovascular health. These antioxidants help protect against oxidative stress and improve blood vessel function, thereby promoting heart health.
3. **Anti-inflammatory Effects:** The presence of specific flavonoids in bilberry leaf, such as kaempferol and myricetin, contributes to its anti-inflammatory properties. These compounds help reduce inflammation throughout the body, which can contribute to overall well-being and support longevity.
4. **Cognitive Support:** Bilberry leaf contains anthocyanins, which have been associated with improved cognitive function and memory. These compounds help enhance blood flow to the brain, reduce oxidative stress, and protect against age-related cognitive decline.

5. **Liver Health:** Certain compounds in bilberry leaf, including catechins and quercetin, possess hepatoprotective properties, supporting the health and function of the liver. They aid in detoxification processes and protect liver cells from damage caused by toxins and free radicals.
6. **Blood Sugar Regulation:** Bilberry leaf has been found to help regulate blood sugar levels due to the presence of compounds like myricetin and quercetin. These antioxidants may improve insulin sensitivity and glucose metabolism, potentially reducing the risk of diabetes and supporting longevity.
7. **Antimicrobial Effects:** The flavonoids in bilberry leaf, such as quercetin and kaempferol, have demonstrated antimicrobial properties against various bacteria and fungi. These compounds may help combat harmful microorganisms and support a healthy immune system.
8. **Digestive Health:** Bilberry leaf contains tannins, which may help promote healthy digestion by reducing inflammation and supporting the intestinal lining. Additionally, the antioxidants in bilberry leaf may protect against gastrointestinal disorders and promote gut health.
9. **Graceful-aging Effects:** The antioxidants found in bilberry leaf, including anthocyanins and quercetin, help neutralize free radicals and reduce oxidative stress, which are known to contribute to the aging process. By combating oxidative damage, bilberry leaf indirectly supports longevity and graceful aging.
10. **Detoxification:** The antioxidants and flavonoids present in bilberry leaf aid in the body's natural detoxification processes. They help neutralize toxins, reduce inflammation, and support liver function, promoting overall detoxification and well-being.

While bilberry leaf is generally considered safe to consume, there are a few important warnings and contradictions to consider. Individuals taking anticoagulant or antiplatelet medications, such as warfarin or aspirin, should exercise caution when using bilberry leaf, as it may enhance the effects of these medications and increase the risk of bleeding. People with diabetes who are taking medications to control blood sugar levels, such as insulin or oral hypoglycemic agents, should also be cautious, as bilberry leaf may potentiate the effects of these medications and lead to low blood sugar levels. Additionally, individuals with known allergies to plants in the Ericaceae family, which includes blueberries and cranberries, may also be allergic to bilberry leaf. It is recommended to consult with your herbalist/practitioner prior to using bilberry leaf during pregnancy or lactation.

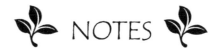
NOTES

BLACK COHOSH

Black cohosh, scientifically known as Actaea racemosa, is a perennial plant native to North America. It has a rich history of traditional use among indigenous peoples, who recognized its medicinal properties. Black cohosh was widely used by Native American tribes, including the Cherokee, Iroquois, and Algonquin, for various women's health concerns and as a general tonic. The plant derives its name from the dark color of its roots, which are believed to resemble the appearance of a cohosh, a traditional Algonquian word meaning "rough." Black cohosh is renowned for its potential health benefits, particularly in relation to women's health, and has gained recognition as a popular herbal remedy.

Now, let's explore ten extensive health and longevity benefits associated with black cohosh:

1. **Menopausal Relief:** Black cohosh is commonly used to alleviate menopausal symptoms such as hot flashes and night sweats. It may be attributed to the presence of compounds like triterpene glycosides, including actein and cimicifugoside, which possess estrogenic effects and may help balance hormone levels. It should be noted that black cohosh does not exhibit estrogenic effects like hormone replacement therapy (HRT).
2. **Bone Health:** Black cohosh may contribute to bone health due to its isoflavones, such as formononetin and biochanin A, which have been shown to exhibit bone-protective properties and support bone density.
3. **Anti-inflammatory Effects:** Black cohosh contains compounds like salicylic acid, isoferulic acid, and caffeic acid, which have demonstrated anti-inflammatory effects, potentially helping to reduce inflammation in the body.
4. **Cardiovascular Health:** Some studies suggest that black cohosh may positively impact cardiovascular health by promoting vasodilation and reducing blood pressure. The antioxidant activity of phenolic compounds found in black cohosh, such as ferulic acid and caffeic acid, may contribute to these effects.
5. **Liver Health:** Black cohosh has been shown to possess hepatoprotective properties and support liver health by promoting liver detoxification processes.
6. **Mood Support:** Black cohosh may have a positive impact on mood and emotional well-being. The presence of serotonin modulators, such as N-methylserotonin and serotonin-N-carboxylic acid methyl ester, may contribute to its potential antidepressant effects.

7. **Muscle-relaxing Effects:** Black cohosh's alkaloids, flavonoids (quercetin, kaempferol), and salicylic acid derivatives collectively contribute to its potential muscle relaxation effects. Alkaloids provide anti-spasmodic effects, flavonoids offer antioxidant and anti-inflammatory properties, and salicylic acid derivatives may impart mild analgesic effects.
8. **Menstrual Support:** For women experiencing menstrual discomfort, such as cramps, bloating, and lower abdominal pain, the application of black cohosh-infused creams to the lower abdomen may offer a soothing and calming effect. The potential anti-inflammatory and muscle-relaxing properties of black cohosh compounds might contribute to reducing the intensity of these symptoms, providing a more manageable and comfortable experience.
9. **Antimicrobial Effects:** Black cohosh exhibits antimicrobial properties. Isoferulic acid and caffeic acid derivatives found in black cohosh have shown inhibitory effects against various bacteria and fungi.
10. **Graceful-aging Effects:** Ultimately, the pro-aging effects of black cohosh manifest in an improved quality of life. By addressing menopausal discomforts, bone health, inflammation, and emotional well-being, black cohosh empowers individuals to experience aging in a more holistic and fulfilling manner.

> While black cohosh is generally considered safe to consume, there are certain medical contradictions and warnings that should be considered. Individuals with estrogen-sensitive conditions, such as breast, ovarian, or uterine cancer, should avoid black cohosh, as it may have estrogenic effects. Black cohosh may also interact with medications that affect the liver, such as hepatotoxic drugs or hormone therapies, potentially exacerbating liver-related side effects. Individuals with a history of blood clotting disorders or taking anticoagulant medications should consult with a healthcare professional before using black cohosh, as it may have mild antiplatelet effects and could potentially increase the risk of bleeding. Individuals sensitive or allergic to aspirin (acetylsalicylic acid) may also have a potential sensitivity or adverse reaction to black cohosh due to the presence of salicylic acid derivatives in black cohosh. Salicylic acid is chemically related to aspirin and can cause similar reactions in individuals sensitive to aspirin. Therefore, individuals with known aspirin sensitivity should exercise caution when considering the use of black cohosh. Pregnant and breastfeeding individuals should avoid black cohosh due to its potential effects on hormone levels and limited safety data in these populations.

BLACK PEPPERCORN

Black peppercorn, scientifically known as Piper nigrum, is a flowering vine native to the tropical regions of India. For centuries, black peppercorns have been valued as a prized spice, coveted for their pungent aroma and distinctive flavor. They have been traded across ancient trade routes and have played a significant role in culinary traditions worldwide. Black peppercorns are derived from the dried fruit of the pepper plant and are widely used in both savory and sweet dishes. Beyond their culinary uses, black peppercorns also possess an impressive array of potential health benefits.

Now, let's explore ten extensive health and longevity benefits associated with black peppercorn:

1. **Digestive Health:** Black peppercorns stimulate the production of digestive enzymes, aiding in digestion and promoting a healthy gastrointestinal system. They may help alleviate digestive discomfort, bloating, and constipation.
2. **Antioxidant Powerhouse:** Black peppercorns contain potent antioxidants that help protect cells from oxidative damage caused by free radicals. Antioxidants play a crucial role in reducing inflammation and supporting overall health.
3. **Enhanced Nutrient Absorption:** The piperine compound found in black peppercorns has been shown to enhance the bioavailability and absorption of various nutrients, including vitamins and minerals. It can increase the body's ability to utilize essential nutrients effectively.
4. **Respiratory Health:** Piperine possess expectorant properties that may help alleviate respiratory congestion, coughs, and cold symptoms. They may also provide relief from sinusitis and nasal congestion.
5. **Anti-inflammatory Effects:** Piperine exhibits anti-inflammatory properties that may help reduce inflammation in the body. It may be beneficial for managing inflammatory conditions such as arthritis.
6. **Cognitive Function:** Black peppercorns have been associated with cognitive enhancement. The piperine content may help improve memory, attention, and overall cognitive performance.

7. **Kidney Health:** Piperine has shown potential in promoting kidney health by supporting renal function and reducing the risk of kidney stones. It may assist in maintaining proper fluid balance and preventing urinary tract infections.
8. **Cardiovascular Health:** Black peppercorns have been linked to cardiovascular benefits. Piperine may help lower cholesterol levels, reduce blood pressure, and promote healthy blood circulation, thereby supporting heart health.
9. **Antimicrobial Effects:** The active compounds in black peppercorns possess antibacterial and antimicrobial properties, which may help fight against various pathogens and promote a healthy immune system. It's important to mention that these effects are more pronounced in the whole peppercorn form or black pepper extracts rather than ground pepper. The grinding and processing of black peppercorns may reduce the concentration of active compounds and, therefore, their antimicrobial potential.
10. **Anti-cancer Effects:** Preliminary studies suggest that black peppercorns may have anti-cancer properties. Piperine has been shown to inhibit the growth of certain cancer cells and may have the potential as an adjuvant therapy in cancer treatment.

While black pepper is generally considered safe to consume, there are certain medical contradictions and warnings that should be considered. Individuals with gastroesophageal reflux disease (GERD) or peptic ulcers may experience increased stomach acid production and irritation when consuming black pepper. Individuals taking anticoagulant medications, such as warfarin, should exercise caution as black pepper may interact with these medications and increase the risk of bleeding. Black pepper may also interact with certain medications metabolized by the liver, such as cyclosporine and phenytoin, potentially affecting their effectiveness. Individuals with known allergies to black pepper or other plants in the Piperaceae family, such as long pepper (Piper longum), may experience allergic reactions and should avoid its consumption. While black pepper is generally considered safe to consume as a spice, pregnant and breastfeeding individuals should consult with their herbalist/practitioner for personalized advice regarding its safety during pregnancy and lactation, especially when considering high-dose supplements.

BLACK WALNUT

Black walnut, scientifically known as Juglans nigra, boasts a fascinating history and origin that spans across North America. This large, deciduous tree is native to the eastern regions of the United States and parts of Canada. The name "black walnut" originates from the dark, almost black-colored husks that encase the edible nuts. Revered by Native American tribes for centuries, the black walnut holds cultural significance as both a valuable food source and a resource for crafting. The nutritious nuts were a staple in their diet, and the wood of the tree was used to create intricate and durable crafts, including bowls, carvings, and furniture. Black walnut hulls have a natural staining ability, which has been utilized as a natural dye by Indigenous peoples and early settlers. Not only are the nuts of the black walnut tree consumed, but the bark, hulls, and leaves are also utilized for their medicinal properties.

Now, let's explore ten extensive health and longevity benefits associated with black walnut:

1. **Cardiovascular Health:** Black walnuts are rich in omega-3 fatty acids, such as alpha-linolenic acid (ALA), which can support heart health by reducing inflammation and promoting healthy blood lipid levels. They also contain antioxidants like ellagic acid, quercetin, and vitamin E that help protect against oxidative stress and maintain cardiovascular function.
2. **Brain Health:** The presence of omega-3 fatty acids, along with antioxidants like juglone and vitamin E in black walnuts, may support brain health and cognitive function. Omega-3 fatty acids are essential for brain development and function, while antioxidants help combat oxidative damage and neurodegenerative processes.
3. **Liver Health:** Juglone is a compound with potential liver-protective properties and has been studied for its ability to promote liver detoxification processes, supporting overall liver health.
4. **Antioxidant Powerhouse:** Black walnuts are rich in antioxidants like ellagic acid, quercetin, and vitamin E. These antioxidants scavenge free radicals, protecting cells from oxidative damage and potentially reducing the risk of chronic diseases.
5. **Bone Health:** Black walnuts contain minerals essential for bone health, including calcium, magnesium, and phosphorus. These nutrients, along with antioxidants like vitamin E, support bone density and strength, promoting graceful aging and longevity.

6. **Antimicrobial Effects:** Black walnuts contain compounds like tannins that possess antimicrobial activity against various bacteria, fungi, and parasites. These properties may help combat infections and promote overall immune health.
7. **Anti-inflammatory Effects:** The presence of omega-3 fatty acids, vitamin E, and other antioxidants in black walnuts contributes to their potential anti-inflammatory effects. These compounds help reduce inflammation in the body, which is associated with various chronic diseases, and support longevity.
8. **Digestive Health:** Black walnuts contain compounds that have been traditionally used for their potential antiparasitic and antifungal properties, which may support digestive health. Juglone, tannins, and other active compounds in black walnuts may help maintain a healthy gut environment.
9. **Skin Health:** The antioxidants and fatty acids present in black walnuts, such as vitamin E and omega-3 fatty acids, support skin health by reducing oxidative stress and inflammation. These compounds contribute to the maintenance of healthy skin and may slow down the aging process.
10. **Anti-cancer Effects:** Some studies suggest that compounds found in black walnuts, including juglone, ellagic acid, and quercetin, possess anti-cancer properties. These compounds may help inhibit the growth of cancer cells and support overall longevity.

> While black walnuts are generally considered safe to consume, there are certain medical contradictions and warnings to be aware of. Black walnut belongs to the Juglandaceae family, which includes other plants such as English walnut and pecan. Cross-reactivity may occur in individuals with nut allergies, so it is important to be aware of any potential sensitivities. Black walnut may interact with certain medications, such as blood thinners, anticoagulants, and antiplatelet drugs, potentially increasing the risk of bleeding. It is important to consult with a healthcare professional if you are taking these medications. It is advised to avoid using black walnut during pregnancy or lactation unless otherwise stipulated by your herbalist/practitioner.

BLACKBERRY LEAF

Blackberry leaf, scientifically known as Rubus fruticosus, boasts a rich history and origin in different parts of the world. This deciduous shrub is native to Europe, but it also thrives in North America, Asia, and Africa. Over time, blackberry leaves have been utilized for numerous purposes. Traditional folk medicine often employed infusions of these leaves in teas or used them topically as poultices to soothe minor skin irritations and promote skin health. The ancient Greeks and Romans held blackberries in high regard, attributing them to diverse symbolic associations and incorporating them into both culinary and medicinal practices. Blackberry leaves have also played a role in folklore and mythology, with their dark purple-black fruits symbolizing fertility and abundance.

Now, let's explore ten extensive health and longevity benefits associated with Blackberry leaf:

1. **Cardiovascular Health:** Blackberry leaves contain flavonoids, such as quercetin and rutin, which have antioxidant properties that help protect against cardiovascular diseases and promote heart health.
2. **Anti-inflammatory Effects:** The presence of ellagic acid in blackberry leaves contributes to their anti-inflammatory properties, which may help alleviate inflammation-related conditions, including arthritis and inflammatory bowel diseases.
3. **Digestive Health:** Tannins found in blackberry leaves can support digestive health by aiding in the management of diarrhea, reducing intestinal inflammation, and promoting the healing of gastric ulcers.
4. **Antioxidant Powerhouse:** Blackberry leaves are rich in antioxidants, such as anthocyanins and vitamin C, which combat free radicals and oxidative stress, supporting overall cellular health and potentially slowing down the aging process.
5. **Respiratory Health:** The leaves of blackberry plants contain quercetin and vitamin C, which have been associated with improving lung function, reducing respiratory inflammation, and supporting respiratory health.
6. **Detoxification:** Blackberry leaves contain compounds like chlorogenic acid and polyphenols, which possess detoxifying properties and may support the body's natural detoxification processes.

7. **Immune System Support:** The presence of vitamin C in blackberry leaves, along with various antioxidants, can enhance immune function and protect against infections by supporting the body's defense mechanisms.
8. **Liver Health:** Blackberry leaves contain hepatoprotective compounds like cyanidin-3-glucoside, which may help protect the liver from damage caused by toxins and oxidative stress.
9. **Antimicrobial Effects:** Blackberry leaves contain compounds like gallic acid and ellagic acid, which have antimicrobial properties and may help fight against certain pathogens, supporting the body's defense against infections.
10. **Cognitive Support:** The presence of flavonoids in blackberry leaves, such as kaempferol and quercetin, has been associated with potential cognitive benefits, including improved memory and brain health.

> While blackberry leaf is generally considered safe to consume, there are a few important contradictions and warnings to consider. Individuals taking diuretic medications, such as hydrochlorothiazide, should exercise caution when consuming blackberry leaf, as it may enhance the diuretic effect. Additionally, individuals with a known allergy to berries or other plants from the Rosaceae family, such as strawberries or raspberries, may also be allergic to blackberry leaf and should avoid its consumption. Pregnant and breastfeeding women should consult with their herbalist/practitioner before using blackberry leaf in large therapeutic doses for prolonged periods.

BLADDERWRACK

Bladderwrack, also known as Fucus vesiculosus, is a type of seaweed that grows along the coasts of the North Atlantic and North Pacific oceans. This brown alga has a long history of traditional use in various cultures, particularly in coastal regions where it has been harvested for its medicinal properties. Bladderwrack thrives in rocky intertidal zones and is characterized by its air-filled sacs, which give it a distinctive appearance. Over the centuries, bladderwrack has been valued for its potential health benefits, thanks to its rich nutritional profile and bioactive compounds.
Now, let's explore ten extensive health and longevity benefits associated with bladderwrack:

1. **Thyroid Health:** Bladderwrack is a natural source of iodine, an essential mineral required for the production of thyroid hormones. Iodine deficiency can lead to thyroid imbalances, and bladderwrack's iodine content helps support optimal thyroid function.
2. **Joint Health:** Bladderwrack contains antioxidants like fucoidan, which has shown anti-inflammatory properties. Fucoidan may help reduce inflammation and support joint health.
3. **Digestive Health:** Bladderwrack contains soluble fiber, which acts as a prebiotic, nourishing beneficial gut bacteria. Healthy gut bacteria contribute to digestive health and immune function.
4. **Immune System Support:** Bladderwrack is rich in vitamins C and E, as well as antioxidants like beta-carotene. These nutrients and antioxidants help support a healthy immune system and protect against oxidative stress.
5. **Cardiovascular Health:** The high content of omega-3 fatty acids, such as eicosapentaenoic acid (EPA), in bladderwrack may help support cardiovascular health by reducing inflammation and improving lipid profiles.
6. **Anti-inflammatory Effects:** Bladderwrack contains phlorotannins, which possess anti-inflammatory properties. These compounds may help reduce chronic inflammation, which is associated with various diseases and aging.
7. **Skin Health:** Bladderwrack is rich in antioxidants like vitamin C, vitamin E, and various polyphenols. These antioxidants help protect the skin from free radical damage and promote a healthy complexion.

8. **Detoxification:** Bladderwrack contains alginates, a type of fiber that can bind to heavy metals and toxins in the digestive system, aiding in their removal from the body.
9. **Bone Health:** Bladderwrack contains minerals such as calcium, magnesium, and iron, which are essential for maintaining strong and healthy bones.
10. **Antimicrobial Effects:** Bladderwrack contains several compounds, including fucoidan and phlorotannins, which have demonstrated antimicrobial and antiviral properties. These properties may help combat certain pathogens and support overall immune health.

While bladderwrack is generally considered safe to consume and offers potential health benefits, there are certain medical contradictions and warnings that should be considered. While bladderwrack is a natural source of iodine, individuals with hyperthyroidism or other thyroid disorders should consult with their herbalist/practitioner before using bladderwrack to ensure proper iodine needs are met. It is important to ensure appropriate iodine intake for those with thyroid conditions, but this should be done under supervision. Individuals with known allergies or sensitivities to seaweed or iodine should avoid bladderwrack. Bladderwrack may also interact with certain medications, such as anticoagulants or antiplatelet drugs, which could impact blood clotting. Additionally, bladderwrack can contain varying levels of heavy metals, including arsenic, so it is important to obtain it from reputable sources to minimize the risk of contamination. Consuming bladderwrack during pregnancy and lactation is not generally recommended unless otherwise advised by your herbalist/practitioner.

BLESSED THISTLE

Blessed thistle, scientifically known as Cnicus benedictus, is a medicinal plant native to the Mediterranean region and parts of Europe. It has a long history of traditional use, dating back to ancient times, and was highly regarded for its numerous health benefits. Blessed thistle is a thistle-like plant with distinctive yellow flowers and spiny leaves. It is known for its bitter taste and has been used in herbal medicine for various purposes. The plant gets its name, "blessed," from the belief that it possesses healing properties and is considered a "blessing" for health.

Now, let's explore ten extensive health and longevity benefits associated with blessed thistle:

1. **Liver Health:** Blessed thistle contains compounds such as cnicin and polyacetylenes that support liver function and promote detoxification processes, helping to eliminate toxins from the body.
2. **Digestive Health:** Blessed thistle is known for its bitter properties, which stimulate digestive secretions and aid in digestion. The herb contains bitter compounds like sesquiterpene lactones, including cnicin, which support digestive health.
3. **Immune System Support:** Blessed thistle is rich in antioxidants such as flavonoids, including apigenin and luteolin, which possess immune-enhancing properties. These antioxidants help neutralize harmful free radicals and support a healthy immune response.
4. **Anti-inflammatory Effects:** Blessed thistle contains compounds like polyphenols, including chlorogenic acid and caffeic acid, which exhibit anti-inflammatory properties. These compounds may help reduce inflammation and support overall well-being.
5. **Gallbladder Health:** Blessed thistle is believed to stimulate the production and flow of bile, a substance produced by the liver and stored in the gallbladder. Bile plays a crucial role in digestion, aiding in the breakdown and absorption of fats.
6. **Skin Health:** Blessed thistle contains antioxidants such as flavonoids and phenolic acids, which help protect the skin from oxidative stress and promote a youthful appearance. These compounds may support skin health and contribute to a radiant complexion.
7. **Antimicrobial Effects:** Blessed thistle contains sesquiterpene lactones, including cnicin, which have demonstrated antimicrobial activity against various pathogens, including bacteria and fungi. These compounds may help combat microbial infections.

8. **Cardiovascular Health:** Blessed thistle is a source of polyphenols, including catechins and quercetin, which have been associated with cardiovascular benefits. These compounds may support heart health by reducing oxidative stress and promoting healthy blood circulation.
9. **Graceful-aging Effects:** The antioxidants present in blessed thistle, including flavonoids, phenolic acids, and polyphenols, help protect cells from oxidative damage, which is associated with aging processes. These antioxidants may contribute to overall longevity and well-being.
10. **Hormonal Balance:** Blessed thistle is believed to offer potential benefits for supporting hormonal balance in the body, particularly in women. While it may not be a significant source of phytoestrogens, blessed thistle's active compounds are thought to have properties that could positively influence menstrual health and help alleviate menopausal symptoms.

> Blessed thistle is generally considered safe to consume. However, there are a few important warnings and contradictions to keep in mind. Individuals with allergies to plants in the Asteraceae/Compositae family, such as ragweed, daisies, or marigolds, may also be allergic to blessed thistle and should avoid its use. Additionally, individuals with hormone-sensitive conditions, such as breast, ovarian, or uterine cancer, should exercise caution as blessed thistle may have estrogenic effects. It is not recommended to use blessed thistle if you are taking anticoagulant or antiplatelet medications, as it may increase the risk of bleeding. As for pregnancy and lactation, there is limited information available, so it is advisable to consult with your herbalist/practitioner before using blessed thistle during these periods.

BLUE VERVAIN

Blue vervain, scientifically known as Verbena hastata, is a perennial herbaceous plant native to North America. Its name is derived from the Latin word "verbenae," meaning sacred bough, due to its historical use in ancient rituals and ceremonies. This herb has a rich cultural and medicinal history, dating back centuries to the indigenous tribes of America. The blue vervain plant typically grows in wet meadows, marshes, and along stream banks, reaching heights of up to 5 feet. It boasts slender spikes of delicate blue-violet flowers that bloom from June to September, attracting various pollinators such as butterflies and bees.

Now, let's explore ten extensive health and longevity benefits associated with blue vervain:

1. **Anti-inflammatory Effects:** Blue vervain contains flavonoids such as apigenin and luteolin, which possess anti-inflammatory properties and may help reduce inflammation in the body.
2. **Liver Health:** Blue vervain contains bitter compounds like verbenalin and aucubin, which support liver function and may aid in detoxification processes.
3. **Digestive Health:** The bitter constituents in blue vervain, including verbenalin, promote healthy digestion by stimulating digestive secretions and supporting proper nutrient absorption.
4. **Stress Relief:** Blue vervain is traditionally used as a nervine, with compounds like verbenalin and hastatoside believed to have calming effects on the nervous system, promoting relaxation and reducing stress.
5. **Immune System Support:** Blue vervain contains phenolic compounds like verbascoside and verbenalin, which possess antioxidant properties and may help support a healthy immune system.
6. **Respiratory Health:** Blue vervain has a long history of traditional use for respiratory conditions. It is believed that compounds found in blue vervain, such as verbascoside and hastatoside, may contribute to its beneficial effects on respiratory health. These compounds are thought to provide expectorant properties, helping to alleviate cough and congestion.
7. **Cardiovascular Health:** Blue vervain contains flavonoids such as verbenalin, which may help support cardiovascular health by reducing oxidative stress and inflammation.

8. **Anxiety Relief:** Blue vervain has traditionally been used to alleviate anxiety, with compounds like verbenalin and hastatoside potentially contributing to its anxiolytic effects.
9. **Antimicrobial Effects:** Blue vervain contains volatile oils and tannins that have shown antimicrobial properties, potentially helping to inhibit the growth of certain pathogens.
10. **Antioxidant Powerhouse:** Blue vervain is a rich source of phenolic compounds, including verbascoside, luteolin, and apigenin, which exhibit antioxidant activity and help protect against oxidative stress.

> While blue vervain is generally considered safe to consume, there are certain medical contradictions and precautions to consider. It is important to be cautious if you have known allergies or sensitivities to plants in the Verbenaceae family, which include vervain species such as Verbena officinalis and lemon verbena (Aloysia citrodora). Individuals with low blood pressure (hypotension) should also exercise caution when using blue vervain, as it may further lower blood pressure levels. If you are taking medications for sedation or anti-anxiety purposes, it is recommended to consult with a healthcare professional before combining them with blue vervain, as it may potentiate the effects of these medications. Pregnant women should avoid blue vervain due to its historical use in stimulating uterine contractions and promoting menstruation, potentially posing a risk to pregnancy. Consult with your herbalist/practitioner prior to using this herb if you are breastfeeding.

BOLDO LEAF

Boldo leaf, scientifically known as Peumus boldus, are native to the central regions of Chile and parts of Peru. With its small, leathery leaves and aromatic scent, this evergreen tree has a long history of traditional use among indigenous cultures in South America. Boldo leaves have been highly regarded for their potential medicinal properties and have been used for centuries to promote health and well-being. The leaves contain various beneficial compounds that contribute to their extensive health benefits.

Now, let's explore ten extensive health and longevity benefits associated with boldo leaf:

1. **Digestive Health:** Boldo leaves have been traditionally used to support digestive health. They may help stimulate the production of digestive enzymes, improve digestion, and alleviate symptoms of indigestion, bloating, and gas.
2. **Detoxification:** Boldo leaves are believed to have hepatoprotective properties, supporting liver health and aiding in the detoxification process. They may assist in the elimination of toxins from the body and promote optimal liver function.
3. **Gallbladder Health:** Boldo leaves contain boldine, a bioactive alkaloid known for its choleretic properties, meaning it stimulates the production and release of bile from the liver into the gallbladder. Bile plays a crucial role in the digestion of fats by emulsifying them, aiding their absorption. By promoting bile flow, boldo leaves can support gallbladder function and contribute to the healthy digestion of fats.
4. **Anti-inflammatory Effects:** Boldo leaves contain compounds with anti-inflammatory properties, which may help reduce inflammation in the body and alleviate symptoms associated with inflammatory conditions such as arthritis.
5. **Antimicrobial Effects:** Boldo leaves contain essential oils rich in constituents like limonene, cineole, and p-cymene, which possess antimicrobial activity. These antimicrobial properties of boldo leaves may contribute to bolstering immune health and providing defense against infections.
6. **Antiparasitic Effects:** Boldo leaves have been traditionally used to combat parasitic infections. They may have antiparasitic properties, helping to eliminate intestinal parasites and promote intestinal health.

7. **Antioxidant Powerhouse:** Boldo leaves are rich in antioxidants, which help protect the body against free radicals and oxidative stress. They may contribute to overall cellular health and longevity.
8. **Urinary Tract Health:** Boldo leaves have diuretic properties, promoting urine production and supporting urinary tract health. They may help alleviate symptoms of urinary tract infections and assist in maintaining a healthy urinary system.
9. **Respiratory Health:** Boldo leaves may offer respiratory benefits. They have been used to alleviate symptoms of respiratory conditions such as coughs, bronchitis, and congestion.
10. **Nervous System Support:** Boldo leaves have been used to promote relaxation and support the nervous system. They may help reduce anxiety and nervous tension and promote a sense of calm.

While boldo leaf is generally safe for consumption in small quantities, there are specific medical contradictions and precautions to consider. Individuals with gallbladder disorders, bile duct obstruction, or liver disease should consult with their healthcare provider before using boldo leaf, as it may stimulate bile flow and exacerbate these conditions. Boldo leaf contains a compound called ascaridole, which may have toxic effects in large amounts or with prolonged use. Therefore, it is recommended to use boldo leaf for short-term periods and under the guidance of your herbalist/practitioner. Boldo leaf may interact with certain medications, such as anticoagulants (blood thinners) and anticonvulsants. Pregnant women and breastfeeding mothers should avoid boldo leaf due to conflicting information on the safety of this herb during these times.

BONESET

Boneset, scientifically known as Eupatorium perfoliatum, has a rich history deeply rooted in North American herbal medicine. Native to the eastern and central regions of the United States and Canada, this perennial plant earned its common name from its historical use in treating breakbone fever (dengue fever), as its powerful properties were believed to alleviate the excruciating pain associated with the illness. Indigenous peoples and early settlers recognized the therapeutic potential of boneset, often preparing it as infusions or poultices to treat various ailments, including fevers and respiratory conditions. Today, it continues to be valued in herbal remedies and alternative medicine for its potential immune-boosting and fever-reducing properties.

Now, let's explore ten extensive health and longevity benefits associated with boneset:

1. **Immune System Support:** Boneset contains powerful antioxidants, such as flavonoids and phenolic compounds, which help bolster the immune system and protect against harmful free radicals.
2. **Respiratory Health:** Boneset's expectorant properties, attributed to compounds such as eupafolin, eupatoriopicrin, and polysaccharides, help relieve congestion and promote healthy respiratory function. It can provide relief for coughs, colds, and bronchial conditions by easing airway constriction, facilitating mucus expulsion, and supporting a healthy inflammatory response.
3. **Digestive Health:** Boneset's bitter properties, attributed to compounds such as sesquiterpene lactones and flavonoids, play a vital role in stimulating digestive processes. These bitter constituents interact with taste receptors on the tongue, triggering a cascade of events that enhance digestive function. The stimulation of digestive enzymes and gastric secretions helps break down food more efficiently, leading to improved nutrient absorption.
4. **Laxative Effects:** Boneset has mild laxative properties and has been used to alleviate constipation.
5. **Anti-inflammatory Effects:** The herb's anti-inflammatory compounds, including sesquiterpene lactones and polysaccharides, contribute to reduced inflammation in the body.
6. **Pain Relief:** Boneset's analgesic properties, including sesquiterpene lactones and alkaloids like tremetol and pyrrolizidine alkaloids, make it a potential pain reliever for conditions like arthritis, muscle aches, and headaches.

7. **Skin Health:** The herb's antimicrobial and anti-inflammatory properties make it a valuable ingredient in topical preparations for skin conditions like wounds, burns, and insect bites. Boneset contains tannins such as catechins and gallic acid which may help inhibit the growth of bacteria, fungi, and other pathogens that can contribute to skin infections.
8. **Diaphoretic Effect:** Boneset's diaphoretic properties are attributed to several of its constituents, including sesquiterpene lactones and flavonoids. These compounds are believed to stimulate the sweat glands and promote sweating, which, in turn, can help reduce fever and facilitate the elimination of toxins from the body.
9. **Antimicrobial Effects:** Active compounds in boneset, such as tannins and essential oils, exhibit antimicrobial effects, helping to combat various pathogens, including bacteria and fungi.
10. **Malaria and Dengue Fever Treatment:** Historically, boneset was used as a treatment for malaria and dengue fever.

> While boneset is generally safe to consume in small quantities and for short durations, it is important to exercise caution and be aware of certain medical contradictions and precautions. Large quantities of boneset should be avoided, as it contains pyrrolizidine alkaloids that may have hepatotoxic effects if used in high doses or for prolonged periods. Individuals with liver or kidney diseases, as well as those with a history of liver damage, should approach the use of boneset with caution. Additionally, individuals with known allergies to plants in the Asteraceae/Compositae family, such as ragweed, marigolds, and daisies, may be at risk of experiencing allergic reactions to boneset. It is essential to consult with a healthcare professional before using boneset if you have specific medical conditions or are taking medications that may interact with the herb, particularly anticoagulants or antiplatelet drugs. Pregnant and breastfeeding women should generally avoid the use of boneset unless otherwise directed by their herbalist/practitioner.

BORAGE

Borage, scientifically known as Borago officinalis, is a flowering plant native to the Mediterranean region but now cultivated worldwide. This herbaceous plant is characterized by its bright blue star-shaped flowers and hairy leaves. Borage has a rich history of traditional use dating back centuries, with its origins traced to ancient Greece and Rome. It has long been recognized for its culinary and medicinal properties and is highly regarded in herbal medicine practices. Borage is known for its abundance of beneficial compounds that contribute to its extensive health benefits.

Now, let's explore ten extensive health and longevity benefits associated with borage:

1. **Anti-inflammatory Effects:** Borage contains triterpenoid compounds such as beta-amyrin and lupeol, which have been shown to possess anti-inflammatory effects. These compounds contribute to the plant's ability to alleviate inflammation in the body. Studies have demonstrated that beta-amyrin and lupeol can inhibit the production of pro-inflammatory molecules, such as cytokines and prostaglandins, in immune cells. These compounds interfere with the inflammatory signaling pathways, reducing the production of inflammatory mediators and modulating the immune response. The anti-inflammatory effects of beta-amyrin and lupeol contribute to the protection of tissues and organs from damage caused by chronic inflammation. By reducing inflammation, these compounds help prevent oxidative stress, tissue damage, and the progression of inflammatory diseases.
2. **Skin Health:** Borage oil, derived from borage seeds, is rich in gamma-linolenic acid (GLA), an omega-6 fatty acid. It has been used to promote skin health, improve moisture retention, and soothe dry, irritated skin conditions like eczema and dermatitis.
3. **Bone Health:** Borage is a source of minerals such as calcium and magnesium, essential for maintaining healthy bones and preventing bone-related conditions like osteoporosis.
4. **Graceful-aging Effects:** Borage contains a variety of antioxidants, including vitamin E, flavonoids like quercetin and kaempferol, phenolic acids such as rosmarinic acid, and gamma-linolenic acid (GLA). These antioxidants help combat free radicals and protect the skin from oxidative damage, promoting a more youthful appearance and contributing to pro-aging effects. They work by preserving cell health, maintaining the integrity of cell membranes, and reducing the risk of oxidative stress.

5. **Hormonal Balance:** Borage contains GLA, which may help regulate hormonal balance in the body, particularly in women. It has been used to alleviate symptoms of premenstrual syndrome (PMS) and menopause and support overall hormonal well-being.
6. **Cardiovascular Health:** Borage is rich in antioxidants, including vitamin C and flavonoids, which contribute to cardiovascular health. These compounds may help reduce oxidative stress, promote healthy blood circulation, and support heart function.
7. **Mood Support:** Borage has been used to uplift mood and promote emotional well-being. Its GLA content may play a role in supporting neurotransmitter function and maintaining a positive outlook.
8. **Adrenal Support:** GLA has been suggested to support adrenal health through its various properties, including exhibiting anti-inflammatory properties, which may help reduce inflammation that can affect adrenal function. As a precursor to prostaglandins, GLA plays a role in hormone regulation, including cortisol, a key hormone produced by the adrenal glands. Additionally, GLA has been associated with anti-stress effects, promoting relaxation and potentially alleviating the burden on the adrenal glands caused by chronic stress.
9. **Digestive Health:** Borage contains specific compounds that aid in digestive support, including gamma-linolenic acid (GLA) and bitter constituents like sesquiterpene lactones. GLA helps regulate inflammation in the digestive tract, promoting healthy digestion. The bitter constituents stimulate digestive secretions, improving digestion and alleviating discomfort such as bloating and gas. Together, these compounds in borage support digestive health and provide relief for digestive issues.
10. **Immune System Support:** Borage contains specific antioxidants that contribute to its immune-boosting properties, including gamma-tocopherol (a form of vitamin E), ascorbic acid (vitamin C), and various phenolic compounds such as rosmarinic acid and caffeic acid derivatives. These antioxidants help strengthen the immune system by neutralizing harmful free radicals and reducing oxidative stress.

While borage is generally safe for consumption, there are certain medical contradictions and precautions to be aware of. Borage contains pyrrolizidine alkaloids, which can be toxic to the liver in high doses or with prolonged use, so it is important to avoid excessive or prolonged consumption of borage extracts or supplements. Making tea using borage is less concentrated and a safer option to exercise. Individuals with liver disease or impaired liver function should consult with their healthcare provider prior to using this herb. Borage may also interact with certain medications, such as diuretics, anticoagulants, and antiplatelet drugs, so it is advisable to consult with a healthcare professional before using borage if you are taking any of these medications. Women who are pregnant or lactating should consult with their herbalist/practitioner prior to using borage.

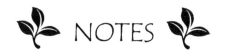

BOSWELLIA

Boswellia, also known as Indian frankincense, is a resinous extract derived from the Boswellia serrata tree native to India, North Africa, and the Middle East. It has a rich history dating back thousands of years in traditional Ayurvedic and herbal medicine systems. The resin from the Boswellia tree has been highly valued for its therapeutic properties and has been used for centuries to promote health and well-being. Boswellia possesses a range of beneficial compounds that contribute to its extensive health benefits.

Now, let's explore ten extensive health and longevity benefits associated with Boswellia:

1. **Anti-inflammatory Effects:** Boswellia contains boswellic acids, such as AKBA (3-O-acetyl-11-keto-beta-boswellic acid), which possess potent anti-inflammatory properties by inhibiting specific enzymes involved in the inflammatory response.
2. **Joint Health:** Boswellia has been traditionally used to support joint health and ease discomfort associated with conditions like osteoarthritis. Its anti-inflammatory properties, specifically the boswellic acids, may contribute to these benefits.
3. **Respiratory Health:** Boswellia has been used for respiratory conditions like asthma and bronchitis. It may help reduce inflammation in the airways, potentially alleviating symptoms. Boswellic acids and other active compounds are believed to play a role in these effects.
4. **Digestive Health:** Boswellia has been suggested to support digestive health by reducing inflammation in the gastrointestinal tract. It may help with conditions like inflammatory bowel disease (IBD). The anti-inflammatory properties of boswellic acids are believed to be involved in these effects.
5. **Liver Health:** Certain active compounds in Boswellia, such as β-boswellic acid, have shown potential hepatoprotective effects by supporting liver function and reducing oxidative stress.
6. **Skin Health:** Boswellia has been used in topical applications for various skin conditions, including wounds, burns, and acne. Its anti-inflammatory and antimicrobial properties may help in wound healing and combating skin infections.
7. **Cognitive Support:** Boswellia may support cognitive function by reducing neuroinflammation. Its active compounds, such as AKBA, may play a role in preserving brain health and potentially protecting against neurodegenerative diseases.

8. **Cardiovascular Health:** Boswellia may contribute to cardiovascular health by reducing inflammation and oxidative stress, which are associated with cardiovascular diseases. The antioxidant properties of Boswellia's active compounds, including boswellic acids, may play a role in these benefits.
9. **Antimicrobial Effects:** Boswellia exhibits antimicrobial effects against various pathogens, including bacteria and fungi. The specific active compounds in Boswellia, such as incensole acetate, contribute to its anti-pathogenic properties.
10. **Antioxidant Powerhouse:** Boswellia contains antioxidants, including terpenes and flavonoids, which help neutralize harmful free radicals, reducing oxidative stress and potentially supporting longevity.

While Boswellia is generally considered safe to consume, there are certain medical contradictions and warnings that should be considered. Individuals with known allergies or sensitivities to Boswellia or other plants in the Burseraceae family should avoid its consumption, as it may trigger allergic reactions. Additionally, individuals with bleeding disorders or those taking anticoagulant or antiplatelet medications should exercise caution, as Boswellia may have mild anticoagulant properties and could potentially increase the risk of bleeding. Boswellia may also interact with certain medications, such as nonsteroidal anti-inflammatory drugs (NSAIDs), and should be used with caution in combination with these drugs. Women who are pregnant or lactating should consult with their herbalist/practitioner prior to using Boswellia.

BRAHMI LEAF (BACOPA)

Brahmi leaf, scientifically known as Bacopa monnieri, is an herb native to the wetlands of Asia, particularly India, Nepal, and Sri Lanka. With a history spanning thousands of years, Brahmi has been revered in Ayurvedic medicine for its numerous health benefits and cognitive-enhancing properties. The herb gets its name from "Brahma," the Hindu god of creation, and is often referred to as the "Herb of Grace" or "Memory Herb" due to its reputation for supporting brain function and memory. Brahmi leaf contains bioactive compounds that contribute to its extensive health benefits.

Now, let's explore ten extensive health and longevity benefits associated with Brahmi leaf:

1. **Cognitive Support:** Brahmi leaf contains bacosides, a group of bioactive compounds that have shown potential for enhancing cognitive function, memory, and learning ability. These compounds work by supporting the release of nitric oxide, improving blood flow to the brain, and enhancing the activity of neurotransmitters involved in learning and memory processes, such as acetylcholine. Brahmi leaf is widely used for its cognitive-enhancing properties, promoting mental clarity and overall cognitive performance.
2. **Adaptogenic Effects:** Brahmi leaf possesses adaptogenic properties, primarily attributed to its content of bacosides. These bioactive compounds have been associated with stress reduction by modulating the body's stress response. Adaptogens work by regulating the production of stress hormones like cortisol, helping to restore balance and promote a sense of calm and relaxation.
3. **Neuroprotection:** Brahmi leaf contains several flavonoids and saponins that contribute to its neuroprotective properties. Specific flavonoids found in Brahmi include apigenin, luteolin, and quercetin, which possess antioxidant and anti-inflammatory effects. These compounds help reduce oxidative stress and inflammation in the brain, protecting against age-related neurodegenerative conditions. Brahmi leaf also contains saponins like bacosides, which have shown potential in enhancing cognitive function and promoting neuronal health. The combined actions of these flavonoids and saponins in Brahmi leaf support its neuroprotective claims by combating oxidative damage, reducing inflammation, and supporting overall brain health.

4. **Anti-inflammatory Effects:** Brahmi leaf's anti-inflammatory properties stem not only from bacosides but also from other compounds present, such as alkaloids (brahmine, herpestine), triterpenoids (bacosides), and sterols (beta-sitosterol, stigmasterol). Together, these compounds work in synergy to regulate inflammatory pathways, suppress the release of pro-inflammatory molecules, and diminish overall inflammation in the body. The collective action of bacosides and these additional compounds underscores the potential of Brahmi leaf as a natural anti-inflammatory agent, offering relief from conditions associated with inflammation.
5. **Anxiety Relief:** Bacosides in Brahmi leaf may have anxiolytic effects, assisting in reducing anxiety symptoms and promoting calmness.
6. **Liver Health:** Brahmi leaf contains specific alkaloids that contribute to its liver-supporting properties. These alkaloids include brahmine and herpestine. Together with the saponins (bacosides A and B), they promote liver health by aiding in detoxification processes and protecting liver cells from oxidative damage.
7. **Cardiovascular Health:** Brahmi leaf contains triterpenoid compounds like betulinic acid, as well as polyphenols such as catechins, apigenin, luteolin, and quercetin, which contribute to its potential cardio-protective effects. These compounds work synergistically to support heart health by reducing oxidative stress, inflammation, and the risk of cardiovascular diseases. The combination of betulinic acid and polyphenols in Brahmi leaf promotes healthy blood circulation, helps maintain the integrity of blood vessels, and supports overall cardiovascular well-being.
8. **Anti-diabetic Effects:** The active compounds, such as saponins (bacosides) and alkaloids (brahmine, herpestine), are compounds that have been suggested to enhance insulin sensitivity, improve glucose metabolism, and reduce oxidative stress.
9. **Antimicrobial Effects:** The active compounds in Brahmi leaf, such as bacosides and alkaloids, have demonstrated antimicrobial properties against various pathogens, potentially supporting the body's defense against infections.
10. **Antioxidant Powerhouse:** Brahmi leaf is rich in antioxidants like flavonoids, alkaloids, and polyphenols, which scavenge free radicals and protect against oxidative damage, ultimately supporting overall health and longevity.

While brahmi leaf is generally considered safe to consume, there are a few important warnings and contradictions to consider. Individuals taking medications for thyroid disorders, such as levothyroxine, should use this herb with caution, as it may interfere with the effectiveness of the medication. Individuals with bradycardia or low heart rate should avoid this herb, as it may further decrease heart rate. It is important to note that brahmi is generally considered safe during pregnancy and lactation, but it is always best to consult with your herbalist/practitioner before incorporating this herb into your health regimen during these periods to ensure the proper amounts are being used.

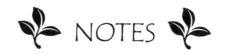

NOTES

BURDOCK ROOT

Burdock root, scientifically known as Arctium lappa, is a plant that belongs to the Asteraceae family. Native to Europe and Asia, it has a long history of use in traditional Chinese, Japanese, and Western herbal medicine. Burdock root is revered for its medicinal properties and has been utilized for centuries to promote health and well-being. The plant grows in abundance in various climates and is recognizable for its large, heart-shaped leaves and prickly burrs. Burdock root contains a variety of bioactive compounds that contribute to its extensive health benefits.

Now, let's explore ten extensive health and longevity benefits associated with burdock root:

1. **Liver and Kidney Health:** Burdock root is known to contain antioxidants, including quercetin, phenolic acids, and lignans, which contribute to liver health and aid in detoxification processes. These antioxidants assist in the elimination of toxins from the body, supporting the liver's function. Additionally, burdock root has traditionally been used to support kidney health and has diuretic properties, which may further aid in the body's natural detoxification processes.
2. **Anti-inflammatory Effects:** The active compound in burdock root, arctigenin, has been shown to possess anti-inflammatory properties, helping to reduce inflammation in the body. This can be attributed to its ability to inhibit the production of pro-inflammatory cytokines.
3. **Skin Health:** Burdock root is rich in antioxidants, including phenolic acids and quercetin, which may help protect the skin against oxidative stress and support overall skin health. It may also help alleviate skin conditions like acne, eczema, and psoriasis due to its anti-inflammatory and antimicrobial properties.
4. **Digestive Health:** Inulin, a type of soluble fiber found in burdock root, acts as a prebiotic, providing nourishment for beneficial gut bacteria. This promotes a healthy gut microbiome and supports digestive health.
5. **Cardiovascular Health:** Burdock root contains potassium, a mineral that supports heart health by regulating blood pressure and promoting proper heart rhythm. Its antioxidants, such as quercetin, may also have beneficial effects on blood vessel health.

6. **Blood Sugar Regulation:** Burdock root contains fiber, polyphenols, and antioxidants that may help regulate blood sugar levels by slowing down the absorption of carbohydrates and enhancing insulin sensitivity.
7. **Antimicrobial Effects:** Burdock root contains several compounds, including arctiin and arctigenin, which have demonstrated antimicrobial properties against various bacteria and fungi. These properties may help fight off harmful pathogens in the body.
8. **Immune System Support:** Burdock root is rich in antioxidants such as quercetin and luteolin, which can strengthen the immune system by neutralizing free radicals and reducing oxidative stress, thereby supporting overall immune function.
9. **Graceful-aging Effects:** Burdock root contains antioxidants that help protect against cellular damage caused by free radicals. By reducing oxidative stress, these antioxidants may indirectly support graceful aging processes.
10. **Anti-cancer Effects:** Some studies have suggested that certain compounds in burdock root, including arctigenin and lignans, may exhibit anti-cancer properties by inhibiting the growth of cancer cells and inducing apoptosis (programmed cell death). However, further research is needed to fully understand these effects.

While burdock root is generally considered safe to consume, there are certain medical contradictions and precautions to be aware of. Individuals with known allergies to daisies, ragweed, or other plants in the Asteraceae/Compositae family may also be allergic to burdock root and should avoid its consumption. Individuals taking diuretic medications, such as furosemide or hydrochlorothiazide, should exercise caution as burdock root has diuretic properties and may enhance the effects of these medications, potentially leading to electrolyte imbalances. Burdock root may also interact with medications that are metabolized by the liver, such as cytochrome P450 substrates, and it is recommended to consult a healthcare professional before using it in conjunction with these medications. It is advisable to consult with your herbalist/practitioner prior to using burdock root during pregnancy or lactation.

BUTTERBUR ROOT

Butterbur root, scientifically known as Petasites hybridus, is an herbaceous perennial plant with a long history of use in traditional medicine. It is native to Europe and parts of Asia and North America. Butterbur derives its name from the traditional use of its large leaves to wrap butter during warm weather to prevent it from melting. The plant has been highly regarded for its medicinal properties, particularly in supporting respiratory health and relieving allergies.

Now, let's explore ten extensive health and longevity benefits associated with butterbur root:

1. **Migraine Relief:** Butterbur root has been shown to help reduce the frequency and severity of migraines. Active compounds called petasins found in butterbur root exhibit anti-inflammatory effects that may help alleviate migraine symptoms.
2. **Allergy Relief:** Butterbur root has demonstrated effectiveness in reducing symptoms of seasonal allergies. The active ingredient petasin is believed to inhibit the release of histamine and leukotrienes, which are involved in allergic reactions.
3. **Respiratory Health:** Butterbur root has been used to support respiratory health and relieve symptoms of asthma and bronchitis. The active compounds, petasins, and flavonoids in butterbur root possess anti-inflammatory and bronchodilatory properties.
4. **Anti-inflammatory Effects:** Butterbur root contains various flavonoids, including quercetin and kaempferol, which exhibit potent anti-inflammatory properties. These antioxidants help reduce inflammation in the body, which may contribute to overall longevity.
5. **Liver Health:** Butterbur root has been found to have hepatoprotective effects, supporting liver health. The active compound, petasin, may help protect the liver against oxidative stress and inflammation.
6. **Antioxidant Powerhouse:** Butterbur root contains various antioxidants, including flavonoids and phenolic compounds, which help neutralize free radicals and reduce oxidative stress in the body. This antioxidant activity may contribute to pro-aging benefits.
7. **Urinary Tract Health:** Butterbur root has diuretic properties that may support urinary tract health. It may help increase urine flow and promote the elimination of toxins from the body.

8. **Graceful-aging Effects:** Butterbur root's antioxidant and anti-inflammatory properties, along with its potential to support various organ systems, can indirectly contribute to graceful aging by promoting overall health and well-being.
9. **Digestive Health:** Butterbur root has a history of traditional use for easing gastrointestinal discomfort. The active compounds, such as petasins, contribute to its potential in relaxing smooth muscles and alleviating spasms in the digestive tract.
10. **Antimicrobial Effects:** Some studies suggest that butterbur root extracts may exhibit antimicrobial properties against certain bacteria and fungi, which may support the body's defense against pathogens.

> While butterbur root is generally considered safe to consume in small quantities, there are certain medical contradictions and warnings that should be considered. Butterbur contains pyrrolizidine alkaloids (PAs), which can be toxic to the liver when consumed in large amounts over extended periods. Therefore, it is crucial to use butterbur under the guidance and supervision of your herbalist. Individuals with liver disease or liver impairment should avoid using butterbur unless otherwise directed by your herbalist/practitioner. Additionally, individuals with a known allergy to plants in the Asteraceae family, such as ragweed, daisies, or marigolds, may also experience allergic reactions to butterbur. Butterbur may interact with certain medications, particularly those metabolized by the liver. It is advised to consult with a healthcare professional before using butterbur if you are taking medications that are processed by the liver, such as certain antihistamines, anti-seizure medications, or cholesterol-lowering drugs. The safety of butterbur during pregnancy and lactation is uncertain, and it is generally recommended to avoid its use during these periods due to the lack of sufficient safety data.

CALENDULA FLOWERS

Calendula flowers, scientifically known as Calendula officinalis, have a rich and fascinating origin that dates back centuries. Belonging to the Asteraceae family, this vibrant and versatile flower has been cherished and utilized for its numerous health benefits throughout history. Originating in the Mediterranean region, calendula flowers have long been cultivated for their beauty and medicinal properties. Ancient civilizations, including the Egyptians, Greeks, and Romans, recognized the therapeutic potential of this extraordinary plant. The name "calendula" is derived from the Latin word "calendae," which means "little calendar," possibly referencing the flower's tendency to bloom on the first day of each month. In folklore and traditional medicine, calendula flowers were believed to possess magical properties and were used to promote healing, enhance skin health, and support overall well-being. Today, modern research continues to unveil the remarkable health and longevity benefits offered by calendula flowers, making them a valuable ingredient in natural remedies, skincare products, and herbal medicine.

Now, let's explore ten extensive health and longevity benefits associated with calendula flowers:

1. **Anti-inflammatory Effects:** Calendula contains flavonoids, such as quercetin and rutin, which possess anti-inflammatory properties. These compounds help reduce inflammation in the body, supporting various organ systems and promoting overall health.
2. **Anti-Radiation Effects:** Calendula unveils its remarkable potential as a natural anti-radiation tool. Laden with potent antioxidants, including carotenoids like lutein and beta-carotene, as well as flavonoids such as quercetin and kaempferol, calendula stands as a formidable defense against the harmful effects of radiation exposure. These antioxidants work tirelessly to counteract the destructive impact of free radicals induced by radiation, safeguarding cellular integrity and promoting resilience in the face of radiation-related challenges. Calendula's role in radiation protection makes it a valuable asset in efforts to mitigate the consequences of exposure to ionizing radiation.
3. **Antimicrobial Effects:** Calendula exhibits antimicrobial properties thanks to compounds like calendulosides, flavonoids, and essential oils. These properties make it effective against certain pathogens, helping to combat infections and support overall health.

4. **Wound Healing:** Calendula contains triterpenoids and oleanolic acid, which have wound-healing properties. These compounds promote tissue repair, reduce inflammation, and stimulate the production of collagen, supporting the healing process.
5. **Antiviral Effects:** Calendula contains flavonoids and triterpenoids, such as quercetin and triterpene saponins, which contribute to its antiviral effects. These compounds have demonstrated inhibitory activity against certain viruses in laboratory studies.
6. **Digestive Health:** Calendula contains mucilage, a soothing compound that supports digestive health. It may help alleviate stomach discomfort, protect the stomach lining, and support healthy digestion.
7. **Liver Health:** Calendula contains flavonoids, such as quercetin and isorhamnetin, which support liver health and promote detoxification processes. These compounds help protect the liver from oxidative stress and support its natural cleansing functions.
8. **Immune System Support:** Calendula's antioxidants, including flavonoids and carotenoids, support immune system function. They help strengthen the immune response, combat pathogens, and protect against cellular damage.
9. **Eye Health:** The carotenoids found in calendula, such as lutein and zeaxanthin, have been associated with improved eye health. Lutein and zeaxanthin are known to accumulate in the macula, a part of the retina responsible for central vision. Their presence in the macula supports its health and function, contributing to clear vision. Additionally, these carotenoids have been suggested to reduce the risk of age-related vision problems, such as macular degeneration and cataracts.
10. **Skin Health:** Calendula's antioxidant compounds, including flavonoids like quercetin and kaempferol, along with carotenoids such as lutein and beta-carotene, contribute to its potential benefits for skin health. These plant compounds possess both antioxidant and anti-inflammatory properties, helping to protect the skin against oxidative stress and reduce inflammation. By doing so, calendula may promote a healthier appearance and overall well-being of the skin.

While calendula is generally considered safe to consume, there are certain medical contradictions and precautions to consider. Individuals with known allergies to plants in the Asteraceae/Compositae family, such as ragweed, daisies, or marigolds, may also be allergic to calendula and should avoid its use. Additionally, individuals with bleeding disorders or those taking anticoagulant medications, such as warfarin, should exercise caution due to the potential for calendula to have mild anticoagulant properties. Calendula may also have estrogenic effects, so individuals with hormone-sensitive conditions, such as breast or uterine cancer, should avoid or use calendula with caution. Women who are pregnant or breastfeeding should consult with their herbalist/practitioner prior to using calendula during these times.

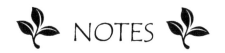

NOTES

CALIFORNIA POPPY

California poppy, scientifically known as Eschscholzia californica, holds a captivating origin deeply rooted in the landscapes of the western United States. This delicate and vibrant flower, often associated with the golden fields of California, has a rich history intertwined with Native American traditions and early settlers. Native to the Pacific coastal region and parts of Mexico, California poppy has long been revered for its ethereal beauty and medicinal properties. Its name pays homage to the renowned Baltic German botanist Johann Friedrich von Eschscholtz, who first documented the plant during an expedition in the early 19th century. This resilient wildflower, with its feathery blue-green foliage and radiant orange or yellow blossoms, has become an iconic symbol of the American West. Beyond its visual allure, California poppy offers a host of health and longevity benefits, as recognized by traditional herbal medicine and contemporary research.

Now, let's explore ten extensive health and longevity benefits associated with California poppy:

1. **Sleep Support:** California poppy contains compounds like eschscholtzine and californidine, which are believed to have sedative effects, promoting relaxation and potentially aiding in sleep.
2. **Nervous System Support:** The presence of protopine in California poppy may contribute to its potential benefits for the nervous system, supporting cognitive function and mood regulation.
3. **Pain Relief:** Active compounds like protopine and allocryptopine found in California poppy have mild analgesic properties that may help alleviate pain.
4. **Liver Health:** Some constituents, including allocryptopine and protopine, found in California poppy, may aid in supporting liver health by aiding detoxification processes and promoting the healthy functioning of this vital organ.
5. **Graceful-aging Effects:** The presence of specific compounds like protopine and eschscholtzine in California poppy may contribute to its potential graceful aging effects by supporting overall cellular health and longevity.
6. **Anti-inflammatory Effects:** The presence of protopine and californidine in California poppy suggests potential anti-inflammatory activity, which can support overall health and longevity.

7. **Respiratory Health:** The eschscholtzines in California poppy exhibit expectorant properties that may aid in alleviating coughs and promoting respiratory well-being.
8. **Cardiovascular Health:** Allocryptopine, an active compound in California poppy, may contribute to cardiovascular health by promoting healthy blood vessel function.
9. **Immune System Support:** The presence of californidine in California poppy may have immune-modulating effects, supporting the optimal function of the immune system.
10. **Digestive Health:** The protopine found in California poppy, may have mild antispasmodic properties, potentially providing relief from digestive discomfort.

While California poppy is generally considered safe to consume, it is important to be aware of some precautions and contradictions. Individuals taking sedative medications, such as benzodiazepines or barbiturates, should exercise caution when using California poppy due to potential interactions. Additionally, individuals with known allergies to plants in the Papaveraceae family should avoid using this herb. It is also recommended to avoid using this herb during pregnancy or lactation unless specifically advised by your herbalist/practitioner.

CAMU CAMU BERRY (POWDER)

Camu camu berries are a small tropical fruit known as Myrciaria dubia and has a captivating origin deeply rooted in the lush Amazon rainforests of South America. Native to the countries of Peru, Brazil, Colombia, and Venezuela, this small round fruit holds a rich history and cultural significance among indigenous communities. The camu camu tree thrives in the nutrient-rich soil near riverbanks and flooded areas, producing abundant clusters of vibrant red or purple berries. Traditionally, the indigenous people of the Amazon have cherished this fruit for its powerful medicinal properties and as a vital source of nutrition. The fruit's name, "camu camu," is derived from the native Quechua language, which translates to "little fruit." In recent years, camu camu has gained global recognition for its exceptional nutritional profile, particularly its extraordinary vitamin C content. Camu camu powder, derived from freeze-dried camu camu berries, has become a popular superfood supplement, offering an array of health and longevity benefits.

Now, let's explore ten extensive health and longevity benefits associated with camu camu berries:

1. **Immune System Support:** Camu camu berry is renowned for its exceptionally high vitamin C content, which helps strengthen the immune system, boost the production of white blood cells, and protect against infections.
2. **Antioxidant Powerhouse:** The abundant antioxidants in camu camu berry, including flavonoids and anthocyanins, help combat free radicals, reduce oxidative stress, and protect cells from damage, supporting overall health and longevity.
3. **Anti-inflammatory Effects:** Camu camu berry contains natural anti-inflammatory compounds that may help alleviate inflammation-related conditions, such as arthritis, joint pain, and inflammatory bowel disease.
4. **Collagen Synthesis:** Vitamin C in camu camu berry plays a crucial role in collagen synthesis, contributing to the health and integrity of skin, connective tissues, and blood vessels. It supports healthy skin, promotes wound healing, and may help reduce the appearance of wrinkles.
5. **Mood Support:** The high vitamin C content in camu camu berry supports brain health and the synthesis of neurotransmitters, potentially enhancing mood, reducing anxiety and depression symptoms, and supporting mental well-being.

6. **Eye Health:** Camu camu berry contains potent antioxidants like vitamin C and anthocyanins, which help protect the eyes from oxidative stress, promote healthy vision, and reduce the risk of age-related eye diseases.
7. **Cardiovascular Health:** The antioxidant and anti-inflammatory properties of camu camu berry may contribute to cardiovascular health by reducing the risk of heart disease, lowering blood pressure, and improving blood circulation.
8. **Detoxification:** Camu camu berry contains natural detoxifying compounds that support liver health and aid in the elimination of toxins from the body, promoting overall detoxification and cleansing.
9. **Graceful-aging Effects:** The potent antioxidants in camu camu berry help combat the effects of aging caused by free radicals, promoting youthful-looking skin, reducing the appearance of wrinkles, and supporting overall vitality.
10. **Energy Boost:** Camu camu berry provides a natural energy boost due to its rich vitamin C content, which helps improve energy levels, reduce fatigue, and enhance physical performance.

While the consumption of camu camu berry is generally considered safe, there are certain medical contradictions to be aware of. Individuals with iron overload disorders, such as hereditary hemochromatosis, should consult with a healthcare professional before consuming camu camu berry, as it is known to be a good source of dietary iron. Camu camu berry may also interact with certain medications, particularly blood-thinning medications such as warfarin, due to its high vitamin C content, which can enhance the effects of these medications and increase the risk of bleeding. It is important to consult with a healthcare professional if you are taking any medications, especially blood thinners, before incorporating camu camu berry into your diet. This berry is generally considered safe to consume during pregnancy and lactation.

CARDAMOM

Cardamom, known for its distinct aroma and flavor, is a spice derived from the seeds of plants belonging to the Zingiberaceae family. The origin of cardamom can be traced back to the lush forests of the Western Ghats in southern India, where it has been cultivated for centuries. This tropical region provides the ideal climate for the growth of cardamom plants, which thrive in warm, humid conditions. Cardamom powder, made by grinding the dried seeds of cardamom pods, has long been valued not only for its culinary uses but also for its numerous health and longevity benefits. Throughout history, cardamom has played a significant role in traditional medicine systems, including Ayurveda and Chinese medicine. Its medicinal properties have been recognized and cherished for centuries. In Ayurveda, cardamom is considered a powerful aromatic herb with a balancing effect on the body and mind. It is traditionally used to support digestion, respiratory health, and overall well-being. In Chinese medicine, cardamom is believed to have warming properties and is often used to promote healthy digestion, alleviate stomach discomfort, and invigorate the spleen and stomach meridians. It is considered a valuable herb in harmonizing the flow of Qi (vital energy) within the body.

Now, let's explore ten extensive health and longevity benefits associated with cardamom:

1. **Digestive Health:** Cardamom contains volatile oils, such as cineole, which may help improve digestion by increasing the secretion of digestive enzymes. It also contains compounds like terpenes, which have been shown to possess gastroprotective effects, protecting the stomach lining from damage.
2. **Liver Health:** Cardamom has been shown to support liver health by enhancing liver detoxification processes. The active compounds in cardamom, such as terpinene and limonene, have hepatoprotective properties, protecting the liver from damage caused by toxins.
3. **Respiratory Health:** Cardamom's volatile oils, including cineole, exhibit expectorant properties that may help promote the expulsion of mucus and relieve congestion. It may benefit individuals with respiratory conditions like bronchitis and asthma.
4. **Oral Health:** Cardamom contains compounds with antimicrobial properties, such as cineole and limonene, which may help combat oral pathogens and prevent tooth decay. It may also freshen breath due to its pleasant aroma.

5. **Anti-inflammatory Effects:** The active compounds in cardamom, including terpenes and flavonoids, exhibit anti-inflammatory effects. These compounds may help reduce inflammation in the body, potentially benefiting conditions like arthritis and inflammatory bowel diseases.
6. **Cardiovascular Health:** Cardamom contains minerals like potassium and magnesium, which are essential for maintaining heart health. It also contains antioxidants like alpha-pinene, which have been associated with a lower risk of heart disease by reducing oxidative stress and inflammation.
7. **Antimicrobial Effects:** The essential oils in cardamom, such as eucalyptol, possess antimicrobial properties. These properties may help inhibit the growth of certain bacteria and fungi, supporting the body's defense against pathogens.
8. **Cognitive Support:** Cardamom contains compounds like alpha-pinene, which have been associated with potential cognitive benefits. These compounds may have neuroprotective effects and support brain health, including memory and focus.
9. **Antispasmodic Effects:** Cardamom has been traditionally used as a natural remedy for abdominal discomfort and muscle spasms. Compounds like cineole have demonstrated antispasmodic properties, providing relief from gastrointestinal issues.
10. **Graceful-aging Effects:** Some studies suggest that the antioxidants found in cardamom, such as alpha-pinene and limonene, may have graceful aging effects by reducing oxidative stress and supporting cellular health.

While cardamom is generally considered safe to consume, there are certain medical contradictions and precautions that should be considered. Individuals with bleeding disorders or those taking anticoagulant medications should be cautious, as cardamom has mild blood-thinning properties that could increase the risk of bleeding. Cardamom may also interact with anticoagulants, antidiabetic drugs, and antihypertensive medications. It is advisable for individuals taking these medications to consult with a healthcare professional before incorporating cardamom into their routine. Additionally, individuals with known allergies to plants in the ginger family, such as turmeric or ginger itself, may also be allergic to cardamom and should avoid its use. Lastly, it's important to note that excessive consumption of cardamom may lead to gastrointestinal discomfort or allergic reactions in some individuals if consumed in large quantities. Cardamom is generally considered safe to consume during pregnancy or lactation if used in culinary amounts.

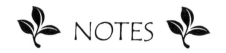

NOTES

CINNAMON

Cinnamon, derived from the bark of trees belonging to the Cinnamomum genus, is a beloved spice with a rich history that spans thousands of years. The origin of cinnamon can be traced back to the ancient civilizations of Egypt, where it was highly prized and often used in embalming rituals and as a fragrant offering to the Gods. This precious spice soon found its way to other parts of the world, including China, India, and the Middle East, where it became an essential ingredient in culinary traditions and traditional medicine. It's important to note the major differences between two commonly known varieties: cassia and Ceylon cinnamon. Cassia cinnamon, also known as Chinese cinnamon, is the more readily available and affordable type. It is characterized by its strong, spicy flavor and dark reddish-brown color. On the other hand, Ceylon cinnamon, often referred to as "true" cinnamon, is considered the premium variety. It is lighter in color, has a subtly sweet and delicate flavor, and is predominantly grown in Sri Lanka. While both varieties share some similarities in terms of taste and aroma, Ceylon cinnamon is generally regarded as superior due to its milder flavor and lower levels of coumarin, a compound that has a bit of controversy around it.

Now, let's explore ten extensive health and longevity benefits associated with cinnamon:

1. **Anti-inflammatory Effects:** Cinnamon contains antioxidants such as polyphenols, particularly cinnamaldehyde, which have anti-inflammatory properties. These compounds help reduce inflammation throughout the body, potentially supporting longevity by lowering the risk of chronic diseases.
2. **Antioxidant Powerhouse:** Cinnamon is rich in antioxidants, including phenolic compounds and flavonoids. These antioxidants help neutralize harmful free radicals, protecting cells from oxidative damage and promoting overall health and longevity.
3. **Digestive Health:** Cinnamon may aid in digestion by stimulating digestive enzymes, reducing inflammation in the gastrointestinal tract, and soothing digestive discomfort.
4. **Respiratory Health:** Cinnamon's anti-inflammatory properties specifically benefit the respiratory system. The antioxidants and anti-inflammatory compounds found in cinnamon have the potential to ease respiratory symptoms, offering support for lung health and overall respiratory well-being.

5. **Blood Sugar Regulation:** Cinnamon has been shown to help regulate blood sugar levels by improving insulin sensitivity and reducing insulin resistance. Specific compounds, such as cinnamaldehyde, may contribute to these effects, supporting metabolic health and potentially reducing the risk of age-related diseases.
6. **Cardiovascular Health:** Cinnamon may have cardioprotective effects by improving lipid profiles and reducing total cholesterol, LDL cholesterol, and triglyceride levels. This benefit may be attributed to the presence of cinnamaldehyde and other phenolic compounds that support heart health.
7. **Cognitive Support:** Some studies suggest that cinnamon can enhance cognitive function and memory. Polyphenols, such as cinnamaldehyde, may play a role in these effects by promoting neuroprotective mechanisms and reducing oxidative stress in the brain.
8. **Antimicrobial Effects:** Cinnamon possesses antimicrobial properties, potentially inhibiting the growth of various pathogens. Cinnamaldehyde and other compounds found in cinnamon have been shown to have broad-spectrum antimicrobial effects against bacteria, fungi, and viruses, supporting the body's defense against infections.
9. **Liver Health:** Cinnamon has been associated with liver-protective effects. Its compounds, including cinnamaldehyde, may support liver function, enhance detoxification processes, and protect against liver damage, promoting overall longevity.
10. **Anti-cancer Effects:** Some studies suggest that cinnamon may have anti-cancer properties. Its antioxidant and anti-inflammatory effects, attributed to compounds like cinnamaldehyde and polyphenols, may help prevent DNA damage, inhibit tumor growth, and support longevity by reducing the risk of certain cancers.

While cinnamon is generally considered safe to consume, there are a few important warnings and contradictions to keep in mind. Individuals taking anticoagulant medications, such as warfarin, should exercise caution, as cinnamon may have blood-thinning effects. Additionally, individuals with liver disease or those taking certain medications that are metabolized by the liver, such as statins or antifungal drugs, should consult their healthcare provider before consuming cinnamon. Cinnamon is generally considered safe to consume during pregnancy and lactation when used in normal culinary amounts. Consult with your herbalist/practitioner before using cinnamon in large therapeutic doses during these times.

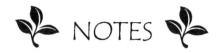

NOTES

CAT'S CLAW

Cat's claw, scientifically known as Uncaria tomentosa, commonly referred to as "Una de Gato" in Spanish, is a woody vine native to the rainforests of Central and South America, particularly the Amazon basin. It has a long history of traditional use among indigenous peoples in these regions for its medicinal properties. The name "cat's claw" is derived from the vine's curved thorns, which resemble the claws of a cat. The indigenous tribes of the Amazon rainforest have revered cat's claw for its therapeutic benefits and have used it for centuries to address various health concerns. Today, cat's claw is recognized worldwide for its potential health-promoting properties and is known for being Mother Nature's antibiotic.

Now, let's explore ten extensive health and longevity benefits associated with cat's claw:

1. **Anti-inflammatory Effects:** Cat's claw contains various compounds, including alkaloids, flavonoids, and tannins, which possess anti-inflammatory properties. These compounds, such as oxindole alkaloids (including mitraphylline), help reduce inflammation and support longevity by potentially lowering the risk of chronic diseases associated with inflammation.
2. **Antioxidant Powerhouse:** Cat's claw is rich in antioxidants, including phenolic compounds and flavonoids such as quercetin and catechins. These antioxidants help neutralize harmful free radicals, protecting cells from oxidative damage and promoting overall graceful aging and longevity.
3. **Immune System Support:** Cat's claw has immune-stimulating properties that help enhance the body's natural defense mechanisms. It contains specific compounds, such as pentacyclic oxindole alkaloids (POAs), which may support immune function, potentially contributing to longevity by reducing the risk of infections and diseases.
4. **Adaptogenic Effects:** Cat's claw is considered an adaptogen, meaning it may help the body adapt to stress and promote overall well-being. Active compounds like POAs and quinovic acid glycosides contribute to its adaptogenic properties.
5. **Joint and Bone Health:** Cat's claw has been traditionally used to support joint health and alleviate joint discomfort. Its anti-inflammatory effects and antioxidant compounds may help reduce inflammation in the joints, supporting longevity by promoting healthy joint function.

6. **Digestive Health:** Cat's claw has been used to support gastrointestinal health. Its active compounds, including tannins, alkaloids, and glycosides, may help reduce inflammation in the digestive tract, support gut health, and promote longevity by maintaining optimal digestive function.
7. **Brain Health:** Cat's claw contains beta-sitosterol, a plant sterol that may have neuroprotective effects. Beta-sitosterol has been studied for its potential benefits in supporting brain health, including reducing neuroinflammation and oxidative stress, and supporting memory and cognitive function.
8. **Detoxification:** Cat's claw may support detoxification processes in the body. Its antioxidant compounds and alkaloids may help neutralize toxins, support liver function, and promote the elimination of harmful substances, contributing to overall longevity.
9. **Cardiovascular Health:** Cat's claw has been associated with potential cardiovascular benefits. Its antioxidant properties and compounds like quercetin and catechins may help protect against oxidative stress, support healthy blood vessels, and promote cardiovascular well-being.
10. **Antimicrobial Effects:** The tannins and alkaloids found in cat's claw, such as prodelphinidins, catechin gallate, mitraphylline, isopteropodine, pteropodine, uncarine F, isomitraphylline, and rhynchophylline, contribute to its anti-pathogenic properties. Prodelphinidins and catechin gallate, which are types of tannins, possess antimicrobial effects, helping inhibit the growth of harmful microorganisms. Mitraphylline, isopteropodine, pteropodine, uncarine F, isomitraphylline, and rhynchophylline are alkaloids that work together with the tannins to support the body's defense against pathogens. These compounds have demonstrated antimicrobial properties including anti-bacterial and antiviral properties, which may help combat various pathogens. Many of these compounds in cat's claw have caught the attention of science for its powerful anti-pathogenic properties.

While cat's claw is generally considered safe to consume, there are some medical contradictions and precautions to consider. Individuals who have undergone organ or tissue transplants or are taking immunosuppressant medications should consult with a healthcare professional prior to using cat's claw, as it may interfere with the effectiveness of these medications. Cat's claw may also have a blood-thinning effect, so individuals taking anticoagulant or antiplatelet medications should avoid using cat's claw to mitigate potential interactions. Individuals with bleeding disorders, upcoming surgeries, or scheduled dental procedures should exercise caution due to the potential risk of increased bleeding. Safety during pregnancy and lactation is not well-established, and it is advisable for pregnant or breastfeeding individuals to avoid using cat's claw unless otherwise advised by their herbalist/practitioner.

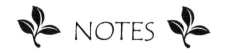

CAYENNE PEPPER

Cayenne pepper, also known as red chili pepper or Capsicum annuum, is a fiery spice that has its origins in the Americas. Native to Central and South America, cayenne pepper has been used for centuries in various culinary and medicinal practices. The name "cayenne" is derived from the city of Cayenne in French Guiana, where this pungent spice was first encountered by European explorers. The popularity of cayenne pepper quickly spread worldwide due to its distinct flavor and potent medicinal properties. Today, it is a staple ingredient in many cuisines and is widely recognized for its potential health benefits.

Now, let's explore ten extensive health and longevity benefits associated with cayenne pepper:

1. **Pain Relief:** Cayenne pepper contains an active compound called capsaicin, which has been used topically to relieve pain and reduce inflammation. It can provide relief for conditions like arthritis, muscle pain, and nerve pain.
2. **Cardiovascular Health:** Research suggests that cayenne pepper may have beneficial effects on heart health. It may help improve circulation, lower blood pressure, reduce cholesterol levels, and prevent the formation of blood clots, thereby supporting cardiovascular function and reducing the risk of heart-related diseases.
3. **Digestive Health:** Cayenne pepper stimulates digestion and increases the production of digestive enzymes and hydrochloric acid, aiding in the breakdown of food. It may help alleviate indigestion, promote healthy bowel movements, and reduce symptoms of gastrointestinal discomfort.
4. **Weight Management:** Cayenne pepper has thermogenic properties, meaning it can promote fat burning. It may help support weight loss efforts by boosting calorie expenditure and suppressing appetite.
5. **Respiratory Health:** The heat and spiciness of cayenne pepper may help alleviate congestion and promote the clearing of the respiratory tract. It may provide relief from symptoms associated with sinusitis, colds, and allergies.
6. **Immune System Support:** Cayenne pepper contains high levels of vitamin C, which is known for its immune-boosting properties. It can enhance the function of the immune system, protect against common illnesses, and contribute to overall well-being.

7. **Anti-inflammatory Effects:** The capsaicin in cayenne pepper exhibits potent anti-inflammatory properties. It may help reduce inflammation in the body, alleviate symptoms of inflammatory conditions, and support joint health.
8. **Antimicrobial Properties:** Cayenne pepper contains capsaicin, a compound that gives it its heat. Capsaicin is thought to have antimicrobial properties that may help combat certain types of microorganisms, including parasites.
9. **Antioxidant Powerhouse:** Cayenne pepper is rich in antioxidants, such as vitamin A and vitamin C, which help protect the body's cells from damage caused by free radicals. This antioxidant activity contributes to overall health and can support graceful aging.
10. **Nutrient Absorption:** Cayenne pepper stimulates the production of gastric juices, promoting optimal digestion and nutrient absorption. It may also help prevent digestive issues like gas, bloating, and stomach ulcers.

While cayenne pepper is generally considered safe to consume, there are certain medical contradictions and precautions to consider. Individuals with a known allergy or hypersensitivity to capsicum, the active compound in cayenne pepper, should avoid its consumption to prevent allergic reactions. Cayenne pepper may interact with certain medications, including anticoagulants (such as warfarin) and antiplatelet drugs, increasing the risk of bleeding. It may also interact with blood pressure medications, such as calcium channel blockers and ACE inhibitors, potentially affecting blood pressure levels. Individuals on medication for diabetes should use caution when consuming cayenne pepper, as it may enhance the effects of these medications and cause low blood sugar levels. Cayenne pepper may cause irritation or discomfort when applied topically. It is advisable to avoid contact with sensitive areas or broken skin. Consuming cayenne pepper as a culinary spice while pregnant is generally considered safe. Women who are breastfeeding should avoid cayenne pepper as it could irritate the baby.

CELERY SEED

Celery seed, derived from the wild celery plant known as Apium graveolens, has a rich history that dates back centuries. Believed to have originated in the Mediterranean region, celery has been cultivated and valued for its medicinal properties since ancient times. The use of celery seed can be traced back to ancient Egypt, where it was highly regarded for its therapeutic benefits. The ancient Greeks and Romans also recognized the health-promoting qualities of celery seed, using it to treat a variety of ailments. Today, celery seed continues to be cherished for its numerous health benefits and age-reversal properties.

Now, let's explore ten extensive health and longevity benefits associated with celery seed:

1. **Anti-inflammatory Effects:** Celery seed contains various antioxidants, including apigenin, luteolin, and quercetin, which possess anti-inflammatory properties. These compounds help reduce inflammation in the body, potentially supporting longevity by lowering the risk of chronic diseases.
2. **Antioxidant Powerhouse:** Celery seed is rich in antioxidants, such as phenolic acids and flavonoids, including caffeic acid and apigenin. These antioxidants help neutralize free radicals, protecting cells from oxidative stress and supporting overall health.
3. **Cardiovascular Health:** Celery seed may support cardiovascular health by lowering blood pressure and reducing cholesterol levels. Active compounds like phthalides and coumarins, including 3-n-butylphthalide (3nB), contribute to these effects, potentially supporting heart health and longevity.
4. **Liver Health:** Celery seed has been associated with liver-protective effects. The presence of antioxidants, such as caffeic acid, helps support liver function, enhances detoxification processes, and protects against liver damage, promoting overall longevity.
5. **Digestive Health:** Celery seed may aid in digestion by stimulating digestive enzymes, promoting gut motility, and reducing inflammation in the gastrointestinal tract. Compounds like apigenin and quercetin contribute to these digestive benefits.
6. **Antimicrobial Effects:** Celery seed exhibits antimicrobial properties, potentially inhibiting the growth of certain pathogens. Active compounds like apigenin and luteolin have been shown to possess broad-spectrum antimicrobial effects, supporting the body's defense against infections.

7. **Respiratory Health:** The anti-inflammatory properties of celery seed extend to the respiratory system. Compounds like apigenin and luteolin may help reduce inflammation in the airways, potentially alleviating respiratory symptoms and promoting lung health.
8. **Adaptogenic Effects:** Celery seed is considered an adaptogen, which means it may help the body cope with stress. The antioxidants and bioactive compounds in celery seed, including apigenin and quercetin, support the body's ability to adapt and maintain overall well-being.
9. **Joint Health:** Celery seed may support joint health by reducing inflammation and providing relief from arthritis symptoms. Compounds like apigenin and caffeic acid contribute to these effects, potentially supporting joint longevity.
10. **Anti-cancer Effects:** Some studies suggest that celery seed may have anti-cancer properties. The presence of antioxidants, such as apigenin and quercetin, may help protect against DNA damage, inhibit tumor growth, and support longevity by reducing the risk of certain cancers.

While celery seed is generally considered safe to consume, it is important to note a few warnings and contradictions. Individuals taking blood-thinning medications such as warfarin should exercise caution when using celery seed due to its potential anticoagulant effects. Individuals with kidney disease or those taking diuretic medications should consult a healthcare professional before incorporating large quantities of celery seed into their diet, as it can increase urine production. Celery seed is considered safe to consume during pregnancy and lactation.

CHAGA MUSHROOM

Chaga mushroom, scientifically known as Inonotus obliquus, has a rich history deeply rooted in traditional medicine and folklore. Originating in regions of Siberia, Russia, and Northern Europe, Chaga has been utilized for centuries by indigenous cultures for its medicinal properties. In traditional Russian, Siberian, and Scandinavian folk medicine, Chaga was highly regarded as a powerful natural remedy, consumed as a tea or decoction to support overall health. With its unique growth patterns on birch trees in cold climates, Chaga's rarity and value have contributed to its reputation as the "King of Mushrooms" or the "Diamond of the Forest." Today, Chaga's popularity has spread worldwide, and it is sought after for its potential health benefits, making it a prominent ingredient in various health products. Its historical legacy and ongoing scientific research continually highlight the remarkable properties of Chaga, ensuring its place in the realm of natural healing.

Now, let's explore ten extensive health and longevity benefits associated with Chaga mushroom:

1. **Antioxidant Powerhouse:** Chaga mushroom is renowned for its high antioxidant content, particularly melanin and polyphenols. These antioxidants help protect cells from damage caused by free radicals, reducing the risk of chronic diseases and supporting overall well-being.
2. **Immune System Support:** Chaga mushroom contains bioactive compounds that stimulate and modulate the immune system, helping to enhance its response against infections, viruses, and harmful pathogens. It may strengthen the body's defense mechanisms and support immune system function.
3. **Anti-inflammatory Effects:** The betulinic acid and other compounds found in Chaga mushroom exhibit potent anti-inflammatory properties, which may help reduce inflammation and alleviate symptoms associated with inflammatory conditions like arthritis and inflammatory bowel disease.
4. **Liver Health:** Chaga mushroom has a long history of use in supporting liver health and detoxification. It may help protect the liver from oxidative damage, promote optimal liver function, and aid in the elimination of toxins.
5. **Cardiovascular Health:** Research suggests that Chaga mushroom may have beneficial effects on cardiovascular health. It may help lower cholesterol levels, reduce blood pressure, improve circulation, and support heart function.

6. **Adaptogenic Effects:** Chaga mushroom is considered an adaptogen, meaning it helps the body adapt to stressors and maintain homeostasis. It may support the body's stress response, promote mental and physical resilience, and improve overall vitality.
7. **Digestive Health:** Chaga mushroom has been used traditionally to support digestive health and alleviate gastrointestinal issues. It may help soothe inflammation in the digestive tract, promote healthy gut flora, and aid in digestion.
8. **Anti-cancer Effects:** Chaga mushroom contains various compounds, such as betulinic acid and polysaccharides, which have demonstrated anti-cancer properties in studies. It may help inhibit the growth of cancer cells, stimulate the immune system's response to cancer, and reduce the risk of certain types of cancer.
9. **Skin Health:** Chaga mushroom's antioxidant and anti-inflammatory properties contribute to its potential benefits for skin health. It may help improve skin tone, reduce the appearance of wrinkles, and protect against oxidative damage caused by environmental factors.
10. **Antimicrobial Effects:** Chaga mushroom contains various bioactive compounds, such as polysaccharides, triterpenoids, and phenolic compounds, that contribute to its antiviral activity. These compounds have demonstrated the ability to inhibit the growth and replication of certain viruses. The mechanisms by which Chaga mushroom exerts its antiviral effects are multifaceted. It can interfere with viral attachment and entry into host cells, inhibit viral replication, and modulate the host immune response. Chaga mushroom's polysaccharides, in particular, have been found to stimulate the activity of immune cells, such as natural killer cells and macrophages, which play a crucial role in combating viral infections.

While Chaga mushroom is generally considered safe to consume, there are certain medical contradictions and precautions to be aware of. Individuals with bleeding disorders or those taking anticoagulant medications, such as warfarin or aspirin, should exercise caution as Chaga mushroom may have anticoagulant properties and increase the risk of bleeding. It may also interact with immunosuppressant medications, potentially compromising their effectiveness. Individuals with known allergies to mushrooms should avoid Chaga mushroom to prevent allergic reactions. It is important to note that Chaga mushroom belongs to the same family as other mushrooms, such as shiitake and reishi, so individuals with known allergies to these mushrooms may also be allergic to Chaga. Pregnant or breastfeeding individuals should consult with their herbalist/practitioner before using Chaga mushroom.

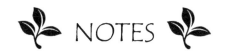
NOTES

CHAMOMILE

Chamomile, derived from the Greek words "khamai," meaning "on the ground," and "melon," meaning "apple," is a fascinating herb with a long and rich history. Belonging to the Asteraceae family, chamomile is renowned for its delicate, daisy-like flowers and its profound therapeutic properties. With origins tracing back to ancient Egypt, where it was revered as a sacred herb, chamomile has been cherished and utilized by various cultures throughout history. This herb has a diverse range of health benefits, aiding in relaxation and digestion and promoting overall well-being.

Now, let's explore ten extensive health and longevity benefits associated with chamomile:

1. **Sleep Support:** Chamomile contains the flavonoid apigenin, which binds to specific receptors in the brain, promoting a calming effect and aiding in relaxation and sleep.
2. **Anxiety and Stress Relief:** Chamomile is rich in apigenin, a flavonoid that helps modulate neurotransmitters and reduce the activity of stress-inducing hormones like cortisol, thus alleviating anxiety and stress.
3. **Digestive Health:** Chamomile contains bisabolol, a compound with anti-inflammatory properties that soothes the digestive tract. It also contains flavonoids like apigenin and luteolin, which aid in reducing inflammation and alleviating gastrointestinal symptoms.
4. **Immune System Support:** Chamomile tea is abundant in antioxidants such as flavonoids, quercetin, and luteolin, which provide immune-boosting benefits by scavenging harmful free radicals and supporting the body's defense mechanisms.
5. **Antioxidant Powerhouse:** Chamomile contains phenolic compounds like caffeic acid and rutin, which act as potent antioxidants, neutralizing oxidative stress and protecting against chronic diseases and aging.
6. **Skin Health:** Chamomile's active compounds, including alpha-bisabolol and chamazulene, possess anti-inflammatory and antioxidant properties, aiding in soothing skin irritations, reducing redness, and promoting wound healing.
7. **Detoxification:** Chamomile acts as a mild diuretic, promoting urine production and supporting the elimination of toxins from the body. It also stimulates bile production, aiding in the digestion and absorption of fats.

8. **Anti-radiation Effects:** Chamomile, with its impressive array of natural compounds, emerges as a potent anti-radiation tool. Among these compounds, apigenin takes the lead in fortifying the body's defenses against radiation exposure. Its radioprotective properties play a pivotal role in mitigating the harmful effects of ionizing radiation. By bolstering cellular integrity and resilience, chamomile contributes significantly to safeguarding against radiation-induced damage, making it a valuable asset in the quest for radiation protection.
9. **Anti-inflammatory Effects:** Chamomile contains compounds like chamazulene, alpha-bisabolol, and apigenin, which possess anti-inflammatory properties. These compounds help alleviate chronic inflammation linked to various diseases and premature aging.
10. **Antimicrobial Effects:** Chamomile exhibits broad-spectrum antimicrobial activity due to compounds like chamazulene and alpha-bisabolol. This supports the body's defense against bacteria, fungi, and viruses, promoting overall health.

While chamomile is generally considered safe to consume, there are important medical contradictions and precautions to be aware of. Individuals with known allergies to plants in the daisy family, including ragweed, chrysanthemums, and marigolds, may experience allergic reactions to chamomile. Chamomile can interact with certain medications, such as anticoagulants, sedatives, and blood pressure medications, potentially affecting their effectiveness. It is advisable to consult with a healthcare professional if you are taking any medications or have any existing health conditions before incorporating chamomile into your diet or health regimen. Chamomile may have sedative effects and can cause drowsiness, so it is important to exercise caution when driving or operating machinery after consuming chamomile. Pregnant or lactating individuals should exercise caution and seek the advice of their herbalist/practitioner before consuming chamomile in large quantities during these times.

CHAPARRAL LEAF

Chaparral leaf, also known as Larrea tridentata or creosote bush, is a plant native to the arid regions of North America, particularly the southwestern United States and Mexico. It is a resilient and hardy plant that has been used by indigenous peoples for centuries due to its medicinal properties. Chaparral leaf has a long history of traditional use as a natural remedy, and it continues to be valued for its potential health benefits. The plant itself is characterized by its small, waxy leaves and distinctive resinous scent.

Now, let's explore ten extensive health and longevity benefits associated with chaparral leaf:

1. **Antioxidant Powerhouse:** Chaparral leaf contains various antioxidants, including nordihydroguaiaretic acid (NDGA), which is its primary active compound. NDGA has strong free-radical scavenging properties, protecting the body's cells from oxidative damage and supporting overall health. It's important to note that nordihydroguaiaretic acid (NDGA) may have potential liver-toxic properties if taken in large quantities or for prolonged periods.
2. **Anti-inflammatory Effects:** NDGA present in chaparral leaf exhibits potent anti-inflammatory effects. It inhibits the production of pro-inflammatory compounds, helping to alleviate inflammation associated with chronic diseases and promoting longevity.
3. **Cardiovascular Health:** Chaparral leaf may have positive effects on cardiovascular health. Some studies suggest that NDGA may help lower blood pressure, reduce LDL cholesterol levels, and improve overall heart health, indirectly supporting longevity.
4. **Anti-cancer Effects:** Some studies suggest that chaparral leaf may possess anti-cancer properties. NDGA has been found to inhibit the growth of certain cancer cells and induce apoptosis (programmed cell death). However, further research is needed to fully understand its effectiveness.
5. **Immune System Support:** Chaparral leaf contains compounds that may help boost the immune system. NDGA has been shown to enhance immune response by promoting the production of immune cells and supporting their activity against pathogens.
6. **Respiratory Health:** Chaparral leaf has a long history of use in supporting respiratory health. It contains expectorant properties that may help soothe coughs, reduce congestion, and support overall respiratory function.

7. **Antimicrobial Effects:** Chaparral leaf possesses antimicrobial properties, which may help inhibit the growth of certain bacteria, fungi, and viruses. These properties are attributed to NDGA, which has been shown to have broad-spectrum antimicrobial effects.
8. **Skin Health:** Topical application of chaparral leaf extract may have beneficial effects on the skin. It may help soothe skin irritations, reduce inflammation, and potentially support wound healing, thanks to the presence of NDGA and other active compounds.
9. **Blood Sugar Regulation:** Chaparral leaf has been traditionally used to support healthy blood sugar levels. Some studies have indicated that NDGA may have hypoglycemic effects, helping to regulate blood sugar levels. However, further research is needed in this area.
10. **Digestive Health:** Chaparral leaf has been used to promote digestive health. It may help alleviate digestive issues such as indigestion and bloating. NDGA present in chaparral leaf exhibits anti-ulcerogenic properties, potentially supporting a healthy digestive system.

While chaparral leaf is generally considered safe to consume, it is important to be aware of certain medical contradictions and precautions associated with its use. The herb may interact with medications metabolized by the liver, such as statins, anticoagulants, and immunosuppressants. Individuals with pre-existing liver disease should exercise caution when using chaparral leaf due to the potential hepatotoxicity associated with its active compound, nordihydroguaiaretic acid (NDGA). While rare, prolonged consumption of large quantities of chaparral leaf may have liver-toxic effects. It is advisable to consult with your herbalist to establish safe quantities and a consumption schedule. Additionally, it is important to be aware of allergy warnings, as cross-reactivity with plants in the Asteraceae family, such as ragweed, daisies, and marigolds, is possible. Therefore, individuals with known allergies to these plants should approach chaparral leaf with caution. The use of chaparral leaf during pregnancy or lactation should be avoided.

CHASTEBERRY (VITEX)

Chasteberry, also known as Vitex agnus-castus, is a herb with a rich history and diverse uses. Its origins can be traced back to the Mediterranean region, where it has been used for centuries in traditional medicine. Chasteberry has been associated with various cultural and historical references throughout time. In ancient Greece, it was believed to be sacred to the goddess Hera and was used by women to maintain chastity, hence its name. The herb has been mentioned in the writings of renowned Greek physicians, including Hippocrates and Dioscorides, who recognized its medicinal properties. Over the years, chasteberry has gained popularity for its ability to support women's health and hormonal balance. It has been used to alleviate symptoms of menstrual disorders, such as irregular periods, premenstrual syndrome (PMS), and menopause. Today, chasteberry continues to be valued for its potential health benefits and is widely studied for its effects on reproductive health and overall well-being.

Now, let's explore ten extensive health and longevity benefits associated with chasteberry:

1. **Hormonal Balance:** chasteberry acts on the hypothalamus to increase the release of luteinizing hormone (LH) while inhibiting the release of follicle-stimulating hormone (FSH) from the pituitary gland. This shift in hormone secretion promotes the production of progesterone and helps to balance estrogen levels.
2. **Breast Tenderness Support:** Chasteberry has been found to have a regulatory effect on prolactin secretion. It acts on the hypothalamus and pituitary gland, which are responsible for controlling hormone production in the body. By influencing the activity of these glands, chasteberry helps restore the balance of prolactin levels, preventing excessive secretion. By reducing prolactin levels, chasteberry contributes to the alleviation of breast tenderness and swelling.
3. **Skin Health:** Chasteberry's hormonal balancing effects can improve skin health, reducing acne breakouts and promoting a clear complexion.
4. **Menopausal Relief:** Chasteberry may provide relief from menopausal symptoms such as hot flashes, night sweats, and mood swings. The herb's ability to modulate hormone levels, particularly by increasing progesterone and balancing estrogen levels, may help alleviate these bothersome symptoms.

5. **Fertility Support:** One of the key ways chasteberry supports fertility is by regulating ovulation. It acts on the hypothalamus and pituitary gland, which are involved in the control of hormone production and the menstrual cycle. Chasteberry helps maintain a balance between the hormones that are necessary for healthy ovulation, such as luteinizing hormone (LH), follicle-stimulating hormone (FSH), and progesterone. By promoting the proper timing and release of these hormones, chasteberry helps regulate the ovulation process.
6. **Mood Support:** Chasteberry may influence neurotransmitters in the brain, including dopamine. Dopamine is a neurotransmitter associated with feelings of pleasure, motivation, and reward. By modulating dopamine activity, chasteberry may have mood-stabilizing effects and help alleviate symptoms of anxiety and depression that can occur alongside hormonal imbalances.
7. **Adrenal Support:** Chasteberry exerts its adrenal-supporting effects through its influence on the hypothalamic-pituitary-adrenal (HPA) axis, which is responsible for regulating the body's stress response. The herb helps modulate the release of stress hormones such as cortisol, promoting a balanced stress response and reducing the negative impact of chronic stress on the adrenal glands. By supporting adrenal function, chasteberry may help enhance resilience to stress, improve energy levels, and promote a sense of well-being.
8. **Digestive Health:** Chasteberry can aid in relieving digestive discomfort, including bloating, cramping, and indigestion.
9. **Anti-inflammatory Effects:** Chasteberry exhibits notable anti-inflammatory effects attributed to its rich content of flavonoids and iridoids. Flavonoids, including orientin, isovitexin, and casticin, along with iridoids such as aucubin and agnuside, contribute to the herb's anti-inflammatory properties. These bioactive compounds work by modulating the activity of inflammatory mediators and enzymes involved in the inflammatory process, ultimately reducing inflammation throughout the body. By regulating the production of pro-inflammatory molecules and promoting the release of anti-inflammatory substances, chasteberry helps alleviate symptoms associated with inflammatory conditions. It is particularly beneficial for individuals dealing with ailments such as arthritis, menstrual pain, and other inflammatory disorders.

10. **Antimicrobial Effects:** Chasteberry may possess antimicrobial properties, providing protection against certain pathogens, including bacteria and fungi. Certain bioactive compounds present in chasteberry, such as flavonoids, alkaloids, and essential oils, contribute to its antimicrobial activity. These compounds help inhibit the growth and spread of pathogenic microorganisms, supporting the body's defense against infections.

> While chasteberry is generally considered safe to consume, it is important to be aware of potential medical contradictions and interactions with certain conditions and medications. Individuals with hormone-sensitive conditions, such as breast cancer and ovarian cancer, should exercise caution when using chasteberry, as it may affect hormone levels. Additionally, chasteberry may interact with medications that affect hormone regulation, such as oral contraceptives, hormone replacement therapies, or medications for hormone-sensitive conditions. It is recommended to consult with a healthcare professional before using chasteberry in such cases. Allergy warnings should be noted for individuals who may have sensitivities to plants in the Verbenaceae family which chasteberry belongs. Other plants in the same family include lemon verbena and blue vervain. Pregnant or breastfeeding individuals are advised to avoid chasteberry due to its potential hormonal effects unless otherwise directed by their herbalist/practitioner.

NOTES

CHICORY ROOT

Chicory root, scientifically known as Cichorium intybus, is a versatile and widely consumed plant with a rich history spanning centuries. It is native to Europe and Asia and has been cultivated for both culinary and medicinal purposes since ancient times. The chicory plant is characterized by its vibrant blue flowers and elongated leaves, but it is the root of the plant that holds significant value. The root of chicory is dried, roasted, and ground to create a flavorful coffee substitute or used as a dietary supplement. Along with its earthy taste, chicory root is renowned for its potential health benefits, making it a popular ingredient in traditional medicine practices and modern herbal remedies.

Now, let's explore ten extensive health and longevity benefits associated with chicory root:

1. **Digestive Health:** Chicory root is rich in inulin, a prebiotic fiber that serves as food for beneficial gut bacteria. It may help promote healthy digestion, improve gut health, and support regular bowel movements.
2. **Liver Health:** The compounds present in chicory root, such as sesquiterpene lactones, have been shown to have hepatoprotective properties, aiding in the protection and detoxification of the liver.
3. **Blood Sugar Regulation:** Chicory root contains compounds that may help regulate blood sugar levels by increasing insulin sensitivity and reducing glucose spikes after meals. It may be beneficial for individuals with diabetes or those at risk of developing the condition.
4. **Gallbladder Health:** Chicory root holds a distinctive role in promoting gallbladder health. Its unique blend of compounds, including inulin, fosters the optimal functioning of the gallbladder. Inulin, a soluble dietary fiber, aids in the emulsification of fats and supports the gallbladder's role in digestion by facilitating the release of bile. This contribution to gallbladder function enhances digestive efficiency and overall digestive comfort, making chicory root a valuable ally in maintaining gallbladder wellness.
5. **Anti-inflammatory Effects:** Chicory root possesses anti-inflammatory properties, which may help reduce inflammation throughout the body and alleviate symptoms associated with inflammatory conditions like arthritis.

6. **Antioxidant Powerhouse:** Chicory root is a rich source of antioxidants, including phenolic compounds and flavonoids, which may help neutralize free radicals and protect cells from oxidative damage.
7. **Bone Health:** Chicory root contains essential minerals such as calcium, magnesium, and phosphorus, which are vital for maintaining strong and healthy bones. Regular consumption of chicory root may contribute to bone density and reduce the risk of osteoporosis.
8. **Cardiovascular Health:** The fiber content in chicory root may help lower cholesterol levels, particularly LDL (bad) cholesterol, thereby supporting cardiovascular health and reducing the risk of heart disease.
9. **Anti-cancer Effects:** Some studies have indicated that chicory root may possess anti-cancer properties attributed to its bioactive compounds like chicoric acid and polyphenols. However, more research is needed to fully understand its effectiveness in cancer prevention and treatment.
10. **Cognitive Support:** Chicory root has been studied for its potential cognitive-enhancing effects. Some compounds present in chicory root may help improve memory and cognitive performance and protect against age-related cognitive decline.

While chicory root is generally considered safe to consume, there are certain medical contradictions and precautions that should be considered. Chicory root may interact with certain medications, including anticoagulants or antiplatelet drugs, such as warfarin or aspirin, as it may possess mild blood-thinning properties. Therefore, it is important for individuals taking these medications to consult with a healthcare professional before consuming chicory root. This root may interfere with the absorption of certain antibiotics, such as tetracycline, due to its high content of inulin. It is advisable to separate the consumption of chicory root from antibiotic doses by a few hours. Individuals with known allergies to the Asteraceae/Compositae family, which includes ragweed, chrysanthemums, marigolds, and daisies, may also experience allergic reactions to chicory root. Pregnant and breastfeeding women should consult with their herbalist/ practitioner prior to using chicory root.

CHIPOTLE POWDER

Chipotle powder is a flavorful and versatile spice that has its origins in Mexico. It is made from smoke-dried jalapeño peppers, giving it a distinct smoky and spicy flavor profile. The word "chipotle" originates from the Nahuatl language, where "chili" means "smoked pepper." The process of smoking the peppers not only imparts a unique taste but also enhances their shelf life. Chipotle powder has gained popularity in various cuisines around the world for its robust flavor and ability to add depth and complexity to dishes. Beyond its culinary uses, chipotle powder also possesses a range of potential health and longevity benefits, making it a valuable addition to a well-rounded diet.

Now, let's explore ten extensive health and longevity benefits associated with chipotle powder:

1. **Antioxidant Powerhouse:** Chipotle powder contains various antioxidants, including capsaicin, vitamin C, and carotenoids. These antioxidants help neutralize harmful free radicals, reducing oxidative stress and promoting cellular health.
2. **Respiratory Health:** Capsaicin, the active compound in chipotle peppers, acts as a natural decongestant and may help relieve nasal congestion. It may also assist in reducing inflammation in the respiratory system, supporting respiratory health.
3. **Immune System Support:** Chipotle powder is rich in vitamin C, which plays a vital role in supporting immune function. Vitamin C enhances the production of white blood cells, strengthens the immune response, and protects against pathogens and chronic diseases.
4. **Cardiovascular Health:** Capsaicin helps reduce inflammation, improve blood flow, and support healthy blood pressure levels, indirectly contributing to heart health and longevity.
5. **Digestive Health:** Chipotle powder stimulates the secretion of digestive enzymes, aiding in the breakdown of food and improving nutrient absorption. Additionally, capsaicin has been shown to have gastroprotective properties, supporting the stomach lining and preventing the formation of ulcers.
6. **Pain Relief:** Capsaicin in chipotle powder has analgesic properties and may help alleviate pain. It works by desensitizing nerve receptors and reducing the transmission of pain signals, providing temporary relief from conditions such as arthritis and muscle soreness.

7. **Detoxification:** Chipotle powder contains various antioxidants and bioactive compounds that support detoxification processes in the body. These compounds help neutralize toxins, enhance liver function, and assist in the elimination of harmful substances from the body.
8. **Metabolic Function Support:** Capsaicin plays a crucial role in supporting metabolic function through its ability to enhance thermogenesis. This fascinating process involves the generation of heat within the body, which subsequently boosts calorie expenditure.
9. **Eye Health:** Chipotle powder contains carotenoids, such as lutein and zeaxanthin, which are beneficial for eye health. These compounds help protect against age-related macular degeneration and cataracts, supporting visual function and overall eye health.
10. **Anti-inflammatory and Antimicrobial Effects:** Capsaicin exhibits anti-inflammatory and antimicrobial effects. These properties contribute to reducing inflammation in the body and inhibiting the growth of certain bacteria and fungi, supporting overall health and longevity.

While chipotle powder is generally considered safe to consume, there are certain medical contradictions and precautions to consider. Individuals with known allergies or sensitivities to peppers or spicy foods should avoid chipotle powder. Chipotle powder's capsaicin content can interact with certain medications. It may interfere with the anticoagulant effects of medications like warfarin or aspirin, increasing the risk of bleeding. Individuals taking these medications should consult their healthcare provider before consuming chipotle powder or any other capsaicin-containing products. Additionally, capsaicin may interact with medications metabolized by the liver's cytochrome P450 enzymes, potentially affecting their efficacy. It is important to discuss potential drug interactions with a healthcare professional if taking medications that fall under this category. In addition to known allergies or sensitivities to peppers or spicy foods, individuals with allergies to other members of the Solanaceae family, such as tomatoes, potatoes, or bell peppers, may also experience allergic reactions to chipotle powder. During pregnancy, it is generally considered safe to consume chipotle powder in very small amounts as a culinary spice. Consult with your herbalist/practitioner prior to consuming chipotle powder during lactation.

CHRYSANTHEMUM FLOWERS

Chrysanthemum flowers, with their striking beauty and rich cultural significance, have a fascinating origin deeply rooted in ancient Chinese history. Believed to have originated in China around the 15th century BC, these exquisite blooms have since captivated people worldwide, adorning gardens, artwork, and various cultural ceremonies. The chrysanthemum's prominence in Chinese culture is evident in its association with joy, longevity, and vitality. Revered as one of the "Four Gentlemen" in Chinese art alongside plum, orchid, and bamboo, chrysanthemums hold a special place in traditional Chinese medicine for their remarkable health benefits. These vibrant flowers, known as "mums" or "chrysanths," are not only a feast for the eyes but also offer an abundance of wellness advantages. From enhancing the immune system to promoting liver health, chrysanthemum flowers have been cherished for centuries as a natural remedy for a wide range of ailments.

Now, let's explore ten extensive health and longevity benefits associated with chrysanthemum flowers:

1. **Eye Health:** In addition to lutein and zeaxanthin, chrysanthemum also contains other beneficial compounds, such as cryptoxanthin and beta-carotene, which contribute to its eye health benefits. These carotenoids support the health of the retina and may help protect against other eye conditions, such as cataracts and glaucoma.
2. **Anti-inflammatory Effects:** Chrysanthemum contains flavonoids, including apigenin, which possess anti-inflammatory properties. These compounds help reduce inflammation throughout the body, supporting the health of organs and body systems affected by chronic inflammation.
3. **Antimicrobial Effects:** Chrysanthemum possesses antimicrobial properties. Its specific antimicrobial effects may be attributed to various compounds, such as flavonoids and phenolic acids. These compounds help inhibit the growth of bacteria, fungi, and viruses, supporting the body's defense against pathogens and promoting overall health.
4. **Stress Relief:** Chrysanthemum has calming properties and is often consumed to alleviate stress and anxiety. Its active compounds, such as apigenin and flavonoids, help reduce the activity of stress hormones like cortisol, promoting relaxation and mental well-being.

5. **Liver Health:** Chrysanthemum contains compounds such as chlorogenic acid and luteolin, which have hepatoprotective properties. They help protect the liver from oxidative stress, detoxify harmful substances, and support liver function.
6. **Respiratory Health:** Chrysanthemum has been traditionally used to alleviate respiratory conditions. Its active compounds, such as caffeic acid and flavonoids, help soothe inflamed airways, reduce coughing, and provide relief from symptoms of respiratory disorders like asthma and bronchitis.
7. **Cardiovascular Health:** Chrysanthemum contains flavonoids, including quercetin and kaempferol, which help improve heart health. These antioxidants reduce oxidative stress, lower blood pressure, improve blood circulation, and promote healthy cholesterol levels.
8. **Immune System Support:** Chrysanthemum is rich in antioxidants, including flavonoids, phenolic acids, and vitamin C. These compounds help strengthen the immune system, neutralize free radicals, and protect against infections and diseases.
9. **Digestive Health:** Chrysanthemum is known to have digestive benefits. It helps soothe the digestive system, reduce inflammation, and alleviate symptoms of gastrointestinal disorders like indigestion and bloating, indirectly supporting digestive health and nutrient absorption.
10. **Detoxification:** Chrysanthemum contains compounds like caffeic acid and flavonoids, which support detoxification processes in the body. These antioxidants help eliminate toxins, heavy metals, and free radicals, contributing to overall well-being and indirectly supporting longevity.

While chrysanthemum is generally considered safe to consume, there are a few medical contradictions and precautions to keep in mind. Individuals with bleeding disorders or taking anticoagulant medications should exercise caution when using chrysanthemum, as it may have mild blood-thinning properties. This herb could potentially enhance the effects of anticoagulant medications, leading to an increased risk of bleeding. Chrysanthemum may also interact with certain medications, such as sedatives, tranquilizers, and medications metabolized by the liver. It is recommended to consult with a healthcare professional if you are taking any medications to determine if there are any potential interactions or adjustments needed. It is important to note that individuals with known allergies or hypersensitivity to plants in the Asteraceae/Compositae family, such as ragweed, daisies, and marigolds, may also experience allergic reactions when exposed to chrysanthemum. The use of chrysanthemum during pregnancy or lactation should be avoided unless under the guidance of your herbalist/practitioner.

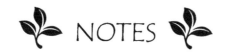

NOTES

CLEAVERS

Cleavers, also known as Galium aparine, is a unique herb with a rich history and a myriad of health benefits. Native to Europe, North America, and Asia, cleavers has been used for centuries in traditional herbal medicine systems around the world. Its name comes from the Latin word "cleave," meaning "to adhere," referring to the herb's remarkable ability to cling to surfaces and fabrics. Cleavers has a long-standing reputation as a medicinal herb, and its usage can be traced back to ancient civilizations such as the Greeks, Romans, and Native Americans. This herb is characterized by its small, hooked bristles that allow it to attach itself to objects, making it easily identifiable in the wild. Cleavers is renowned for its cleansing and purifying properties, and its numerous health benefits have made it a cherished herb among herbalists and natural health enthusiasts. From supporting the lymphatic system to promoting skin health, cleavers offers a wealth of health and longevity benefits.

Now, let's explore ten extensive health and longevity benefits associated with cleavers:

1. **Lymphatic Support:** Cleavers have a strong affinity for the lymphatic system, assisting in the detoxification process. Its active compounds, including iridoid glycosides such as asperuloside, help stimulate lymphatic drainage, promoting the removal of toxins and waste products from the body.
2. **Diuretic Effects:** Cleavers possess diuretic properties, promoting increased urine production and aiding kidney function. This herb supports kidney health and helps eliminate toxins and waste products from the body.
3. **Anti-inflammatory Effects:** Cleavers contain flavonoids, such as quercetin and kaempferol, which possess anti-inflammatory properties. These compounds help reduce inflammation in various body systems, contributing to overall health and longevity.
4. **Skin Health:** Cleavers have traditionally been used for various skin conditions due to their soothing and anti-inflammatory effects. Active compounds like tannins and flavonoids help alleviate skin irritations, rashes, and inflammation, promoting healthy skin.
5. **Antioxidant Powerhouse:** Cleavers are rich in antioxidants, including phenolic acids such as caffeic acid and chlorogenic acid. These antioxidants help neutralize harmful free radicals, reducing oxidative stress and protecting cells from damage.

6. **Detoxification:** Cleavers contain compounds such as coumarins, flavonoids, and lignans that support liver function and assist in detoxification processes. These compounds aid in the removal of toxins and waste products from the body.
7. **Urinary Tract Health:** Cleavers have traditionally been used to support urinary tract health. While the specific mechanisms are not fully understood, it is believed that cleavers' constituents help maintain a healthy urinary system, promoting its overall well-being.
8. **Immune System Support:** Cleavers possess immune-enhancing properties attributed to its various bioactive constituents. Flavonoids, alkaloids, and phenolic acids found in cleavers support immune function, protecting the body against pathogens.
9. **Digestive Health:** Cleavers' mucilaginous properties help soothe the digestive tract and support healthy digestion. Cleavers also possess antimicrobial properties that help control harmful bacteria in the gut.
10. **Antimicrobial Effects:** Cleavers exhibit antimicrobial properties thanks to its active compounds, such as asperuloside. These compounds help inhibit the growth of bacteria and other pathogens.

While cleavers are generally considered safe to consume, there are certain medical contradictions and precautions to consider. Individuals with known allergies or hypersensitivity to cleavers or any other plants in the Rubiaceae family should avoid its use. Cleavers may interact with certain medications, including anticoagulants or antiplatelet drugs, due to its potential blood-thinning properties, which could increase the risk of bleeding. It is advisable for individuals taking these medications to consult with a healthcare professional before using cleavers. Additionally, individuals with low blood pressure or hypotension should exercise caution, as cleavers may further decrease blood pressure. Cleavers might interfere with the effectiveness of certain medications for diabetes by lowering blood sugar levels, so individuals with diabetes should monitor their blood sugar levels closely when using cleavers. It's best to cycle the usage of cleavers as prolonged use may diminish its effects. Consult with your herbalist/practitioner regarding the cycling schedule that would be best suited for you. Those who are pregnant and/or lactating should consult with their herbalist/practitioner prior to using cleavers.

CLOVES

Cloves, scientifically known as Syzygium aromaticum, have a fascinating origin deeply rooted in ancient civilizations and spice trade routes. These aromatic flower buds, derived from the evergreen clove tree, have been utilized for centuries in various cultures for their distinct flavor, fragrance, and medicinal properties. Originating in the Moluccas, a group of islands in Indonesia, cloves quickly gained prominence due to their unique qualities and were highly sought after by traders and explorers. Today, cloves are widely used as a versatile spice in cuisines around the world, and their therapeutic potential continues to captivate researchers and health enthusiasts alike. Beyond their delightful taste and aroma, cloves offer a wide array of health and longevity benefits, making them a valuable addition to our well-being arsenal.

Now, let's explore ten extensive health and longevity benefits associated with cloves:

1. **Oral Health:** Cloves contain eugenol, a potent compound with antimicrobial properties. Eugenol helps combat bacteria in the mouth, promoting oral health and preventing tooth decay, gum disease, and bad breath. It also acts as a natural analgesic, providing temporary relief from toothaches.
2. **Anti-inflammatory Effects:** Cloves are rich in eugenol, which possesses significant anti-inflammatory properties. Eugenol helps reduce inflammation throughout the body, supporting joint health and potentially preventing chronic diseases associated with inflammation.
3. **Digestive Health:** Cloves contain essential oils, including eugenol, which promote healthy digestion. Eugenol stimulates the production of digestive enzymes, aids in nutrient absorption, and alleviates digestive discomfort such as bloating and flatulence.
4. **Bone Health:** Cloves contain minerals like manganese and calcium, which are essential for maintaining strong bones. These minerals, along with the anti-inflammatory properties of cloves, contribute to bone health and may help prevent conditions like osteoporosis.
5. **Blood Sugar Regulation:** Cloves contain compounds that aid in regulating blood sugar levels. Eugenol and other active components enhance insulin sensitivity and assist in glucose metabolism, potentially benefiting individuals with diabetes or those at risk of developing the condition.

6. **Antioxidant Powerhouse:** Cloves are a great source of antioxidants, including phenolic compounds like eugenol, gallic acid, and quercetin. These antioxidants help neutralize harmful free radicals, reducing oxidative stress and protecting cells from damage.
7. **Liver Health:** The antioxidants in cloves aid in liver detoxification processes. Cloves enhance the activity of liver enzymes, promoting the elimination of toxins and supporting overall liver health.
8. **Immune System Support:** Cloves contain notable amounts of vitamin C, a potent immune booster. Vitamin C supports the production of white blood cells, strengthening the immune system and its ability to fight against pathogens.
9. **Respiratory Health:** Clove oil possesses expectorant properties, making it beneficial for respiratory conditions such as coughs, colds, and bronchitis. Eugenol acts as a bronchodilator, helping to ease breathing and reduce inflammation in the respiratory tract.
10. **Antimicrobial Effects:** Cloves possess potent antimicrobial and antifungal activity. Eugenol, along with other compounds in cloves, helps inhibit the growth of bacteria, fungi, and yeast, supporting overall health and preventing infections.

While cloves are generally considered safe to consume, there are certain medical contradictions and precautions to consider. Individuals with bleeding disorders or those scheduled for surgery should exercise caution, as cloves may have blood-thinning effects. It is advised to discontinue clove consumption at least two weeks before any surgical procedures. Cloves may also interact with anticoagulant medications, such as warfarin, increasing the risk of bleeding. Individuals with liver disorders should use cloves with caution, as high doses may potentially exacerbate liver conditions. Individuals with known allergies or sensitivities to clove or other spices in the same family (Myrtaceae) should avoid cloves to prevent adverse reactions. It's generally considered safe for pregnant and lactating women to use clove in small culinary amounts.

COMFREY LEAF

Comfrey leaf, scientifically known as Symphytum officinale, is an herbaceous perennial plant that has been revered for centuries due to its remarkable medicinal properties. Originating in Europe and parts of Asia, this herb has a rich history dating back to ancient Greece and Rome, where it was commonly used as a healing herb. Comfrey leaf derives its name from the Latin word "confervere," meaning "to knit together," highlighting its traditional use in promoting the mending of bones, wounds, and other bodily tissues. Today, comfrey leaf is widely cultivated and appreciated for its extensive range of topical skin benefits. Its versatile nature allows for various applications, including its usage in traditional medicine, natural skincare, and even as a nutrient-rich organic fertilizer.

Now, let's explore ten extensive health and longevity benefits associated with comfrey leaf:

1. **Wound Healing:** Comfrey leaf contains allantoin, which supports cell growth and accelerates wound healing.
2. **Anti-inflammatory Effects:** Comfrey leaf contains rosmarinic acid and other compounds that help reduce inflammation and soothe skin irritations.
3. **Skin Moisturization:** The mucilage content in comfrey leaf provides a soothing and moisturizing effect on the skin.
4. **Anti-itch Relief:** Comfrey leaf's anti-inflammatory properties may help alleviate itching and provide relief from skin conditions like eczema and insect bites.
5. **Skin Health:** Allantoin in comfrey leaf promotes the regeneration of skin cells, aiding in the recovery of damaged or irritated skin.
6. **Scar Reduction:** Comfrey leaf is believed to have properties that can support cell growth and tissue repair, which may contribute to reducing the appearance of scars. When applied topically, the active compounds in comfrey leaf, such as allantoin, work to promote the regeneration of skin cells. This can aid in the healing process of damaged or irritated skin, potentially helping to minimize the formation of scar tissue.
7. **Acne Support:** Comfrey leaf's antibacterial properties, along with its ability to soothe inflammation, make it beneficial in addressing acne and reducing breakouts.
8. **Dry Skin Relief:** The moisturizing properties of comfrey leaf help hydrate and nourish dry skin, restoring its natural balance.

9. **Sunburn Relief:** Comfrey leaf contains compounds such as rosmarinic acid that possess anti-inflammatory properties, which may help alleviate symptoms associated with sunburn. The anti-inflammatory action of comfrey leaf works by reducing the production of inflammatory mediators and suppressing the activity of enzymes involved in the inflammatory process. This helps to calm and soothe the skin, reducing redness, swelling, and discomfort caused by sunburn.
10. **Minor Burn Treatment:** Comfrey leaf can be used topically to soothe minor burns and promote healing.

Please note that while comfrey leaf has potential topical benefits, it is important to exercise caution and seek guidance from your herbalist before using it internally. Prior to applying comfrey leaf externally, it is advisable to perform a patch test on a small area of skin to check for potential allergic reactions or sensitivities. While comfrey leaf is generally considered safe for topical use, it should not be ingested unless specifically directed by your herbalist. This herb contains certain alkaloids that can be toxic to the liver if consumed for prolonged periods. Therefore, internal use of comfrey leaf is not recommended. Additionally, individuals taking certain medications, such as blood thinners or liver medications, should avoid using comfrey leaf due to possible interactions. If you are pregnant or lactating, it is advised to consult with your herbalist/practitioner prior to using this herb in any capacity.

COMFREY ROOT

Comfrey root, derived from the plant known as Symphytum officinale, has a fascinating background and history as a herbal remedy with a wide array of health benefits. This herbaceous perennial plant has a rich and enduring legacy that can be traced back to ancient civilizations such as Greece and Rome. Throughout history, comfrey root has been highly regarded for its exceptional healing properties. It was commonly used in traditional medicine to address various ailments and promote overall well-being. The herb gained popularity due to its remarkable ability to support the healing of wounds, fractures, and sprains. Its traditional uses also extended to the treatment of respiratory conditions, gastrointestinal disorders, and skin conditions. Comfrey root was particularly valued for its topical applications. It was used externally to soothe and heal wounds, burns, and skin irritations. The herb was known for its capacity to promote tissue regeneration and reduce inflammation, making it a trusted remedy for addressing skin-related concerns.

Now, let's explore ten extensive health and longevity benefits associated with comfrey root:

1. **Wound Healing:** Comfrey root contains allantoin, a compound that promotes cell proliferation and wound healing by stimulating tissue growth and reducing inflammation. It helps accelerate the healing process of abrasions, and minor burns.
2. **Skin Repair:** Allantoin in comfrey root aids in repairing damaged skin by promoting the formation of new skin cells. It can be beneficial for addressing skin conditions like dryness, cracking, and roughness.
3. **Joint and Muscle Support:** Comfrey root has been traditionally used to alleviate joint and muscle discomfort. Its anti-inflammatory properties, coupled with compounds like allantoin, help reduce inflammation and provide soothing relief.
4. **Graceful-aging Effects:** The antioxidant properties of comfrey root, including rosmarinic acid, help combat free radicals and oxidative stress, which contribute to premature aging. It supports the skin's elasticity, reducing the appearance of fine lines and wrinkles.
5. **Scar Reduction:** Comfrey root's ability to support tissue regeneration and reduce inflammation makes it beneficial for minimizing the appearance of scars. Regular application of comfrey root preparations may aid in scar healing.

6. **Moisturization:** Comfrey root extracts contain mucilage, a natural substance that helps retain moisture in the skin. This moisturizing effect can be beneficial for individuals with dry or dehydrated skin.
7. **Anti-inflammatory Effects:** Comfrey root contains rosmarinic acid, a potent antioxidant and anti-inflammatory compound. Rosmarinic acid helps reduce inflammation, soothing skin conditions such as eczema, psoriasis, and dermatitis.
8. **Skin Brightening:** Comfrey root contains compounds like allantoin and caffeic acid, which help improve skin tone and promote a brighter complexion. It can assist in reducing the appearance of age spots and hyperpigmentation.
9. **Calming Irritated Skin:** Comfrey root has soothing properties that help calm irritated skin. It can provide relief for skin conditions characterized by redness, itching, or inflammation.
10. **Hair and Scalp Health:** Comfrey root extracts can be beneficial for promoting healthy hair and scalp. Its moisturizing and conditioning properties may help nourish the hair, reduce dryness, and soothe scalp irritation.

While comfrey root is generally not suitable for oral consumption due to its pyrrolizidine alkaloid content, caution should also be exercised when using comfrey root topically. Individuals with open wounds, cuts, or broken skin should avoid topical use to minimize the risk of increased absorption of pyrrolizidine alkaloids and potential liver toxicity. Those with known allergies to plants in the Boraginaceae family should be cautious or avoid comfrey root products to prevent allergic reactions. Individuals with pre-existing liver conditions or impaired liver function should avoid topical use due to the potential cumulative effect of pyrrolizidine alkaloids on liver health. It is advisable for individuals taking medications metabolized by the liver to consult a healthcare professional before using comfrey root topically to prevent potential interactions or exacerbation of medication effects. Regarding pregnancy and lactation, both oral and topical use of comfrey root is not recommended. The presence of pyrrolizidine alkaloids in comfrey root can cross the placenta, potentially impacting fetal development and affecting nursing infants through breast milk. Pregnant and breastfeeding individuals should consult with their herbalist/practitioner before considering the use of comfrey root products topically.

CORDYCEPS MUSHROOM

Cordyceps mushroom (sinensis fungi) has a rich history rooted in traditional Chinese medicine and the high altitudes of the Tibetan plateau. This extraordinary mushroom, known as "the caterpillar fungus," is native to the Himalayan regions of Tibet, Bhutan, and Nepal. Cordyceps mushrooms have a remarkable life cycle that involves infecting and ultimately transforming the bodies of specific insect larvae, resulting in a highly prized medicinal mushroom. Revered for centuries, cordyceps mushroom has gained global recognition for its extensive health and longevity benefits.

Now, let's explore ten extensive health and longevity benefits associated with cordyceps mushroom:

1. **Energy Boost:** Cordyceps contains adenosine, a nucleotide that plays a crucial role in energy production. It also contains cordycepin, a bioactive compound that enhances cellular energy metabolism and improves oxygen utilization, thereby increasing endurance and stamina.
2. **Respiratory Health:** Cordyceps has been traditionally used to promote respiratory health. It contains cordycepic acid, a compound that supports bronchial and lung function. Cordyceps also exhibits anti-inflammatory properties, which may help alleviate symptoms of respiratory conditions like asthma and chronic bronchitis.
3. **Immune System Support:** Cordyceps possesses immune-enhancing properties. It contains polysaccharides, such as beta-glucans, which stimulate immune cell activity, enhance antibody production, and increase the body's resistance to infections and diseases.
4. **Detoxification:** Cordyceps contains compounds like cordycepin and cordycepic acid, which support liver health and aid in detoxification processes. These compounds have been shown to protect the liver from oxidative damage and improve liver function.
5. **Anti-inflammatory Effects:** Cordyceps exhibits potent anti-inflammatory effects due to its various bioactive compounds, including cordycepin and adenosine. These compounds help reduce inflammation in the body, which is a key factor in many chronic diseases and aging processes.

6. **Cardiovascular Health:** Cordyceps has been found to have cardioprotective effects. It contains nucleosides, such as adenosine, which help dilate blood vessels, improve blood flow, and regulate blood pressure. Cordyceps also exhibits cholesterol-lowering properties and supports healthy lipid profiles.
7. **Cognitive Support:** Cordyceps contains active compounds that support brain health and cognitive function. Cordycepin and adenosine play a role in improving brain circulation, increasing oxygen and nutrient supply to brain cells, and protecting against age-related cognitive decline.
8. **Enhances Libido and Sexual Health:** Traditional use of cordyceps includes its reputation as an aphrodisiac and for improving sexual function. Some studies suggest that cordyceps may enhance libido, improve reproductive health, and address certain sexual dysfunctions.
9. **Antimicrobial Effects:** Cordyceps has antimicrobial and antiviral properties that help combat various pathogens. This mushroom contains cordycepin, which exhibits antiviral effects and supports the body's defense against viral infections. Cordyceps also boosts immune function, indirectly aiding in pathogen resistance.
10. **Adaptogenic Effects:** Cordyceps is recognized as an adaptogen due to its unique bioactive compounds that have the ability to influence the body's stress response systems, such as the hypothalamic-pituitary-adrenal (HPA) axis and the sympathetic-adrenal-medullary (SAM) system. These adaptogenic compounds help regulate and balance these stress response systems. Specifically, cordyceps works by normalizing the HPA axis and reducing excessive cortisol levels, thus promoting a more balanced stress response. This adaptogenic action assists the body in achieving and maintaining homeostasis, which is the state of equilibrium and optimal functioning. By supporting the body's response to stress, cordyceps contributes to overall well-being and resilience.

While cordyceps mushroom is generally considered safe to consume, there are certain medical contradictions, precautions, and potential interactions to be aware of. Individuals with bleeding disorders or those taking anticoagulant or antiplatelet medications should exercise caution, as cordyceps may have mild blood-thinning effects, potentially increasing the risk of bleeding or bruising. It is important to consult with a healthcare professional before using cordyceps if you have scheduled surgery or dental procedures. Cordyceps has the potential to interact with certain medications, such as immunosuppressants, anti-diabetic drugs, and antiviral medications. Therefore, it is crucial to discuss the use of cordyceps with your healthcare provider if you are taking any of these medications. Individuals with known allergies or sensitivities to mushrooms or other fungi should avoid cordyceps to prevent allergic reactions. It is also important to note that cordyceps belongs to the same family as other fungi, such as shiitake and maitake mushrooms, so individuals with known allergies to these mushrooms should exercise caution. Cordyceps mushroom is generally considered safe to consume during pregnancy and lactation.

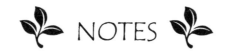

NOTES

CORIANDER SEED

Coriander seed, derived from the Coriandrum sativum plant, has a fascinating history that traces back to ancient times and encompasses diverse cultures and continents. Believed to have originated in the Mediterranean region, this aromatic spice has a longstanding presence in culinary traditions and herbal medicine practices across the globe. Its cultivation can be traced back to ancient Egypt, where it was revered for its culinary and medicinal properties. The seeds, also known as coriander or cilantro seeds, have been utilized for thousands of years in various cuisines, including Indian, Middle Eastern, Mexican, and Asian cuisines, to enhance flavors and add a delightful aroma to dishes. In addition to its culinary significance, coriander seed has been valued for its health benefits in traditional medicine systems. Ancient civilizations such as the Greeks, Romans, and Egyptians recognized its medicinal properties and used it to address various ailments.

Now, let's explore ten extensive health and longevity benefits associated with coriander seed:

1. **Carminative Effects:** Coriander seeds contain compounds like linalool and borneol, which possess carminative properties, aiding in digestion and relieving gas and bloating. They also contain dietary fiber, which helps regulate bowel movements and supports overall digestive health.
2. **Detoxification:** The antioxidants present in coriander seeds, including quercetin, kaempferol, and various phenolic compounds, help protect against oxidative stress and aid in the detoxification processes of the liver, enhancing its functionality.
3. **Anti-inflammatory Effects:** Coriander seeds contain active compounds such as linalool, cineole, and alpha-pinene, which exhibit anti-inflammatory properties. These compounds help reduce inflammation in the body, which is linked to chronic diseases and accelerated aging.
4. **Blood Sugar Regulation:** Coriander seeds contain compounds like quercetin, kaempferol, and flavonoids that have been associated with potential blood sugar-lowering effects. These compounds may help regulate blood sugar levels and improve insulin sensitivity.
5. **Bone Health:** Coriander seeds are a good source of calcium, which is essential for maintaining strong bones and teeth. Additionally, they contain small amounts of other minerals like magnesium and phosphorus, which contribute to bone health.

6. **Cardiovascular Health:** Coriander seeds contain antioxidants like quercetin and phenolic compounds that help reduce oxidative stress and inflammation, contributing to cardiovascular health. They may also help regulate cholesterol levels, indirectly supporting heart health and longevity.
7. **Antimicrobial Effects:** Coriander seeds possess antimicrobial properties due to their active compounds, such as dodecanal and cineole. These compounds help inhibit the growth of bacteria, fungi, and certain viruses, promoting overall health and supporting the body's defense against pathogens.
8. **Skin Health:** Coriander seeds contain antioxidants like vitamin C and various phenolic compounds, which help protect the skin from oxidative damage caused by free radicals. They also exhibit anti-inflammatory properties, potentially aiding in the management of skin conditions such as acne and eczema.
9. **Cognitive Support:** Coriander seeds contain compounds like quercetin and flavonoids that possess neuroprotective properties. These antioxidants help reduce oxidative stress in the brain, potentially improving cognitive function and supporting brain health.
10. **Digestive Health:** Coriander seeds have been traditionally used as a digestive cleanser. They may help eliminate toxins from the body and support the overall detoxification processes of the digestive system.

> While coriander seed is generally considered safe to consume, there are some medical contradictions and precautions to be aware of. Coriander seed may interact with certain medications, particularly anticoagulant or antiplatelet drugs, due to its potential blood-thinning effects, so individuals taking these medications should exercise caution and consult with their healthcare provider. Individuals with known allergies to coriander or related plants in the Apiaceae or Umbelliferae family, including celery, parsley, or carrot, should avoid its consumption to prevent allergic reactions. Coriander seed is generally considered safe to consume in culinary quantities while pregnant or lactating.

CORNFLOWERS

Cornflowers, scientifically known as Centaurea cyanus, are vibrant and enchanting flowers with a captivating history that dates back centuries. Native to Europe and often associated with folklore and symbolism, cornflowers have been cherished for their aesthetic appeal and various medicinal properties. Throughout history, cornflowers have been used in traditional medicine for their soothing properties and as a natural remedy for eye irritations and discomfort. They have also been treasured for their culinary uses, adding a touch of color and flavor to dishes and beverages. Today, cornflowers continue to be appreciated for their visual allure and potential health benefits, making them a beloved flower in both traditional and modern practices.

Now, let's explore ten extensive health and longevity benefits associated with cornflowers:

1. **Anti-inflammatory Effects:** Cornflowers contain flavonoids such as apigenin and luteolin, which exhibit potent anti-inflammatory effects. These compounds help reduce inflammation in the body, supporting the overall health of organs and body systems.
2. **Anxiety and Stress Relief:** Cornflowers possess mild sedative properties, promoting relaxation and helping to relieve stress and anxiety. This benefit can indirectly contribute to overall well-being and support longevity by reducing the negative effects of chronic stress on the body.
3. **Cardiovascular Health:** The presence of anthocyanins in cornflowers, such as cyanidin, provides cardiovascular benefits. These compounds help protect blood vessels, reduce inflammation, and support healthy blood pressure, indirectly promoting heart health and longevity.
4. **Eye Health:** Cornflowers contain anthocyanins, including cyanidin-3-glucoside, which possess antioxidant properties. These compounds help protect the eyes from oxidative damage, supporting eye health and potentially reducing the risk of age-related vision problems.
5. **Antimicrobial Effects:** Cornflowers contain natural antimicrobial and antifungal properties. Active compounds like polyphenols and flavonoids help inhibit the growth of pathogens, including bacteria and fungi, supporting immune health and overall well-being.

6. **Antioxidant Powerhouse:** Cornflowers are rich in antioxidants like cyanidin and quercetin. These antioxidants scavenge harmful free radicals, reducing oxidative stress and protecting cells from damage, which is crucial for promoting longevity.
7. **Digestive Health:** Cornflowers possess soothing properties that benefit the digestive system. The presence of flavonoids in cornflowers helps calm gastrointestinal inflammation, alleviating symptoms associated with digestive disorders.
8. **Skin Health:** Cornflowers are rich in antioxidants and tannins, which provide benefits to the skin. These compounds help protect the skin from damage caused by free radicals, promote skin regeneration, and soothe irritations, contributing to a healthy and youthful complexion.
9. **Respiratory Health:** Cornflowers contain compounds that have the potential to support respiratory health and provide soothing benefits. These compounds, such as flavonoids and other bioactive components, may help alleviate respiratory irritation and promote clearer breathing.
10. **Menstrual Support:** Cornflowers have been known for their potential to alleviate menstrual discomfort and symptoms. The soothing properties of cornflowers, along with their mild analgesic effects, can help ease cramps, reduce bloating, and promote overall comfort during menstruation.

Although cornflowers are generally considered safe to use, it is important to note a few warnings and contradictions. Individuals taking sedatives or medications for hypertension should exercise caution, as cornflowers may have mild sedative and blood pressure-lowering effects. Additionally, if you have known allergies to plants in the Asteraceae family (such as ragweed), it's advisable to avoid cornflowers to prevent any allergic reactions. While cornflowers are generally considered safe during pregnancy and lactation, it's best to consult with your herbalist/practitioner for personalized advice.

CORYDALIS ROOT

Corydalis root, derived from the plant known as Corydalis yanhusuo, has a long history deeply rooted in traditional Chinese medicine. Originating in China, this herb has been used for centuries in various formulations to support pain relief and promote relaxation. Corydalis root has been highly regarded for its analgesic properties and is often used in traditional Chinese remedies for conditions such as menstrual discomfort, headaches, and joint pain. The herb's historical use and reputation have made it an integral part of Chinese herbal medicine, where it continues to be valued for its potential health benefits.

Now, let's explore ten extensive health and longevity benefits associated with corydalis root:

1. **Pain Relief:** Corydalis root contains the alkaloid compound dehydrocorybulbine, which exhibits analgesic properties. dehydrocorybulbine interacts with opioid receptors, providing pain relief and potentially reducing reliance on traditional pain medications.
2. **Cardiovascular Health:** The active compounds tetrahydropalmatine and protopine in corydalis root have been found to have vasodilatory effects, promoting improved blood flow and cardiovascular health.
3. **Liver Health:** Corydalis root contains antioxidants, including tetrahydropalmatine and tetrahydrocoptisine. These antioxidants help protect the liver from oxidative damage and support its detoxification functions.
4. **Anti-inflammatory Effects:** Corydalis root contains protopine, which possesses anti-inflammatory properties. Protopine helps reduce inflammation throughout the body, which is linked to chronic diseases and accelerated aging.
5. **Menstrual Support:** Corydalis root has been traditionally used to support menstrual health and alleviate symptoms associated with menstruation. Its active compounds, such as dehydrocorybulbine, tetrahydropalmatine, and protopine, may help regulate menstrual cycles and reduce discomfort.
6. **Skin Health:** Corydalis root possesses antioxidant properties, which may help protect the skin from oxidative damage caused by environmental factors. Antioxidants in corydalis root, such as tetrahydropalmatine, support skin health and contribute to a youthful appearance.

7. **Respiratory Health:** Corydalis root has traditionally been used to alleviate respiratory conditions such as coughs and bronchitis. Its active compounds, including tetrahydropalmatine, help relax bronchial smooth muscles and promote respiratory health.
8. **Digestive Health:** Corydalis root contains alkaloid compounds like tetrahydropalmatine and tetrahydrocoptisine, which have been shown to promote digestive health. These compounds help soothe the gastrointestinal tract, reduce inflammation, and alleviate symptoms of digestive disorders.
9. **Antimicrobial Effects:** Corydalis root exhibits broad-spectrum antimicrobial activity due to its active compounds. These compounds, including tetrahydropalmatine, help inhibit the growth of bacteria, fungi, and other pathogens, supporting overall health.
10. **Detoxification:** The active compounds tetrahydropalmatine and tetrahydrocoptisine in corydalis root support the liver's detoxification processes. They assist in the elimination of toxins and promote overall detoxification and longevity.

While corydalis root is generally considered safe to consume, it is important to be aware of certain medical contradictions and precautions. Individuals with pre-existing liver or kidney conditions should exercise caution and consult with a healthcare professional before using corydalis root, as it may interact with medications or exacerbate these conditions. Additionally, individuals taking medications such as anticoagulants or antiplatelet drugs should be cautious, as corydalis root may have mild blood-thinning effects. It is advisable to consult with a healthcare provider before using corydalis root if you have scheduled surgery or dental procedures. Individuals with known allergies to plants in the Papaveraceae family, which includes corydalis root, should avoid its consumption to prevent allergic reactions. Pregnant or breastfeeding individuals should consult with their herbalist/practitioner before using corydalis root to ensure safety for both mother and baby.

CURRY POWDER

Curry powder, a fragrant and vibrant spice blend, has a fascinating origin deeply rooted in the culinary traditions of the Indian subcontinent. This iconic blend of spices has evolved over centuries, drawing inspiration from the diverse regional cuisines of India. While there is no singular "authentic" curry powder recipe, it typically comprises a harmonious combination of aromatic spices such as turmeric, coriander, cumin, fenugreek, ginger, and chili peppers. Curry powder not only adds depth, complexity, and a burst of flavors to dishes but also offers an array of health and longevity benefits. Now, let's explore ten extensive health and longevity benefits associated with curry powder:

1. **Anti-inflammatory Effects:** The presence of turmeric in curry powder provides potent anti-inflammatory effects, which may help alleviate inflammation in the body and reduce the risk of chronic diseases.
2. **Antioxidant Powerhouse:** Curry powder contains a variety of spices, including turmeric and cumin, that are rich in antioxidants, offering protection against oxidative stress and cellular damage.
3. **Digestive Health:** The combination of spices in curry powder, such as coriander and cumin, can aid digestion, stimulate enzyme production, and relieve digestive discomfort.
4. **Immune System Support:** The diverse array of spices in curry powder, such as ginger and garlic, possess immune-boosting properties that can strengthen the body's defense against infections and diseases.
5. **Cardiovascular Health:** Some components of curry powder, including turmeric and cardamom, have been associated with heart-protective benefits, such as reducing inflammation, improving cholesterol levels, and promoting healthy blood circulation.
6. **Anti-cancer Effects:** The presence of turmeric in curry powder, with its active compound curcumin, has shown promising anti-cancer properties, potentially inhibiting tumor growth and reducing the risk of certain cancers.
7. **Blood Sugar Regulation:** Spices like cinnamon and fenugreek found in curry powder have been studied for their potential to regulate blood sugar levels, making it beneficial for individuals with diabetes or insulin resistance.

8. **Cognitive Support:** Certain spices found in curry powder, such as turmeric and black pepper, have been linked to improved cognitive function, memory, and brain health.
9. **Appetite Control:** Curry powder contains spices like cayenne pepper and mustard seeds, which have been associated with supporting healthy digestion and appetite control. Cayenne pepper contains capsaicin, a compound that may help stimulate digestion and support a healthy gastrointestinal system. Additionally, mustard seeds contain various antioxidants and bioactive compounds that can contribute to improved digestion. By incorporating curry powder into your meals, you may experience enhanced digestive health and a better sense of appetite control.
10. **Antimicrobial Effects:** Some spices present in curry powder, such as turmeric and garlic, possess antimicrobial properties, potentially helping to fight against bacteria, viruses, and fungi.

> While curry powder is generally considered safe to consume, there are certain warnings and contradictions to consider. Individuals taking specific medications, such as blood thinners (e.g., Warfarin) or antiplatelet drugs, should exercise caution when consuming large amounts of curry powder due to the blood-thinning properties of some of its components, particularly turmeric. It is generally considered safe to consume curry powder during pregnancy and lactation.

DAMIANA

Damiana, scientifically known as Turnera diffusa, is a small shrub native to the subtropical regions of Central and South America. With a history deeply intertwined with indigenous cultures, damiana has been treasured for centuries for its medicinal properties and aphrodisiac qualities. Traditionally, it was used as an aphrodisiac by cultures like the Maya and Aztecs, as well as a relaxant, mood enhancer, and mild diuretic. Beyond its potential medicinal benefits, damiana played a significant role in the spiritual and social practices of these indigenous peoples.

Now, let's explore ten extensive health and longevity benefits associated with damiana:

1. **Enhances Libido and Sexual Health:** Damiana has been traditionally used as an aphrodisiac. It contains flavonoids such as apigenin and quercetin, which may improve sexual function by increasing blood flow, reducing stress, and balancing hormone levels.
2. **Nervous System Health:** Damiana contains compounds like pinocembrin and arbutin, which exhibit neuroprotective properties. These compounds help support the health of the nervous system, enhance cognitive function, and reduce symptoms of anxiety and depression.
3. **Energy Boost:** Damiana contains caffeine-like compounds, such as theobromine, which can provide a natural energy boost. These compounds stimulate the central nervous system, increase alertness, and improve physical performance.
4. **Digestive Health:** Damiana has been used traditionally as a digestive tonic. It contains flavonoids and volatile oils that stimulate digestion, alleviate indigestion, and relieve gastrointestinal disorders such as constipation and bloating.
5. **Urinary Tract Health:** Damiana acts as a diuretic, helping to promote urine production and flush out toxins from the body. This diuretic effect can support the health of the urinary tract and prevent urinary infections.
6. **Antioxidant Powerhouse:** Damiana contains antioxidants, including flavonoids and phenolic compounds, which help protect the body against oxidative stress and damage caused by free radicals. These antioxidants contribute to overall health and longevity.

7. **Antimicrobial Effects:** Damiana possesses antimicrobial properties thanks to its active compounds, such as pinocembrin and arbutin. These compounds help inhibit the growth of bacteria, fungi, and viruses, supporting the body's defense against pathogens.
8. **Respiratory Health:** Damiana has expectorant properties, making it beneficial for respiratory health. It may help relieve coughs, congestion, and respiratory infections.
9. **Skin Health:** Damiana possesses antimicrobial and anti-inflammatory properties that can benefit the skin. It may help soothe skin irritations, reduce redness, and prevent bacterial or fungal infections, supporting overall skin health.
10. **Detoxification:** Damiana stimulates kidney function, aiding in the elimination of toxins from the body. Its diuretic properties help remove waste products, promoting detoxification and supporting the health of vital organs.

While damiana is generally considered safe to consume, there are certain medical contradictions and precautions that should be taken into account. Individuals with hormone-sensitive conditions, such as breast, uterine, or ovarian cancers, should exercise caution due to damiana's potential estrogenic effects. Individuals with diabetes or hypoglycemia should monitor their blood sugar levels closely, as damiana may lower blood glucose levels. It is advisable for individuals with a history of liver disease or liver impairment to consult with a healthcare professional before using damiana, as it may have hepatotoxic effects in high doses. Damiana may also interact with certain medications, particularly those metabolized by the liver. These medications include but are not limited to cytochrome P450 substrates, antidiabetic drugs, and hormone-related medications. The safety of damiana during pregnancy and lactation is not well-established, and it is recommended to avoid its use during these periods due to insufficient evidence on its effects on fetal development and potential transfer into breast milk.

DANDELION LEAF

Dandelion leaf, scientifically known as Taraxacum officinale, is a remarkable herbaceous plant with a fascinating history deeply rooted in European, Asian, and North American cultures. While often regarded as a humble weed, dandelion has been cherished for centuries for its versatile culinary and medicinal properties. This resilient plant has been a part of traditional practices, where its leaves have been highly esteemed for their exceptional nutritional value. Whether enjoyed as a refreshing herbal tea, incorporated into nourishing salads, or utilized in herbal remedies, dandelion leaf has been treasured for its abundant health benefits, thanks to its diverse array of bioactive compounds and remarkable nutrient profile. Now, let's explore ten extensive health and longevity benefits associated with dandelion leaf:

1. **Liver Health:** Dandelion leaf contains antioxidants such as flavonoids (including luteolin and apigenin) and polyphenols, which help protect the liver from oxidative stress. These compounds also stimulate liver detoxification enzymes, supporting the liver's ability to eliminate toxins and promote overall liver health.
2. **Digestive Health:** Dandelion leaf acts as a natural diuretic, increasing urine production and promoting healthy kidney function. It also contains compounds like inulin, which acts as a prebiotic, supporting the growth of beneficial gut bacteria and improving digestion.
3. **Anti-inflammatory Effects:** The flavonoids and polyphenols in dandelion leaf, including luteolin and chlorogenic acid, possess anti-inflammatory properties. These compounds help reduce inflammation in the body, contributing to the management of chronic inflammatory conditions.
4. **Antioxidant Powerhouse:** Dandelion leaf is rich in antioxidants like beta-carotene, vitamin C, and luteolin. These antioxidants help neutralize harmful free radicals, reducing oxidative stress and preventing cellular damage, which is associated with various chronic diseases and aging.
5. **Blood Sugar Regulation:** Dandelion leaf contains compounds like chlorogenic acid, which may help regulate blood sugar levels by inhibiting certain enzymes involved in carbohydrate metabolism. This can be beneficial for individuals with diabetes or those at risk of developing the condition.

6. **Kidney Health:** Dandelion leaf acts as a diuretic, promoting urine production and supporting kidney function. This helps flush out toxins and waste products from the body, aiding in maintaining optimal kidney health.
7. **Anti-radiation Effects:** Dandelion's unique properties extend to its role as a natural anti-radiation ally. Rich in antioxidants, such as vitamins A and C, dandelion contributes to shielding the body from the harmful effects of radiation exposure. These antioxidants actively neutralize free radicals induced by radiation, aiding in the protection of cellular integrity and helping mitigate the consequences of ionizing radiation. Dandelion's potential in radiation protection makes it a valuable asset in efforts to combat radiation-related challenges.
8. **Antimicrobial Effects:** Dandelion leaf exhibits antimicrobial effects due to the presence of various compounds such as taraxacin and chicoric acid. These compounds help inhibit the growth of certain bacteria and fungi, supporting the body's defense against pathogens.
9. **Bone Health:** Dandelion leaf is a good source of calcium, which is essential for maintaining strong and healthy bones. It also contains other bone-supporting minerals like magnesium and potassium, along with vitamin K, which plays a role in bone metabolism.
10. **Immune System Support:** Dandelion leaf is rich in vitamin C, an essential nutrient for immune system function. Vitamin C acts as an antioxidant, helps support immune cell function, and contributes to the overall health and vitality of the immune system.

> While dandelion leaf is generally considered safe to consume, there are some medical contradictions and precautions to consider. Dandelion leaf may interact with certain medications, such as diuretics and lithium, so it is advisable to consult with a healthcare professional before using dandelion leaf if taking these medications. Individuals with an allergy to plants in the Asteraceae family, including daisies, marigolds, and ragweed, may also be allergic to dandelion and should avoid its consumption. The actual dandelion leaf is generally safe to consume while pregnant and lactating. However, your herbalist should be consulted before using a dandelion supplement to ensure it's a good fit for you.

DANDELION ROOT

Dandelion root, scientifically known as Taraxacum officinale, is the underground part of the dandelion plant, a perennial herbaceous plant that is native to Europe, Asia, and North America. Dandelion root has a long history of traditional use in various cultures for its medicinal properties. The roots are typically harvested and dried for use in herbal preparations such as teas, tinctures, or capsules. Dandelion root offers a wide range of health and longevity benefits due to its rich nutritional composition and bioactive compounds.

Now, let's explore ten extensive health and longevity benefits associated with dandelion root:

1. **Liver Health:** Dandelion root contains bitter compounds like taraxacin and sesquiterpene lactones, which stimulate bile production and promote healthy liver function. It also provides essential nutrients such as vitamin A, vitamin C, and iron that support liver detoxification processes.
2. **Digestive Health:** Dandelion root, rich in compounds like inulin and terpenes, plays a crucial role in enhancing digestion by stimulating bile production. Bile, essential for fat breakdown, is facilitated by dandelion root, promoting efficient digestion and nutrient absorption. This stimulation not only aids in preventing bloating and constipation but also supports a healthy gut microbiota.
3. **Immune System Support:** Dandelion root contains vitamins A and C, which are crucial for maintaining a robust immune system. These vitamins act as antioxidants, supporting immune cell function and protecting against infections and disease.
4. **Bone Health:** Dandelion root contains essential minerals like calcium, magnesium, and potassium, which are vital for maintaining strong and healthy bones. These minerals play a role in bone mineralization, density, and overall skeletal health.
5. **Anti-cancer Effects:** Dandelion root contains various compounds with potential anti-cancer effects, including sesquiterpene lactones, luteolin, and beta-sitosterol. These compounds have been shown to inhibit the growth of cancer cells and induce apoptosis (cell death) in certain types of cancer.
6. **Cardiovascular Health:** Dandelion root contains potassium, a mineral that helps regulate blood pressure and maintain heart health. Its antioxidant properties, along with flavonoids like luteolin, help reduce oxidative stress and inflammation, supporting cardiovascular function.

7. **Detoxification:** The diuretic properties of dandelion root help flush out toxins and excess fluids from the body, supporting kidney function and aiding in detoxification processes. It also contains antioxidants, including luteolin and beta-carotene, which help protect against oxidative stress and cellular damage.
8. **Anti-inflammatory Effects:** Dandelion root possesses anti-inflammatory compounds such as sesquiterpene lactones, flavonoids, and polyphenols. These active compounds help reduce inflammation in the body, which is associated with various chronic diseases and premature aging.
9. **Skin Health:** Dandelion root is rich in antioxidants, including vitamin C and beta-carotene, which protect the skin against oxidative stress and promote a youthful appearance. Its antimicrobial properties may also contribute to improved skin health by combating acne-causing bacteria.
10. **Urinary Tract Health:** Dandelion root possesses diuretic properties, which may help promote urinary tract health and prevent urinary tract infections (UTIs). Additionally, its antimicrobial properties may aid in fighting off bacteria responsible for UTIs.

While dandelion root is generally considered safe to consume, there are certain medical contradictions and precautions to be aware of. Individuals taking medications that are metabolized by the liver, such as cytochrome P450 substrates, should consult with their healthcare provider before using dandelion root, as it may interfere with the metabolism of these drugs. Additionally, individuals on anticoagulant or antiplatelet medications should exercise caution, as dandelion root may have mild blood-thinning effects. It is important to note that dandelion root may cause allergic reactions in individuals sensitive to plants in the Asteraceae family, including chamomile, ragweed, and marigold. Dandelion root is generally considered safe to consume in small quantities while pregnant or lactating. Consult with your herbalist/practitioner before consuming large supplemental quantities during these times.

DEVIL'S CLAW

Devil's claw, scientifically known as Harpagophytum procumbens, is a medicinal plant with a fascinating history rooted in the Kalahari Desert of Southern Africa. It owes its name to the distinctive appearance of its fruit, which features claw-like projections that resemble the mythical talons of a devil. For centuries, indigenous tribes in the region have harnessed the therapeutic properties of devil's claw by utilizing its tuberous roots. These roots have been esteemed for their potential to alleviate a range of health conditions and promote overall well-being. In recent times, devil's claw has garnered attention as a natural remedy, sought after for its diverse array of health benefits. This remarkable herb boasts a rich phytochemical composition, which contributes to its remarkable therapeutic potential.
Now, let's explore ten extensive health and longevity benefits associated with devil's claw:

1. **Anti-inflammatory Effects:** Devil's claw contains harpagoside, a bioactive compound with potent anti-inflammatory properties. It inhibits the production of inflammatory mediators, such as cytokines and prostaglandins, making it beneficial for reducing inflammation in various body systems.
2. **Joint Health:** Devil's claw is commonly used to alleviate joint pain and inflammation associated with conditions like osteoarthritis and rheumatoid arthritis. The harpagoside compound in devil's claw acts as a natural pain reliever and supports joint mobility.
3. **Digestive Health:** Devil's claw has been traditionally used to improve digestion and relieve symptoms of indigestion. It stimulates digestive secretions and supports the production of digestive enzymes, aiding in the breakdown and absorption of nutrients.
4. **Liver Health:** Devil's claw contains iridoid glycosides, including harpagide and harpagoside, which exhibit hepatoprotective properties. These compounds support liver function by enhancing detoxification processes and protecting liver cells from oxidative stress. Some of the compounds in this herb may help stimulate bile production.
5. **Skin Health:** The antioxidant properties of devil's claw, including flavonoids and phenolic compounds, help protect the skin from oxidative damage caused by free radicals. Additionally, its anti-inflammatory effects may contribute to the management of skin conditions like eczema and psoriasis.

6. **Cardiovascular Health:** Devil's claw contains flavonoids, such as luteolin and kaempferol, which have been linked to cardiovascular health benefits. These antioxidants help reduce oxidative stress, promote healthy blood flow, and support the maintenance of optimal blood pressure levels.
7. **Pain Relief:** Devil's claw has analgesic properties and is often used to alleviate various types of pain, including headaches, backaches, and muscle pain. The harpagoside compound in devil's claw inhibits pain pathways, providing natural pain relief.
8. **Immune System Support:** Devil's claw contains antioxidants, such as quercetin and kaempferol, that support immune function. These compounds help neutralize free radicals, strengthen the immune system, and protect against infections and diseases.
9. **Antimicrobial Effects:** Devil's claw exhibits antimicrobial activity against various microorganisms, including bacteria and fungi. This property is attributed to the presence of bioactive compounds like harpagoside, which may help protect against pathogenic infections.
10. **Anti-diabetic Effects:** Devil's claw has shown potential in supporting blood sugar control and managing diabetes. Certain compounds found in devil's claw, such as harpagoside and procumbide, may help improve insulin sensitivity and regulate glucose metabolism.

While devil's claw is generally considered safe to consume, there are certain medical contradictions and precautions to consider. People with blood clotting disorders or those taking anticoagulant medications like warfarin should avoid devil's claw due to its potential antiplatelet effects. It is important to note that devil's claw may interact with certain medications, such as nonsteroidal anti-inflammatory drugs (NSAIDs), aspirin, and diabetic medications, potentially leading to adverse effects or interfering with the medications' efficacy. Devil's claw is not recommended for use during pregnancy, as its effects on fetal development are not well-studied. It is also not advised during lactation, as there is limited information regarding its safety for breastfeeding mothers and infants.

DILL WEED

Dill weed, scientifically known as Anethum graveolens, is a fragrant herb indigenous to the Mediterranean region and select areas of Asia. This versatile herb, characterized by its delicate yellow flowers and feathery leaves, has a rich history steeped in culinary and medicinal traditions across various cultures. Throughout the ages, dill weed has played a pivotal role in the culinary world, lending its distinctive flavor to an array of dishes and serving as a key ingredient in pickling recipes. Beyond its culinary prowess, dill weed has found applications in herbal preparations and has been cherished by different cultures for its unique attributes, making it a remarkable herb with a diverse cultural legacy.

Now, let's explore ten extensive health and longevity benefits associated with dill weed:

1. **Digestive Health:** Dill weed is abundant in compounds such as carvone, limonene, and anethofuran, each recognized for their potential to support digestive health. Carvone is believed to possess carminative properties, aiding in the reduction of bloating and discomfort. Limonene has been studied for potential gastroprotective effects. Anethofuran is believed to contribute to the herb's digestive benefits through its potential ability to ease digestive discomfort.
2. **Anti-inflammatory Effects:** Dill weed contains compounds that possess anti-inflammatory properties, potentially helping to reduce inflammation and alleviate associated symptoms.
3. **Antioxidant Powerhouse:** Dill weed is rich in antioxidants, such as flavonoids and polyphenols, which help protect the body against oxidative stress and free radical damage.
4. **Bone Health:** The calcium, magnesium, and vitamin K content in dill weed contribute to its potential benefits for bone health, helping to maintain strong and healthy bones.
5. **Immune System Support:** Dill weed is a natural immune booster, thanks to its immune-enhancing compounds that may help strengthen the body's defense against infections and diseases.
6. **Respiratory Health:** Dill weed has been traditionally used to soothe respiratory conditions like coughs, bronchitis, and asthma, helping to ease congestion and promote easier breathing.
7. **Oral Health:** Dill weed possesses antimicrobial properties that can contribute to oral health by reducing the growth of bacteria in the mouth and freshening breath.

8. **Sleep Support:** Dill weed has mild sedative properties, promoting relaxation, reducing anxiety, and aiding in achieving restful sleep.
9. **Diuretic Effects:** Dill weed acts as a natural diuretic, promoting healthy urine flow, helping to flush out toxins, and supporting kidney function.
10. **Menstrual Support:** Dill weed has been traditionally used to regulate menstrual cycles, reduce menstrual cramps, and alleviate symptoms associated with premenstrual syndrome (PMS).

While dill weed is generally considered safe to consume, there are certain medical contradictions and precautions to be aware of. Individuals with allergies to plants in the Apiaceae family, including celery, carrot, and fennel, may also be allergic to dill weed and should avoid its consumption. Dill weed may interact with certain medications, such as anticoagulants and antiplatelet drugs, due to its potential antiplatelet effects, and individuals taking these medications should exercise caution. Individuals with hormone-sensitive conditions, such as breast, uterine, or ovarian cancers, should avoid dill weed due to its potential estrogenic effects. Dill weed may have mild diuretic properties and interact with certain medications that affect kidney function or blood pressure, so it is advisable to consult with a healthcare professional before using dill weed if taking these medications. Dill weed is generally considered safe to consume in culinary amounts during pregnancy and lactation. Consult with your herbalist/practitioner before consuming large amounts of dill weed for prolonged periods during these times.

DONG QUAI ROOT

Dong quai root, scientifically known as Angelica sinensis, is a perennial herb that has been highly revered in traditional Chinese medicine for centuries. It is native to China, Korea, and Japan and is often referred to as the "female ginseng" due to its profound effects on women's health. Dong quai root has a long history of use as a medicinal herb, particularly for its potential benefits in balancing hormones and promoting overall well-being. Now, let's explore ten extensive health and longevity benefits associated with dong quai root:

1. **Hormonal Balance:** Dong quai root is renowned for its ability to support hormonal balance in women, particularly during menstrual cycles and menopause. It may help regulate menstrual flow, reduce menstrual cramps, and alleviate symptoms of hormonal imbalances.
2. **Menstrual Support:** Dong quai root has been traditionally used to relieve menstrual disorders such as irregular periods, heavy bleeding, and menstrual pain.
3. **Menopausal Support:** Dong quai root may assist in managing menopausal symptoms like hot flashes, night sweats, mood swings, and vaginal dryness.
4. **Blood Circulation:** Dong quai root has potential benefits for blood circulation, promoting healthy blood flow and cardiovascular health.
5. **Immune System Support:** Dong quai root is believed to enhance immune function and increase the body's resistance to infections and diseases.
6. **Anti-inflammatory Effects:** Dong quai root contains compounds with anti-inflammatory effects, potentially reducing inflammation throughout the body and alleviating associated symptoms.
7. **Liver Health:** Dong quai root may support liver health and detoxification processes, aiding in the removal of toxins from the body.
8. **Bone Health:** Dong quai root has been traditionally used to improve bone density and prevent osteoporosis, potentially contributing to long-term skeletal health.
9. **Stress Relief:** Dong quai root is known for its adaptogenic properties, helping the body adapt to stress, promote relaxation, and improve overall well-being.

10. **Skin Health:** Dong quai root is believed to have positive effects on the skin, promoting a clear complexion and supporting overall skin health.

While dong quai root is generally considered safe to consume, there are certain medical contradictions and precautions to be aware of. Individuals with hormone-sensitive conditions, such as breast, uterine, or ovarian cancers, should exercise caution due to dong quai's potential estrogenic effects. Dong quai may interact with certain medications, including anticoagulants and antiplatelet drugs, due to its potential anticoagulant and antiplatelet effects. It may also potentiate the effects of hormone therapies and contraceptives. Individuals with bleeding disorders or who are scheduled for surgery should consult with their healthcare provider before using dong quai. Allergy warnings should be noted, as dong quai belongs to the same family as celery, carrot, and parsley, and individuals with known allergies to these plants may also be allergic to dong quai. It is not recommended to use dong quai during pregnancy as it may stimulate uterine contractions. Individuals who are lactating should consult with their herbalist/practitioner prior to using dong quai root.

DULSE FLAKES

Dulse flakes, scientifically known as Palmaria palmata, are a type of red seaweed that grows along the rocky shores of the North Atlantic and Pacific Oceans. Dulse has a long history of culinary and medicinal use, particularly in coastal regions where it is harvested and consumed for its nutritional and therapeutic properties. Dulse flakes are derived from drying and processing the seaweed, resulting in a versatile and nutrient-rich ingredient. Packed with vitamins, minerals, and antioxidants, dulse flakes offer an array of health and longevity benefits.

Now, let's explore ten extensive health and longevity benefits associated with dulse flakes:

1. **Rich in Essential Minerals:** Dulse flakes are a natural source of essential minerals such as iodine, iron, calcium, potassium, and magnesium, supporting optimal bodily functions and promoting overall health.
2. **Thyroid Health:** The high iodine content in dulse flakes makes them beneficial for maintaining a healthy thyroid gland, which plays a crucial role in regulating metabolism and hormone production.
3. **Heart Health:** Dulse flakes may contribute to heart health by promoting healthy cholesterol levels, supporting normal blood pressure, and reducing the risk of cardiovascular diseases.
4. **Digestive Health:** Dulse flakes contain dietary fiber, which aids in digestion, supports regular bowel movements, and promotes a healthy gut microbiome.
5. **Anti-inflammatory Effects:** Dulse flakes possess anti-inflammatory compounds that may help reduce inflammation in the body, supporting overall well-being and potentially alleviating symptoms of inflammatory conditions.
6. **Antioxidant Powerhouse:** Dulse flakes are rich in antioxidants, such as polyphenols and flavonoids, which help neutralize free radicals, protect against oxidative stress, and reduce the risk of chronic diseases.
7. **Vitality Support:** Dulse flakes provide valuable nutrients that can support energy levels and overall vitality. Dulse contains essential nutrients such as iron, potassium, magnesium, and various B vitamins. These nutrients play important roles in energy metabolism, nerve function, and red blood cell production, which are essential for maintaining energy levels and reducing fatigue.

8. **Bone Health:** Dulse flakes contain minerals that contribute to overall bone health, including calcium, magnesium, and trace amounts of iron. Calcium and magnesium are essential for maintaining strong and healthy bones, while iron plays a role in bone metabolism.
9. **Skin Health:** The antioxidants and minerals in dulse flakes contribute to healthy skin by promoting collagen production, protecting against oxidative damage, and supporting a youthful appearance.
10. **Detoxification:** Dulse flakes are rich in nutrients that help to support detoxification, such as iodine, iron, potassium, magnesium, calcium, vitamin C, and various phytochemical compounds. Dulse is also known for its ability to bind to heavy metals in the body and facilitate their excretion from the body.

While dulse is generally considered safe to consume, there are certain medical contradictions, precautions, and considerations to keep in mind. Individuals with existing kidney conditions or impaired kidney function should exercise caution when consuming dulse due to its naturally occurring potassium content. Individuals taking medications that affect potassium levels, such as certain diuretics or potassium-sparing medications, should be mindful of their dulse consumption to avoid excessive potassium levels in the body. People with allergies to seafood or iodine should also be cautious when consuming dulse, as it may trigger allergic reactions. Safety during pregnancy and lactation is another important consideration. While dulse contains beneficial nutrients, excessive iodine intake during pregnancy can be harmful to the developing fetus. Pregnant or breastfeeding individuals should consult with their herbalist/practitioner to determine safe levels of iodine intake and to ensure the overall safety of consuming dulse during these periods. It is also crucial to source dulse from the Atlantic Ocean to avoid higher levels of contamination from pollutants in the Pacific Ocean.

ECHINACEA ANGUSTIFOLIA LEAF

Echinacea angustifolia, commonly known as Narrow-Leaved Coneflower, is a flowering plant native to North America. It has a long-standing history of use in Native American traditional medicine, where it was revered for its medicinal properties. The plant is easily recognized by its vibrant purple flowers and slender, elongated leaves. Today, Echinacea angustifolia is widely cultivated and valued for its therapeutic benefits. The plant's active compounds, including polysaccharides, flavonoids, and alkamides, contribute to its potential health benefits.

Now, let's explore ten extensive health and longevity benefits associated with Echinacea angustifolia leaf:

1. **Immune System Support:** Echinacea angustifolia leaf contains bioactive compounds, such as polysaccharides, flavonoids, and alkamides, that have been shown to have immunomodulatory effects. These compounds help activate and enhance various components of the immune system, including immune cells and signaling molecules. By stimulating immune responses, Echinacea angustifolia leaf may help the body defend against pathogens and infections.
2. **Seasonal Sickness and Flu Support:** Polysaccharides and alkamides found in Echinacea angustifolia have been studied for their potential effects on the respiratory system. These compounds are believed to reduce inflammation and support the body's natural defense mechanisms in the respiratory tract.
3. **Respiratory Health:** This herb may support respiratory health by promoting clearer airways, reducing inflammation, and assisting with respiratory conditions like bronchitis and sinusitis.
4. **Anti-inflammatory Effects:** Echinacea angustifolia leaf contains active compounds that have been found to possess anti-inflammatory properties. These compounds, including flavonoids, alkamides, and polysaccharides, may help modulate the body's inflammatory response.
5. **Urinary Tract Health:** Echinacea angustifolia leaf is believed to have diuretic properties, supporting the health of the urinary tract and potentially aiding in the treatment of urinary tract infections.
6. **Histamine Regulation:** Histamine is a key player in allergic reactions, and its release leads to various symptoms. Echinacea angustifolia leaf may help regulate histamine release and prevent an excessive histamine response, thereby reducing allergy symptoms.

7. **Modulation of Neurotransmitters:** Echinacea angustifolia leaf may influence the levels and activity of certain neurotransmitters in the brain, such as serotonin and gamma-aminobutyric acid (GABA). These neurotransmitters play a role in regulating mood, anxiety, and stress responses. By modulating their activity, Echinacea angustifolia may help promote a sense of calm and relaxation.
8. **Antiviral Effects:** Echinacea angustifolia leaf possesses potent antiviral effects attributed to key compounds such as polyphenols (flavonoids, phenolic acids), alkamides, and polysaccharides. These constituents demonstrate antioxidant activity and may directly interfere with viral replication, while also supporting immune responses.
9. **Antioxidant Powerhouse:** The antioxidants present in this herb, including flavonoids, phenolic acids, and polysaccharides, play a crucial role in neutralizing harmful free radicals. These unstable molecules can damage cells and contribute to the development of chronic diseases. By scavenging free radicals, the antioxidants in Echinacea angustifolia leaf help mitigate oxidative stress, promoting overall cellular health.
10. **Wound Healing:** Some studies suggest that Echinacea angustifolia leaf may have wound-healing properties. Its bioactive compounds, including polysaccharides, can promote the formation of new tissue and enhance the skin's natural healing processes. This may be beneficial for minor cuts, abrasions, or skin injuries.

While Echinacea angustifolia leaf is generally considered safe to consume, there are certain medical contradictions and precautions to be aware of. Echinacea angustifolia leaf may interact with immunosuppressant medications, such as corticosteroids or medications used after organ transplantation, as it can potentially interfere with their effectiveness. Additionally, Echinacea angustifolia leaf may interact with medications metabolized by the liver, such as certain antiviral, antifungal, or statin medications. Individuals with allergies to plants in the Asteraceae/Compositae family, including ragweed, chrysanthemums, marigolds, and daisies, may also be allergic to Echinacea angustifolia leaf and should avoid its consumption. It is important to note that the use of Echinacea angustifolia during pregnancy or lactation should be done under the guidance of your herbalist/practitioner.

ECHINACEA ANGUSTIFOLIA ROOT

Echinacea angustifolia root, derived from the Echinacea angustifolia plant, is a revered herbal remedy with a rich history deeply rooted in North American traditional medicine. Native American tribes have long recognized the potent medicinal properties of this perennial herb and have utilized Echinacea angustifolia root for its remarkable immune-boosting and healing abilities. The plant's roots have been treasured for generations as a natural remedy to support overall wellness and promote the body's innate defense mechanisms. Today, Echinacea angustifolia root continues to be valued for its historical significance and profound health benefits, making it a sought-after herbal remedy worldwide.

Now, let's explore ten extensive health and longevity benefits associated with Echinacea angustifolia root:

1. **Immune System Support:** Echinacea angustifolia root is renowned for its ability to strengthen the immune system, promoting the body's defense mechanisms against infections and diseases.
2. **Seasonal Sickness and Flu Support:** Using Echinacea angustifolia root during acute sickness and flu can potentially aid in reducing the severity and duration of symptoms, supporting a faster recovery. The active compounds present in Echinacea angustifolia root, such as alkamides and polysaccharides, have been associated with immune-enhancing properties. These compounds may help stimulate the immune system's response, increasing the activity of immune cells and promoting a more efficient defense against seasonal sickness and flu viruses.
3. **Respiratory Health:** The root has been traditionally used to alleviate respiratory conditions, including bronchitis, sinusitis, and allergies, by reducing inflammation and supporting healthy lung function.
4. **Anti-inflammatory Effects:** Echinacea angustifolia root contains compounds with anti-inflammatory properties, potentially reducing inflammation throughout the body and relieving associated symptoms.
5. **Wound Healing:** The root's antimicrobial and immune-enhancing properties may contribute to faster wound healing and tissue regeneration when applied topically or ingested.
6. **Antimicrobial Effects:** Echinacea angustifolia root exhibits antibacterial and antiviral activities, which may help combat various pathogens and support overall health.

7. **Pain Relief:** The analgesic properties of Echinacea angustifolia root are attributed to its various bioactive compounds, including alkamides and polysaccharides. Alkamides are known for their pain-relieving effects and have been found to interact with cannabinoid receptors in the body, which are involved in pain modulation. These compounds may help reduce pain sensations and provide relief from headaches, toothaches, and sore throats.
8. **Skin Health:** Echinacea angustifolia root contains anti-inflammatory compounds that may help reduce inflammation on the skin, leading to a calmer complexion and potentially alleviating symptoms associated with skin conditions.
9. **Digestive Health:** This root contains compounds that have been traditionally believed to stimulate digestion and enhance the production of digestive enzymes, facilitating the breakdown and absorption of nutrients. This may help alleviate gastrointestinal discomfort and promote more efficient digestion.
10. **Graceful-aging Effects:** Echinacea angustifolia root contains antioxidant compounds, such as flavonoids and phenolic acids, which have the potential to neutralize harmful free radicals in the body. Free radicals are unstable molecules that can cause oxidative damage to cells, leading to accelerated aging and an increased risk of chronic diseases.

While Echinacea angustifolia root is generally considered safe to consume, there are certain medical contradictions and precautions to consider. Echinacea angustifolia root may interact with certain medications, including immunosuppressants and medications metabolized by the liver. Individuals with known allergies to plants in the Asteraceae family, which includes ragweed, daisies, and marigolds, may be at an increased risk of developing allergic reactions to Echinacea angustifolia root. It is important to note that the use of Echinacea angustifolia root during pregnancy or lactation should be done under the guidance of your herbalist/practitioner.

ECHINACEA PURPUREA LEAF

Echinacea purpurea, scientifically known as purple coneflower, is a modest yet captivating plant native to North America. With its charming purple petals and distinctive cone-shaped center, it has found a special place in gardens for its simple, natural beauty. But beyond its looks, Echinacea purpurea leaf has a history rooted in practicality and tradition, especially among Native American tribes. Over time, it has quietly earned recognition for its potential health benefits, embodying a connection between nature and well-being. In exploring Echinacea purpurea leaf, we uncover not just its floral charm but also its down-to-earth contributions to herbal remedies and holistic health.

Now, let's explore ten extensive health and longevity benefits associated with Echinacea purpurea leaf:

1. **Immune System Support:** Echinacea purpurea leaf supports the immune system through several mechanisms. It contains bioactive compounds, such as polysaccharides, alkamides, and caffeic acid derivatives, which are believed to stimulate immune cells and enhance their activity. These compounds may help increase the production of immune cells, such as white blood cells, and enhance their ability to recognize and eliminate pathogens. Echinacea purpurea leaf's immune-boosting effects may also involve its ability to modulate cytokine production, which plays a crucial role in immune responses.
2. **Seasonal Sickness and Flu Support:** Echinacea purpurea leaf may aid in reducing the duration and severity of cold and flu symptoms, thereby promoting a faster recovery. Its active compounds, such as polysaccharides and alkamides, are believed to have immune-modulating and antiviral properties, which may help support the body's natural defenses against viral infections.
3. **Anti-inflammatory Effects:** Echinacea purpurea leaf exhibits anti-inflammatory effects due to the presence of various bioactive compounds, including alkamides, polysaccharides, and flavonoids. These compounds have been shown to modulate the production of inflammatory mediators, such as cytokines and prostaglandins, which are involved in the inflammatory response. By inhibiting the release of these inflammatory molecules, Echinacea purpurea leaf may help reduce inflammation and alleviate associated symptoms, such as pain, swelling, and redness.

4. **Respiratory Health:** This herb has been traditionally used to alleviate respiratory conditions such as bronchitis, sinusitis, and asthma, promoting clear airways and improved lung function.
5. **Antioxidant Powerhouse:** This leaf is rich in antioxidants, which help neutralize harmful free radicals, safeguarding cells from oxidative damage and supporting overall well-being.
6. **Wound Healing:** Echinacea purpurea leaf can be used both topically and internally to support wound healing. When applied topically, the herb's antimicrobial properties help inhibit the growth of bacteria and other microorganisms that can lead to infection. By preventing infection, Echinacea purpurea leaf creates a favorable environment for the healing process to occur. Additionally, the herb's bioactive compounds, such as alkamides and polysaccharides, may promote faster tissue regeneration and wound closure. When taken internally, Echinacea purpurea leaf supports the immune system, which plays a crucial role in wound healing.
7. **Digestive Health:** Echinacea purpurea leaf may have beneficial effects on the digestive system, promoting healthy digestion, alleviating gastrointestinal discomfort, and supporting overall gut health.
8. **Skin Health:** Echinacea purpurea leaf's anti-inflammatory and antioxidant properties contribute to healthy skin by reducing inflammation, supporting collagen production, and protecting against environmental damage.
9. **Stress Relief:** This herb may help alleviate stress and anxiety, promoting relaxation and mental well-being. Echinacea purpurea leaf's potential effects on stress relief may be attributed to its ability to modulate the hypothalamic-pituitary-adrenal (HPA) axis, which regulates the body's stress response.
10. **Allergy Relief:** Echinacea purpurea leaf may assist in reducing the severity of allergic reactions by modulating the immune response and mitigating symptoms like nasal congestion and itching.

While Echinacea purpurea leaf is generally considered safe to consume, there are certain medical contradictions and precautions to be aware of. This herb may interact with certain medications, including immunosuppressants and drugs metabolized by the liver. If you are taking any medications, it is essential to consult with your healthcare provider to ensure there are no potential interactions. Individuals with known allergies to plants in the Asteraceae family, such as ragweed, chrysanthemums, or marigolds, may also have an allergic reaction to Echinacea purpurea leaf. It is important to note that the use of Echinacea purpurea leaf during pregnancy or lactation should be done under the guidance of your herbalist/practitioner.

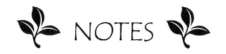

NOTES

ECHINACEA PURPUREA ROOT

Echinacea purpurea root, derived from the Echinacea purpurea plant, has deep roots in the traditions of North American indigenous communities, especially the Plains Indians. Considered sacred by shamans, the root played a vital role in their medicinal practices. Early practitioners viewed this root as a powerful ally for enhanced immune function and overall well-being. Its significance lies not just in its botanical properties but in the profound connection it symbolized between ancient communities and the natural world.

Now, let's explore ten extensive health and longevity benefits associated with Echinacea purpurea root:

1. **Immune System Support:** The roots of Echinacea purpurea contain bioactive compounds, including polysaccharides, alkamides, and caffeic acid derivatives, which are thought to contribute to its medicinal properties. These compounds are believed to stimulate immune cells, enhance their activity, and modulate cytokine production, thereby supporting a robust immune response.
2. **Seasonal Sickness and Flu Support:** Usage of Echinacea purpurea root during acute illness may assist in reducing the duration and severity of symptoms, supporting a faster recovery.
3. **Respiratory Health:** The root has been traditionally used to alleviate respiratory conditions such as bronchitis, sinusitis, and allergies, promoting clear airways and respiratory well-being.
4. **Anti-inflammatory Effects:** Echinacea purpurea root contains compounds with anti-inflammatory properties, potentially reducing inflammation throughout the body and alleviating associated symptoms.
5. **Antiviral Effects:** It is believed that the bioactive compounds present in the root, such as polysaccharides, alkamides, and flavonoids, may contribute to its antiviral effects. These compounds have shown activity against certain viruses in laboratory studies, including influenza viruses and herpes simplex viruses.
6. **Skin Health:** The potential benefits of Echinacea purpurea root for skin health can be attributed to its anti-inflammatory and antimicrobial properties. When used topically, Echinacea purpurea root may help promote healthy skin by reducing inflammation, which can contribute to conditions like acne. Its antimicrobial properties may also help inhibit the growth of certain bacteria that can contribute to skin irritations and infections.

7. **Allergy Relief:** The potential allergy-relieving effects of Echinacea purpurea root are thought to be attributed to its ability to modulate the immune response. When exposed to allergens, the immune system can overreact and trigger the release of inflammatory substances, leading to symptoms like sneezing, itching, and nasal congestion. Echinacea purpurea root contains bioactive compounds, including polysaccharides and flavonoids, which are believed to regulate immune function and reduce the release of these inflammatory substances.
8. **Antioxidant Powerhouse:** This root is rich in antioxidants, which help neutralize harmful free radicals, protecting cells from oxidative stress and supporting overall health.
9. **Wound Healing:** Echinacea purpurea root may aid in wound healing due to its antimicrobial properties, helping to prevent infection and promote faster tissue regeneration.
10. **Digestive Health:** The potential beneficial effects of Echinacea purpurea root on the digestive system are attributed to its various bioactive compounds, such as polysaccharides and phenolic compounds. These compounds have been studied for their anti-inflammatory and antioxidant properties, which may help reduce inflammation in the gastrointestinal tract and protect against oxidative damage. Echinacea purpurea root may also support healthy digestion by stimulating the production of digestive enzymes and enhancing nutrient absorption.

> While Echinacea purpurea root is generally considered safe to consume, there are a few warnings and contradictions to be aware of. It is important to note that this herb may interact with certain medications, such as immunosuppressants and medications metabolized by the liver. Individuals with allergies to plants in the Asteraceae family, such as ragweed, chrysanthemums, or marigolds, may also have an allergic reaction to Echinacea purpurea root. It is important to note that the use of Echinacea purpurea root during pregnancy or lactation should be done under the guidance of your herbalist/practitioner.

ELDERFLOWER

Elderflower, scientifically known as Sambucus nigra, have an enduring connection to European heritage, being historically intertwined with various cultural and folkloric practices. In traditional European herbalism, elderflowers were highly valued for their potential health-promoting properties. Beyond medicinal uses, elderflowers have found a place in culinary traditions, contributing to the creation of elderflower cordials and teas that enhance the flavor and aroma of beverages and dishes. The act of harvesting elderflowers during the summer has transformed into a ritual, symbolizing a profound connection to nature's bounty and serving as a continuation of age-old practices passed down through generations.
Now, let's explore ten extensive health and longevity benefits associated with elderflower:

1. **Immune System Support:** Elderflowers contain various bioactive compounds, including flavonoids and antioxidants, which contribute to their immune-boosting properties. These compounds help stimulate the production and activity of immune cells, such as white blood cells, which play a crucial role in fighting off pathogens and maintaining overall immune health.
2. **Respiratory Health:** The flowers have been traditionally used to relieve respiratory conditions such as coughs and congestion, promoting clear airways and easier breathing.
3. **Anti-inflammatory Effects:** The anti-inflammatory effects of elderflowers can be attributed to their bioactive compounds, including flavonoids and phenolic acids. These compounds have been found to possess anti-inflammatory properties in various studies. They work by inhibiting the activity of inflammatory enzymes and reducing the production of inflammatory molecules in the body, such as cytokines and prostaglandins.
4. **Antioxidant Powerhouse:** The flowers are rich in antioxidants, which help protect cells from oxidative damage caused by free radicals and promote overall health.
5. **Diuretic Effects:** Elderflowers possess diuretic properties, aiding in the elimination of excess water and toxins from the body, supporting kidney function and maintaining fluid balance.
6. **Sleep Support:** The relaxation and sleep-inducing effects of elderflowers are attributed to their natural compounds, including flavonoids and essential oils. These compounds have been found to have sedative and calming properties, which may help reduce anxiety, promote relaxation, and support restful sleep.

7. **Digestive Health:** Elderflowers contain bioactive compounds with antimicrobial properties, including flavonoids and tannins, which may help inhibit the growth of certain pathogenic bacteria in the digestive system. By promoting a healthy balance of gut bacteria and reducing harmful bacteria, elderflowers can contribute to improved digestion and alleviate symptoms such as bloating and indigestion. Additionally, elderflowers have mild laxative effects, which may help regulate bowel movements and promote healthy digestion.
8. **Skin Health:** The flowers' anti-inflammatory and antioxidant properties make them beneficial for promoting healthy skin, reducing inflammation, and soothing skin irritations.
9. **Fever Reduction:** The flowers contain bioactive compounds, including flavonoids and phenolic acids, which are believed to possess antipyretic properties. These compounds may help lower body temperature and provide relief from feverish conditions. Additionally, elderflowers have diaphoretic properties, meaning they can promote sweating, which aids in cooling the body and supporting the body's natural fever response.
10. **Cardiovascular Health:** Elderflowers may help support cardiovascular health by promoting healthy blood circulation and maintaining optimal blood pressure levels.

> While elderflowers are generally considered safe to consume, it is important to be aware of certain medical contradictions and precautions. Individuals with diabetes or those taking medications to lower blood sugar levels should exercise caution when using elderflowers, as they may have a hypoglycemic effect and interact with diabetes medications. Elderflowers may also interact with diuretic medications, as they possess diuretic properties themselves. Individuals with known allergies to plants in the Adoxaceae family, such as elderberries or viburnum, may be at a higher risk of allergic reactions to elderflowers. Pregnant or breastfeeding individuals should consult with their herbalist/practitioner before using elderflowers to ensure their safety during these periods.

ELDERBERRIES

Elderberries, the dark purple berries of the Elder plant (Sambucus nigra), have a long history of medicinal use and are revered for their powerful health benefits. The Elder plant is native to Europe but can also be found in other regions across the globe. The small, juicy berries are rich in nutrients and have been utilized for centuries in traditional medicine.

Now, let's explore ten extensive health and longevity benefits associated with elderberries:

1. **Immune System Support:** Elderberries offer immune system support through their rich antioxidant and vitamin content. Elderberries are particularly high in vitamin C, which is known for its role in supporting immune function.
2. **Seasonal Sickness and Flu Support:** The potential flu-relieving effects of elderberries are attributed to their bioactive compounds, including flavonoids and anthocyanins. These compounds have been shown to have antiviral properties and may inhibit the replication of certain strains of the influenza virus. Additionally, elderberries have immune-modulating effects, which may help strengthen the immune system's response to viral infections.
3. **Antiviral Effects:** Elderberries possess antiviral properties that can inhibit the replication of certain viruses, potentially offering protection against common viral infections.
4. **Antioxidant Powerhouse:** Elderberries are rich in antioxidants, including flavonoids such as anthocyanins, quercetin, and rutin, as well as vitamin C and vitamin E. These antioxidants play a crucial role in neutralizing harmful free radicals in the body, which are unstable molecules that can cause cellular damage and contribute to various health issues.
5. **Anti-inflammatory Effects:** The anti-inflammatory effects of elderberries are attributed to their rich content of bioactive compounds, such as flavonoids and anthocyanins. These compounds have been shown to inhibit the production of inflammatory molecules and enzymes in the body, thereby reducing inflammation and its associated symptoms. By modulating the activity of inflammatory pathways, elderberries may help alleviate conditions characterized by chronic inflammation, such as arthritis, joint pain, and inflammatory bowel diseases.

6. **Cardiovascular Health:** The flavonoids present in elderberries contribute to heart health by reducing the risk of cardiovascular diseases, improving blood circulation, and lowering cholesterol levels.
7. **Digestive Health:** Elderberries contain bioactive compounds, such as flavonoids and anthocyanins, which contribute to their digestive health benefits. These compounds have been found to possess anti-inflammatory properties, helping to reduce inflammation in the digestive system and alleviate digestive discomfort.
8. **Skin Health:** Elderberries' high antioxidant content promotes healthy skin by combating free radicals, reducing signs of aging, and improving skin tone and texture.
9. **Cognitive Support:** The anthocyanins in elderberries may support brain health, potentially improving cognitive function and protecting against age-related cognitive decline.
10. **Respiratory Health:** Elderberries have been traditionally used to ease respiratory conditions such as asthma and bronchitis, providing relief from coughing and congestion.

> While elderberries are generally considered safe to consume, there are a few medical contradictions and precautions to be aware of. Elderberries may interact with certain medications, including immunosuppressants and diabetes medications, so it is important to consult with a healthcare professional. Those with known allergies to plants in the Adoxaceae family, such as elderflowers or viburnum, may also be allergic to elderberries and should avoid their consumption. It is advisable for pregnant or breastfeeding individuals to consult with their herbalist/practitioner before consuming elderberry products to ensure safety during these periods. It is also crucial to note that raw or unripe elderberries contain cyanogenic glycosides, which can release cyanide when ingested. Therefore, it is important to ensure that elderberries are fully ripe and properly prepared before consumption.

ELECAMPANE ROOT

Elecampane root, derived from the Inula helenium plant, is well-known for its medicinal properties, particularly in supporting respiratory health. This perennial herb, native to Europe and certain parts of Asia, has a rich history dating back to ancient times. It is characterized by its tall stalks, vibrant yellow flowers, and aromatic roots. Elecampane root has been used for centuries in traditional herbal medicine, primarily for addressing respiratory conditions such as coughs, bronchitis, and asthma.

Now, let's explore ten extensive health and longevity benefits associated with elecampane root:

1. **Respiratory Health:** Elecampane root is highly valued for its beneficial effects on the respiratory system. It contains bioactive compounds, such as inulin, alantolactone, and helenalin, which have expectorant, antitussive, and bronchodilatory properties. These compounds work together to help soothe coughs, relieve bronchial congestion, and promote clear airways. Elecampane root is often used as an herbal remedy for respiratory conditions like asthma, bronchitis, and allergies, providing relief and supporting overall lung health. It may help loosen and expel mucus, and alleviate symptoms associated with respiratory inflammation.
2. **Expectorant Effects:** The root acts as an expectorant, helping to loosen and expel mucus from the lungs, thereby relieving chest congestion and facilitating easier breathing.
3. **Anti-inflammatory Effects:** Leveraging its rich reservoir of bioactive compounds, elecampane root employs alantolactone and helenalin to skillfully inhibit inflammatory pathways within the body. This strategic approach entails a reduction in the production of pro-inflammatory molecules and the adept modulation of immune responses. With a targeted focus on suppressing excessive inflammation, elecampane root aims to alleviate symptoms commonly associated with inflammatory conditions, including but not limited to arthritis, asthma, and digestive disorders.
4. **Detoxification:** Elecampane root supports liver health and aids in detoxification processes, assisting the body in eliminating toxins and promoting overall well-being.
5. **Skin Health:** Elecampane root may be used topically to help soothe skin irritations such as rashes, eczema, or insect bites. Its anti-inflammatory properties may help reduce redness, swelling, and itching.

6. **Immune System Support:** Elecampane root contains bioactive compounds that have been shown to support immune function, helping to strengthen the body's natural defense mechanisms and protect against infections. These compounds, including inulin, alantolactone, and helenalin, have immunomodulatory effects, meaning they can regulate and enhance immune responses.
7. **Antimicrobial Effects:** Elecampane root exhibits antimicrobial properties due to the presence of bioactive compounds such as sesquiterpene lactones, polyacetylenes, and essential oils. These compounds have been shown to have inhibitory effects against various bacteria and fungi, including common pathogens. Elecampane root's antimicrobial activity helps to inhibit the growth and proliferation of these microorganisms, potentially reducing the risk of infections and supporting the body's natural defense mechanisms.
8. **Digestive Health:** The volatile oils found in elecampane root possess carminative properties, helping to reduce gas and bloating. Overall, elecampane root promotes healthy digestion and supports overall gastrointestinal well-being.
9. **Antioxidant Powerhouse:** Some sesquiterpene lactones exhibit antioxidant properties, helping to neutralize free radicals in the body. This antioxidant activity contributes to cellular health and may play a role in reducing oxidative stress.
10. **Wound Healing:** The antimicrobial properties of elecampane root can make it useful for promoting wound healing. It may help prevent infection and support the natural healing process of minor cuts, scrapes, or burns.

> While elecampane root is generally considered safe to consume, there are certain medical contradictions and precautions to be aware of. Elecampane root may interact with certain medications, including anticoagulants (blood thinners), antidiabetic medications, and immunosuppressants. It is important to consult with a healthcare professional before using elecampane root if you have any of these conditions or are taking any medications. Individuals with known allergies to plants in the Asteraceae/Compositae family, such as ragweed, daisies, or marigolds, may also be allergic to elecampane root and should exercise caution. Those who are pregnant or lactating should consult with their herbalist/practitioner prior to using this root.

ELEUTHERO (SIBERIAN GINSENG)

Eleuthero, scientifically known as Eleutherococcus senticosus, is a remarkable herb commonly referred to as Siberian ginseng. It has a rich history of use in traditional medicine and holds significant value for its potential health benefits. Eleuthero is native to the wild forests of northeastern Asia, specifically regions such as Siberia, China, and Korea. Throughout centuries, it has been treasured and incorporated into various herbal remedies due to its reputed medicinal properties.

Now, let's explore ten extensive health and longevity benefits associated with eleuthero:

1. **Adaptogenic Support:** Eleuthero is well-known for its adaptogenic properties. This remarkable herb contains active compounds, such as eleutherosides and polysaccharides, which support its adaptogenic effects. These compounds are believed to help the body adapt to stress, promote resilience, and restore balance.
2. **Energy Boost:** Eleuthero is often used to enhance physical and mental performance, increase energy levels, and combat fatigue and exhaustion.
3. **Immune System Support:** The herb has immune-boosting effects, supporting the body's natural defense mechanisms and helping to ward off infections and diseases.
4. **Stress Relief:** Eleuthero contains a group of bioactive compounds known as eleutherosides, which are responsible for its adaptogenic properties. These eleutherosides play a crucial role in supporting the body's stress response system and promoting resilience. By interacting with the body's stress pathways, eleutherosides help the body adapt to various stressors, restore balance, and enhance overall well-being.
5. **Cognitive Support:** Eleuthero contains various bioactive compounds, including eleutherosides, polysaccharides, and lignans, which are believed to have neuroprotective and cognition-enhancing properties. These compounds may interact with neurotransmitters and receptors in the brain, potentially influencing cognitive processes.
6. **Adrenal Support:** Eleutherosides, specifically eleutheroside B and eleutheroside E, are considered key active compounds in eleuthero. These compounds are believed to support adrenal gland function and help regulate the body's stress response, which can result in increased energy levels and improved stamina.

7. **Athletic Performance Enhancement:** One of the key factors contributing to these effects is the presence of eleutherosides, including eleutheroside B and eleutheroside E. These compounds have been associated with increased oxygen utilization, improved energy metabolism, and reduced fatigue. By supporting efficient energy production and utilization within cells, eleuthero may enhance endurance and delay the onset of fatigue during physical activity.
8. **Anti-inflammatory Effects:** The herb exhibits anti-inflammatory properties, which may help reduce inflammation in the body and alleviate symptoms associated with inflammatory conditions.
9. **Antioxidant Powerhouse:** Eleuthero is rich in antioxidants that help neutralize free radicals, reducing oxidative stress and protecting against cellular damage.
10. **Hormonal Balance:** Eleuthero contains various bioactive compounds, including eleutherosides, polysaccharides, and lignans, which are believed to interact with the endocrine system and help regulate hormone levels. These compounds may support the hypothalamic-pituitary-adrenal (HPA) axis, a complex system involved in hormone regulation and stress response.

While eleuthero is generally considered safe to consume, there are certain medical contradictions and precautions. Eleuthero may interact with certain medications, including anticoagulants (blood thinners), immunosuppressants, and antidiabetic medications. It is important to consult with a healthcare professional before using eleuthero if you are taking any medications. Additionally, eleuthero may have stimulant effects, and individuals with conditions such as hypertension or anxiety should use it with caution. Individuals with known allergies to plants in the Araliaceae family, such as ginseng or ivy, may also be allergic to eleuthero and should exercise caution. It is generally recommended to avoid using eleuthero during pregnancy and lactation due to potential effects on hormone levels unless otherwise directed by your herbalist/practitioner.

ESSIAC TEA BLEND

Essiac tea is an herbal infusion that has gained popularity for its potential health benefits and holistic healing properties. Its origin can be traced back to a Canadian Ojibwa healer named Rene Caisse in the early 1920s. Essiac tea is a blend of several herbs, including burdock root (Arctium lappa), sheep sorrel (Rumex acetosella), slippery elm bark (Ulmus rubra), Indian rhubarb root (Rheum officinale), which are carefully selected and combined to create a powerful herbal remedy. This unique blend has been used by many individuals seeking alternative approaches to wellness.

Now, let's explore ten extensive health and longevity benefits associated with Essiac tea:

1. **Immune System Support:** Burdock root contains compounds like arctigenin and inulin that have been studied for potential immune-modulating properties. Sheep sorrel contains antioxidants like quercetin and anthraquinones, which have been studied for their immunomodulatory properties. The mucilage in slippery elm bark may help improve the absorption of nutrients in the digestive tract. Proper nutrient absorption is essential for maintaining a strong immune system. Indian rhubarb root contains anthraquinones and tannins, which are believed to possess antimicrobial properties. These compounds may help inhibit the growth of certain bacteria, fungi, or other microorganisms.
2. **Anti-cancer Effects:** Essiac tea is an herbal remedy that has been traditionally used a complementary or alternative therapy for individuals with cancer. The specific mechanisms by which Essiac tea may support those with cancer are not well understood by the scientific community (because studies on this herbal blend are far and few between by design). It should be noted, as anecdotal information, users of Essiac tea have claimed benefits such as tumor reduction, relief from cancer-related symptoms, and immune support.
3. **Skin Health:** Essiac tea has been associated with potential benefits for skin health. The antioxidant and anti-inflammatory properties of the herbs in this blend may help promote a healthy complexion and soothe certain skin conditions.
4. **Urinary Tract Health:** Some traditional uses of Essiac tea include supporting urinary tract health. The herbal blend is believed to help maintain urinary system function and alleviate certain urinary discomforts.

5. **Anti-inflammatory Effects:** Essiac tea possesses anti-inflammatory properties, which may help reduce inflammation in the body and alleviate symptoms associated with inflammatory conditions.
6. **Digestive Health:** The herbal blend in Essiac tea may help promote healthy digestion, soothe gastrointestinal discomfort, and support overall digestive well-being.
7. **Antioxidant Powerhouse:** Essiac tea is believed to have antioxidant properties, protecting cells from oxidative damage caused by free radicals and promoting cellular health.
8. **Liver Health:** The herbs in Essiac tea have been traditionally used to support liver health, promoting liver function and aiding in the detoxification process.
9. **Stress Relief:** Essiac tea is known for its calming and relaxing effects, helping to alleviate stress and anxiety and promote a sense of well-being.
10. **Detoxification:** The blend of herbs in Essiac tea has been traditionally used to support detoxification processes, aiding in the elimination of toxins and waste from the body.

> While Essiac tea is generally considered safe to consume, there are certain medical contradictions and precautions to be aware of. Essiac tea may interact with certain medications, including blood thinners, immunosuppressants, and chemotherapy drugs. Consult with a healthcare provider if you have any of these conditions prior to using Essiac tea. Allergy warnings apply to individuals with known allergies to any of the ingredients in Essiac tea, such as burdock root or rhubarb. Additionally, since Essiac tea contains herbs from the same family as ragweed, individuals with ragweed allergies should exercise caution. It is advisable to consult with your herbalist/practitioner before using Essiac tea during pregnancy or lactation.

EUCALYPTUS LEAF

Eucalyptus leaf, derived from the tall and aromatic eucalyptus trees native to Australia, holds a rich history of traditional use and therapeutic properties. These evergreen trees, belonging to the Myrtaceae family, are renowned for their distinctive fragrance and unique healing abilities. Eucalyptus leaf has been used for centuries by indigenous Australians for its numerous health benefits. The leaves of the eucalyptus tree are steam-distilled to extract the essential oil, which is widely utilized in various medicinal and wellness applications.

Now, let's explore ten extensive health and longevity benefits associated with eucalyptus leaf:

1. **Respiratory Health:** The compounds responsible for the respiratory health benefits of eucalyptus leaf are primarily the essential oils it contains, with the key compound being eucalyptol (also known as cineole). Eucalyptol is known for its expectorant and bronchodilator properties. In addition to eucalyptol, eucalyptus leaf also contains other compounds such as pinene, limonene, and alpha-terpineol, which contribute to its respiratory benefits. These compounds may have antimicrobial and anti-inflammatory properties that can further support respiratory health by reducing inflammation and combating respiratory infections.
2. **Sinus Relief:** Inhalation of eucalyptus leaf essential oil may help alleviate sinus congestion and promote sinus drainage, providing relief from sinus-related discomfort.
3. **Immune System Support:** The antimicrobial properties of eucalyptus leaf make it beneficial for supporting immune system function and helping the body fight against infections.
4. **Skin Health:** Eucalyptus leaf is commonly used in skincare products due to its cleansing and purifying properties, helping to promote clear and healthy skin.
5. **Cognitive Support:** The invigorating aroma of eucalyptus leaf essential oil may help improve focus and mental clarity and enhance overall cognitive function.
6. **Stress Relief:** Eucalyptus leaf is known for its relaxing and soothing effects, which may help reduce stress and anxiety and promote a sense of calm.
7. **Oral Health:** The antimicrobial properties of eucalyptus leaf make it beneficial for maintaining oral hygiene and supporting gum health.

8. **Pain Relief:** Eucalyptol/cineole has been found to possess anti-inflammatory and analgesic properties. It may help reduce inflammation and pain by inhibiting certain enzymes and signaling pathways involved in the inflammatory response. By doing so, eucalyptol/cineole may help alleviate muscle and joint pain, as well as headaches.
9. **Anti-inflammatory Effects:** Eucalyptus leaf possesses anti-inflammatory properties such as eucalyptol/cineole that may help reduce inflammation in the body and alleviate symptoms associated with inflammatory conditions.
10. **Insect Repellent:** Eucalyptus leaf essential oil acts as a natural insect repellent, helping to ward off mosquitoes, ticks, and other pesky insects.

While eucalyptus leaf is generally considered safe to consume, there are some medical contradictions and precautions to be aware of. Eucalyptus leaf can potentially interact with certain medications, including anticoagulants and anticonvulsants, altering their effectiveness or increasing the risk of side effects. Allergy warnings apply to individuals with known allergies to eucalyptus or related plants, such as guava, myrtle, or tea tree. These plants belong to the same family, Myrtaceae. It is also important to note that high doses of eucalyptus leaf products should not be consumed. While eucalyptus leaf is generally safe for topical and inhalation use, ingesting eucalyptus essential oil or applying it directly to the skin should be avoided. Those who are pregnant or breastfeeding should consult with their herbalist/practitioner before using eucalyptus leaf products.

EYEBRIGHT

Eyebright, scientifically known as Euphrasia officinalis, is a small flowering herb that holds a long history of traditional use and medicinal significance. Native to Europe, eyebright has been used for centuries in herbal remedies and natural healing practices. Its name originates from its traditional use in promoting eye health and treating various eye-related conditions. Eyebright's delicate white and yellow flowers, resembling a human eye, have contributed to its reputation as an "eye herb." Apart from its association with ocular health, eyebright possesses numerous health benefits that extend beyond vision care.

Now, let's explore ten extensive health and longevity benefits associated with eyebright:

1. **Eye Health:** Eyebright contains compounds such as aucubin and tannins, which are believed to reduce eye inflammation, soothe eye irritation, and alleviate symptoms of conjunctivitis and dry eyes.
2. **Allergy Relief:** The anti-inflammatory and antihistamine properties of eyebright can be attributed to compounds like flavonoids and iridoid glycosides. These compounds may help relieve symptoms of allergies, including itchy and watery eyes, sneezing, and nasal congestion.
3. **Respiratory Health:** Eyebright has been traditionally used to promote respiratory wellness due to its content of mucilage, tannins, and volatile oils. These components are thought to provide relief from respiratory conditions such as sinusitis, bronchitis, and hay fever.
4. **Anti-inflammatory Effects:** Eyebright contains various compounds, including flavonoids and phenolic acids, which possess anti-inflammatory properties. These compounds may help reduce inflammation throughout the body and alleviate associated symptoms.
5. **Skin Health:** The astringent properties of eyebright are due to its tannin content. Tannins help tighten pores, reduce excess oil, and soothe skin irritation, making eyebright beneficial for maintaining healthy skin.
6. **Headache Relief:** In the context of headaches, the astringent properties of tannins found in eyebright may play a role in constricting blood vessels in the head, potentially reducing blood flow and providing relief from pain.

7. **Digestive Health:** Eyebright's stimulation of digestion and reduction of bloating can be attributed to its content of bitter compounds, such as aucubin and iridoid glycosides. These compounds help support digestive health and relieve gastrointestinal discomfort.
8. **Immune System Support:** Eyebright contains antioxidants like flavonoids and phenolic acids, which are believed to enhance immune function and protect against common infections.
9. **Cognitive Support:** Phenolic acids are another group of compounds present in eyebright and other plants. Some studies suggest that phenolic acids can modulate neurotransmitter activity, improve synaptic plasticity (the ability of brain cells to form new connections), and enhance cognitive processes such as memory and learning.
10. **Antioxidant Powerhouse:** Flavonoids found in eyebright, such as quercetin and luteolin, have been shown to possess potent antioxidant properties, helping to neutralize free radicals and protect cells from oxidative damage. Phenolic acids, including caffeic acid and chlorogenic acid, are another class of antioxidants present in eyebright. These compounds are effective scavengers of free radicals, helping to prevent oxidative stress and maintain cellular health. Phenolic acids can also enhance the activity of other antioxidant enzymes within the body, further boosting the defense against oxidative damage.

While eyebright is generally considered safe to consume, there are certain medical contradictions and precautions to be aware of. Individuals taking medications for blood pressure or anticoagulants should consult with their healthcare provider before using eyebright, as it may interact with these medications and increase the risk of bleeding. Allergy warnings should be noted, as some individuals may have allergic reactions to eyebright, particularly those who are sensitive to plants in the Asteraceae/Compositae family, which includes plants such as ragweed, daisies, and chrysanthemums. Those who are pregnant or lactating should consult with their herbalist/practitioner prior to using eyebright.

FENNEL SEED

Fennel seed, derived from the aromatic flowering plant Foeniculum vulgare, have a rich history that dates back centuries, tracing its origins to the Mediterranean region. This versatile spice has been utilized for its medicinal and culinary properties since ancient times, earning a prominent place in traditional herbal medicine systems like Ayurveda and Traditional Chinese Medicine. Fennel seeds are small, oval-shaped, and possess a distinct licorice-like flavor, which lends a unique and pleasant taste to various culinary preparations. Beyond its culinary applications, fennel seeds offer a plethora of health and longevity benefits.

Now, let's explore ten extensive health and longevity benefits associated with fennel seed:

1. **Digestive Health:** Fennel seeds are renowned for their ability to promote healthy digestion. They possess carminative properties that can alleviate bloating, gas, and indigestion while also stimulating the production of digestive enzymes.
2. **Anti-inflammatory Effects:** Fennel seeds contain compounds with potent anti-inflammatory properties, such as anethole and flavonoids. Regular consumption may help reduce inflammation in the body, potentially benefiting conditions like arthritis and inflammatory bowel disease.
3. **Antioxidant Powerhouse:** Fennel seeds are packed with antioxidants like quercetin and kaempferol, which help protect the body against free radicals, thus reducing oxidative stress and combating cellular damage.
4. **Anti-flatulent Effects:** Anethole is a primary component of the essential oil found in fennel seeds. It possesses carminative properties, meaning it helps to reduce excess gas and alleviate discomfort associated with flatulence. The presence of anethole in fennel seeds helps relax the smooth muscles in the digestive tract, reducing spasms and allowing trapped gas to be released more easily, thereby providing relief from flatulence and related discomfort.
5. **Immune Boost Support:** Fennel seeds contain various phytonutrients that can support immune function. These include flavonoids, such as quercetin and kaempferol, which have antioxidant and anti-inflammatory properties. Flavonoids may help reduce inflammation, enhance immune response, and support the body's defense against pathogens.

6. **Cardiovascular Health:** The presence of potassium, quercetin, kaempferol, and phenolic compounds in fennel seeds can contribute to cardiovascular health. These seeds may help lower blood pressure, reduce cholesterol levels, and support overall heart health.
7. **Hormonal Balance:** Fennel seeds contain phytoestrogens, plant compounds that mimic the effects of estrogen in the body. These phytoestrogens, including anethole and dianethole, exhibit mild estrogenic activity. Interacting with estrogen receptors, they may assist in regulating hormone levels and supporting hormonal balance, particularly in women undergoing hormonal fluctuations during the menstrual cycle or menopause.
8. **Respiratory Health:** The expectorant properties of fennel seeds make them beneficial for respiratory health. They may help soothe coughs, clear congestion, and relieve symptoms of respiratory conditions like bronchitis and asthma.
9. **Oral Health:** Chewing fennel seeds after meals can freshen breath and promote oral health. The antimicrobial properties of fennel seeds may help combat bacteria in the mouth, reducing the risk of cavities and gum disease.
10. **Eye Health:** Fennel seeds contain essential nutrients like vitamin A, which plays a crucial role in maintaining good vision. Regular consumption may help protect against age-related macular degeneration and cataracts.

> While fennel seeds are generally considered safe to consume, there are a few important warnings and contradictions to consider. Individuals taking specific medications, such as anticoagulants (blood thinners), should exercise caution as fennel seeds may have mild anticoagulant effects. Additionally, those with estrogen-sensitive conditions, such as certain types of breast cancer, should avoid excessive consumption of fennel seeds due to their phytoestrogen content. It is always advisable to consult with a healthcare professional if you have any concerns or existing health conditions before incorporating fennel seeds into your diet. It is generally considered safe to consume fennel seeds in culinary amounts when pregnant or lactating. Consult with your herbalist/practitioner prior to using large quantities of fennel seeds therapeutically during these times.

FENUGREEK LEAF

Fenugreek, scientifically known as Trigonella foenum-graecum, and Blue fenugreek, botanically classified as Trigonella caerulea, are two distinct varieties of this versatile herb that hail from diverse corners of the world. Fenugreek, with its origins traced to the Mediterranean region and parts of Asia, has a long history of use in both culinary and traditional medicine practices. Its seeds and leaves have been cherished for centuries as a spice, a digestive aid, and for their potential health benefits, including supporting digestive health and regulating blood sugar levels. In contrast, Blue fenugreek, characterized by its striking blue-green foliage, finds its roots in regions like the Caucasus and parts of Eastern Europe. It holds a unique place in regional cuisines, particularly in Georgian dishes like khachapuri, where its milder flavor adds depth and character to culinary creations. Both standard fenugreek (Trigonella foenum-graecum) and Blue fenugreek (Trigonella caerulea) share some common health benefits due to their similar chemical compositions, including the presence of various phytonutrients and antioxidants. However, there may be subtle differences in health benefits based on their unique characteristics.

Now, let's explore ten extensive health and longevity benefits associated with fenugreek leaf, (blue and standard):

1. **Digestive Health:** Both varieties are known for their potential to support digestive health. They can help alleviate issues like indigestion and bloating. Blue fenugreek, with its milder flavor, may be easier on the stomach for some individuals.
2. **Bone Health:** Rich in calcium, magnesium, and phosphorus, essential minerals for strong bones, fenugreek leaf aids in maintaining bone density and strength. Its abundance of vitamin K contributes to bone mineralization, preventing osteoporosis and promoting bone health. The presence of flavonoids, such as quercetin and kaempferol, and saponins, such as diosgenin, provides antioxidant and anti-inflammatory properties, protecting bones from oxidative damage and inflammation. Fenugreek leaf also contains phytoestrogens like diosgenin and isoflavones, which may help promote bone formation and prevent bone loss in postmenopausal women.
3. **Lactation and Breast Health:** Standard fenugreek is often used to support lactation in breastfeeding mothers and may have a stronger reputation in this regard than Blue fenugreek.

4. **Detoxification:** Fenugreek leaf promotes gentle detoxification due to its high content of soluble fiber known as galactomannan. This unique compound plays a crucial role in supporting the body's detox processes, particularly in the liver. Galactomannan forms a gel-like substance in the digestive tract, which helps to bind and eliminate toxins, heavy metals, and waste products from the body. As a result, fenugreek leaf aids in cleansing the liver and improving its function, which is essential for overall detoxification. By facilitating the removal of harmful substances, fenugreek leaf contributes to a healthier internal environment and supports the body's natural detoxification mechanisms.
5. **Anti-inflammatory Effects:** The anti-inflammatory benefits of fenugreek leaf are attributed to the presence of alkaloids, particularly trigonelline. Trigonelline is a natural compound found in fenugreek leaves that exhibits anti-inflammatory properties. When consumed, trigonelline interacts with certain receptors and enzymes in the body, inhibiting the production of inflammatory molecules and reducing the overall inflammatory response. By reducing inflammation, fenugreek leaf can support joint health and alleviate symptoms of conditions like arthritis and other inflammatory disorders. The anti-inflammatory action of trigonelline may also benefit various body systems and organs, promoting overall well-being and healthy aging.
6. **Brain Health:** Fenugreek leaf contributes to brain health and cognitive function due to its natural choline content. Choline is an essential nutrient that acts as a precursor to acetylcholine, a neurotransmitter crucial for memory, learning, and overall brain function. By providing the body with choline, fenugreek leaf promotes the synthesis of acetylcholine, supporting various cognitive processes. Additionally, fenugreek leaf's potential anti-inflammatory and antioxidant properties may further contribute to brain health by protecting brain cells from oxidative stress and inflammation.
7. **Hormonal Balance:** Fenugreek leaf aids in hormonal balance and adrenal support through its various phytonutrients, such as saponins like diosgenin. These compounds have been linked to promoting hormonal health by influencing the production and regulation of hormones in the body. Diosgenin, in particular, is considered a precursor to certain hormones and may play a role in supporting hormone balance. Including fenugreek leaf in the diet may help promote equilibrium within the endocrine system, which is responsible for hormone secretion and regulation.

8. **Antimicrobial Effects:** Fenugreek leaf possesses antimicrobial properties attributed to its active compounds, such as alkaloids and flavonoids, including trigonelline, galactomannan, and quercetin. These compounds have shown potential in inhibiting the growth and proliferation of various pathogenic microorganisms, including bacteria, viruses, and fungi. Trigonelline, in particular, has been studied for its antimicrobial effects, and it may help combat certain bacteria and fungi. Galactomannan, a soluble fiber present in fenugreek leaf, also contributes to its antimicrobial properties by promoting a healthy gut environment where beneficial gut bacteria can thrive, further supporting the immune system.
9. **Gastrointestinal Health:** Fenugreek leaf contains mucilage, a gel-like substance that provides soothing and protective effects on the digestive system. This mucilage contributes to gastrointestinal health by helping to alleviate irritation and promote overall digestive comfort.
10. **Testosterone Support:** Fenugreek contains active compounds like saponins and protodioscin, which have been linked to enhancing testosterone production. Saponins, in particular, are believed to stimulate the release of luteinizing hormone (LH) in the pituitary gland. LH, in turn, signals the testes in men and ovaries in women to produce more testosterone. In men, increased testosterone levels can have various positive effects, such as improved muscle mass, strength, and physical performance. It may also support overall vitality and energy levels. For women, balanced testosterone levels are crucial for overall hormonal health, as testosterone plays a role in reproductive health, muscle maintenance, and bone density.

While both varieties of fenugreek leaf are generally considered safe to consume when used in culinary amounts, it is essential to be aware of potential medical contradictions and drug interactions. Individuals with certain medical conditions, such as diabetes, should exercise caution, as fenugreek may lower blood sugar levels and could interfere with diabetes medications. Those with bleeding disorders or taking anticoagulant medications should also consult their healthcare provider, as fenugreek may have mild anticoagulant effects. Individuals with allergies to legumes, including chickpeas, peanuts, and green peas, may be at an increased risk of allergic reactions to fenugreek. Although fenugreek leaf is generally considered safe to use during pregnancy in culinary amounts, it is advisable to seek guidance from your herbalist/practitioner if you are breastfeeding to ensure proper dosage and usage.

FENUGREEK SEED

Fenugreek seed, derived from the plant Trigonella foenum-graecum, have a fascinating history that can be traced back to ancient civilizations of the Mediterranean and Western Asia. This herbaceous plant has been cultivated for thousands of years and holds a significant place in traditional medicine and culinary practices around the world. Fenugreek seeds are small, yellowish-brown, and possess a distinct maple-like aroma and flavor. Not only are they a versatile ingredient in various cuisines, but they also offer a wide array of health and longevity benefits.

Now, let's explore ten extensive health and longevity benefits associated with fenugreek seed:

1. **Improved Insulin Sensitivity:** Fenugreek seeds may enhance insulin sensitivity, which is the ability of cells to respond to insulin and effectively transport glucose from the bloodstream into the cells. Compounds present in fenugreek, such as trigonelline, 4-hydroxyisoleucine, and galactomannan fiber, have been associated with improving insulin sensitivity. By enhancing insulin action, fenugreek seeds may help improve glucose metabolism and regulate blood sugar levels.
2. **Digestive Health:** The high fiber content of fenugreek seeds promotes healthy digestion and aids in the prevention of constipation. They can also help soothe gastrointestinal inflammation and relieve stomach ulcers.
3. **Bile Acid Binding:** Fenugreek seeds may also contribute to cholesterol management through bile acid binding. Bile acids, produced by the liver, aid in the digestion and absorption of dietary fats. The soluble fiber in fenugreek seeds can bind to bile acids in the intestines, promoting their excretion. To compensate for the loss of bile acids, the liver utilizes cholesterol to produce more, thereby reducing the levels of cholesterol circulating in the bloodstream.
4. **Breast Milk Production:** Phytoestrogens found in fenugreek seeds can mimic estrogen and promote the release of prolactin, the hormone responsible for milk production. Additionally, saponins present in fenugreek seeds may have lactogenic properties, potentially enhancing milk production. The proteins and enzymes in fenugreek seeds provide essential nutrients and support milk synthesis.

5. **Hormonal Balance:** Fenugreek seeds contain phytoestrogens, plant compounds that mimic estrogen in the body. This may help regulate hormonal imbalances and alleviate symptoms associated with menstruation, menopause, and polycystic ovary syndrome (PCOS).
6. **Anti-inflammatory Effects:** Fenugreek seeds boast robust anti-inflammatory properties attributed to their rich content of compounds, including flavonoids and alkaloids. These bioactive substances synergistically engage in disrupting the release of pro-inflammatory agents in the body. Flavonoids, known for their antioxidant and anti-inflammatory characteristics, play a pivotal role in mitigating inflammation. Alkaloids, another group of compounds present in fenugreek seeds, contribute to this effect by interfering with the pathways that lead to the release of inflammatory substances. This concerted action makes fenugreek seeds a valuable natural remedy for providing significant relief from inflammation, particularly beneficial for conditions such as arthritis.
7. **Respiratory Health:** Fenugreek seeds possess expectorant properties, making them effective in relieving respiratory congestion and coughs. They may help expel mucus and soothe inflamed airways.
8. **Liver Health:** Fenugreek seeds contain antioxidants, including flavonoids and polyphenols, which help combat oxidative stress in the liver. Oxidative stress occurs when there is an imbalance between free radicals and the body's antioxidant defenses. By neutralizing free radicals and reducing oxidative damage, fenugreek seeds may help protect liver cells from injury and damage.
9. **Skin Health:** Fenugreek seeds are known for their potential benefits for the skin. The seeds may help improve skin texture, reduce inflammation, and alleviate conditions like acne, eczema, and dryness. Fenugreek seeds contain flavonoids and saponins that support wound healing. These compounds may help stimulate the production of collagen, a protein important for skin structure and healing.
10. **Antioxidant Powerhouse:** Fenugreek seeds are rich in antioxidants that help combat free radicals and oxidative stress, thereby protecting cells from damage and reducing the risk of chronic diseases.

While fenugreek seeds are generally safe to consume, there are a few important warnings and contradictions to consider. Individuals taking blood-thinning medications, such as warfarin, should exercise caution, as fenugreek seeds may have potential interactions. Additionally, individuals with certain health conditions, such as allergies, asthma, or hypoglycemia, should consult with a healthcare professional before incorporating fenugreek into their diet or health regimen. Pregnant women should consult with their herbalist/practitioner before using fenugreek seeds, although it is generally considered safe during pregnancy. Breastfeeding mothers can safely consume fenugreek seeds to support lactation, but it is advisable to seek guidance from your herbalist/practitioner to ensure proper dosage and usage.

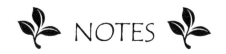

NOTES

FEVERFEW

Feverfew, scientifically known as Tanacetum parthenium, is a flowering plant native to the Balkan Peninsula and has a rich history rooted in traditional herbal medicine. Its name is derived from the Latin word "febrifugia," which means "fever reducer." Feverfew has been used for centuries as a natural remedy for various ailments, and its usage can be traced back to ancient Greek and Roman civilizations. This perennial herb features delicate, daisy-like flowers and leaves with a distinctive aroma.
Now, let's explore ten extensive health and longevity benefits associated with feverfew:

1. **Migraine Relief:** Feverfew's potential to alleviate migraines is attributed to compounds like parthenolide, which exhibit anti-inflammatory and vasodilatory properties. By reducing inflammation and preventing the constriction of blood vessels, feverfew may help reduce the frequency and intensity of migraines.
2. **Anti-inflammatory Effects:** The active compounds in feverfew, including parthenolide and other sesquiterpene lactones, possess anti-inflammatory properties. These compounds help reduce inflammation markers in the body, which can be beneficial for conditions like arthritis, joint pain, and inflammation-related disorders.
3. **Digestive Health:** Feverfew has been traditionally used to promote digestive health and relieve gastrointestinal distress. It may help reduce bloating, indigestion, and symptoms of irritable bowel syndrome (IBS).
4. **Menstrual Support:** Feverfew has been recognized for its potential to alleviate menstrual discomfort and symptoms. It may help reduce cramping, pain, and inflammation associated with menstrual cycles.
5. **Skin Health:** Feverfew's anti-inflammatory properties make it beneficial for managing certain skin conditions. The active compounds, including sesquiterpene lactones and flavonoids, help soothe and reduce redness, irritation, and itchiness associated with conditions like eczema, psoriasis, and dermatitis.
6. **Respiratory Health:** Feverfew has been used traditionally to support respiratory health. Its anti-inflammatory properties may help relieve symptoms associated with asthma, bronchitis, and allergies.

7. **Immune System Support:** Feverfew contains various antioxidants, including flavonoids and terpenes, which may help boost the immune system's defenses. These antioxidants may protect against free radicals, reducing oxidative stress and supporting overall immune health.
8. **Cardiovascular Health:** Feverfew may have a positive impact on cardiovascular health by promoting healthy blood flow, reducing blood pressure, and inhibiting platelet aggregation, thus potentially lowering the risk of heart disease.
9. **Serotonin Modulation:** Parthenolide has been noted to influence the levels of neurotransmitters in the brain, including serotonin. Serotonin is a neurotransmitter known for its crucial role in regulating mood and promoting feelings of well-being. Modulating serotonin levels may have a positive impact on mental well-being by helping to reduce anxiety and stress while promoting relaxation.
10. **Antimicrobial Effects:** Feverfew exhibits antimicrobial properties, showing inhibitory effects against certain bacteria and some fungal pathogens. The active compounds in feverfew, such as sesquiterpene lactones and flavonoids, contribute to its antimicrobial activity. These compounds have been found to inhibit the growth and reproduction of bacterial pathogens. By harnessing its antimicrobial properties, feverfew may assist in combating bacterial infections and supporting overall health.

> While feverfew is generally considered safe to consume, there are certain medical contradictions and precautions to be aware of. Feverfew may interact with certain medications, including blood-thinning medications, antiplatelet drugs, and nonsteroidal anti-inflammatory drugs (NSAIDs). It is crucial to consult with a healthcare professional before incorporating feverfew into your health regimen if you have any underlying medical conditions or are taking medications. Individuals allergic to plants in the Asteraceae family, such as daisies, marigolds, or ragweed, may also be sensitive to feverfew and should avoid its use. Feverfew should not be consumed by pregnant women, as it may stimulate uterine contractions. Women who are lactating should consult with their herbalist/practitioner prior to using feverfew.

FO-TI ROOT

Fo-ti root, scientifically known as Polygonum multiflorum, is an herbaceous perennial plant that holds a prominent place in traditional Chinese medicine (TCM) and has a rich history spanning centuries. Originating from China, fo-ti root is also known by other names such as He Shou Wu, which translates to "Mr. He's Black Hair," referencing the legendary man who reputedly restored his vitality and youthful appearance by consuming this herb. Fo-ti root has gained popularity globally due to its potential health benefits and longevity-promoting effects.

Now, let's explore ten extensive health and longevity benefits associated with fo-ti root:

1. **Graceful-aging Effects:** Fo-ti root is traditionally revered for its pro-aging properties. It is believed to nourish and tonify the body, promoting longevity and vitality.
2. **Hair Health**: Fo-ti root is widely used to support hair health and promote hair growth. The active compounds in fo-ti root, such as antioxidants and certain flavonoids, are believed to help prevent premature graying, strengthen hair follicles, and improve overall hair quality.
3. **Detoxification:** Fo-ti root is known for its hepatoprotective properties. The active compounds, including stilbenes glycosides and anthraquinones, are believed to support liver detoxification processes by assisting in the elimination of toxins, protecting the liver from damage, and improving liver function.
4. **Cardiovascular Health:** Fo-ti root has been used to support cardiovascular health and reduce the risk of heart disease. The active compounds, including stilbenes, flavonoids, and phytosterols, may help regulate cholesterol levels, lower blood pressure, and improve blood circulation.
5. **Immune System Support:** Fo-ti root contains compounds, such as flavonoids and polysaccharides, that may enhance immune system function. Regular consumption of fo-ti root may help strengthen the body's defenses against infections and improve overall immune health.
6. **Cognitive Support:** Fo-ti root is believed to have positive effects on cognitive function and brain health. The active compounds, including stilbenes and other antioxidants, may help improve memory, enhance mental clarity, and support overall cognitive performance.

7. **Enhanced Libido and Sexual Health:** In traditional medicine, fo-ti root is often used to support sexual health and vitality. It is believed to enhance libido, improve fertility, and support reproductive health.
8. **Anti-inflammatory Effects:** Fo-ti root contains compounds with anti-inflammatory properties, such as stilbenes and anthraquinones. Regular consumption of fo-ti root may help reduce inflammation, alleviate joint pain, and support overall joint health.
9. **Adaptogenic Effects:** Fo-ti root is commonly used as an adaptogen, believed to enhance energy levels, improve endurance, and combat fatigue. It may help increase physical stamina and promote overall vitality.
10. **Anti-cancer Effects:** Some studies have suggested that certain compounds found in fo-ti root, such as stilbenes and anthraquinones, may have anti-cancer properties. However, further research is needed to fully understand the potential role of fo-ti root in cancer prevention and treatment.

While fo-ti root is generally considered safe to consume in small quantities, there are certain medical contradictions and precautions to be aware of. Individuals with specific conditions, such as liver disease or dysfunction, should exercise caution when using fo-ti root, as the herb has been associated with potential hepatotoxic effects in large doses. Fo-ti root may also interact with certain medications, such as anticoagulants (blood thinners) and antidiabetic drugs, affecting their efficacy or increasing the risk of bleeding or hypoglycemia. It is important to note that fo-ti root's safety during pregnancy and lactation has not been sufficiently established, so it is advisable for pregnant or breastfeeding individuals to consult with their herbalist/practitioner before using fo-ti root.

GINGER ROOT

Ginger root, scientifically known as Zingiber officinale, is a flowering plant with a rich history deeply rooted in traditional medicine and culinary practices. Originating from Southeast Asia, ginger has been cultivated for over 4,000 years and has spread its influence across various cultures worldwide. The root of the ginger plant is highly prized for its unique flavor, warm aroma, and its remarkable health benefits. Ginger root has been used for centuries as a natural remedy for various ailments, offering a wide array of health and longevity benefits.

Now, let's explore ten extensive health and longevity benefits associated with ginger root:

1. **Digestive Health:** Ginger root is renowned for its ability to soothe digestive discomfort, including nausea, indigestion, and bloating. It stimulates digestion, promotes the release of digestive enzymes, and helps alleviate gastrointestinal distress.
2. **Anti-inflammatory Effects:** Ginger root contains potent anti-inflammatory compounds called gingerols. These compounds may help reduce inflammation in the body, potentially easing symptoms of arthritis, joint pain, and other inflammatory conditions.
3. **Nausea and Morning Sickness Relief:** Ginger root is widely recognized for its antiemetic properties, making it effective in relieving nausea and vomiting, including those associated with motion sickness and pregnancy-related morning sickness.
4. **Immune System Support:** Ginger root is known to possess immune-boosting properties. It may help strengthen the immune system, reduce the risk of infections, and promote overall immune health.
5. **Pain Relief:** Ginger root has analgesic properties and can act as a natural pain reliever. It may help alleviate menstrual cramps, headaches, and muscle soreness.
6. **Post-exercise Recovery Support:** Lactic acid is a byproduct of muscle metabolism and can contribute to muscle soreness. The active compounds gingerol and shogaol in ginger possess anti-inflammatory properties. These compounds may aid in reducing inflammation, promoting efficient circulation, and facilitating the elimination of lactic acid.
7. **Brain Health:** Ginger root may have neuroprotective effects and support brain health. It has been studied for its potential in reducing the risk of neurodegenerative diseases such as Alzheimer's and improving cognitive function.

8. **Anti-cancer Effects:** Some studies have suggested that certain compounds in ginger root may have anti-cancer properties. These compounds may inhibit the growth of cancer cells and promote apoptosis (cell death) in certain types of cancer. However, more research is needed in this area.
9. **Respiratory Health:** Ginger root has traditionally been used to alleviate respiratory conditions such as coughs and bronchitis. Its expectorant properties may help loosen mucus and ease respiratory congestion. Zingerone is a compound in ginger known for its anti-inflammatory properties. It helps soothe respiratory inflammation and alleviate respiratory discomfort.
10. **Antioxidant Powerhouse:** Ginger contains various antioxidants, such as gingerols and shogaols, which help combat oxidative stress and reduce cellular damage caused by free radicals. By reducing oxidative stress, ginger supports the overall health and function of the immune system.

> While ginger is generally considered safe to consume, there are certain medical contradictions and precautions to be aware of. Individuals with specific conditions, such as bleeding disorders, should exercise caution when using ginger, as it may interfere with blood clotting. Ginger may also interact with certain medications, including anticoagulants (blood thinners) and antidiabetic drugs, affecting their efficacy or increasing the risk of bleeding or hypoglycemia. Allergy warnings include the possibility of hypersensitivity reactions to ginger, especially in individuals with known allergies to plants in the Zingiberaceae family, which includes turmeric and cardamom. It's important to note that safety during pregnancy and lactation is controversial, and it is advisable for pregnant or breastfeeding individuals to consult with their herbalist/practitioner before using ginger due to its potential effects on uterine contractions and/or breast milk production.

GINKGO

Ginkgo, scientifically known as Ginkgo biloba, is a unique and ancient tree species with a fascinating origin dating back millions of years. Believed to be one of the oldest living tree species on Earth, ginkgo trees have survived for over 200 million years, with fossils dating back to the time of dinosaurs. Native to China, ginkgo trees have a rich cultural and medicinal history in traditional Chinese medicine. Renowned for its distinct fan-shaped leaves and remarkable resilience, ginkgo has gained global recognition for its potential health and longevity benefits. Now, let's explore ten extensive health and longevity benefits associated with ginkgo:

1. **Cognitive Support:** Ginkgo is believed to improve cognitive function and memory due to its flavonoids, terpenoids and sesquiterpene trilactones. These compounds have antioxidant and neuroprotective properties that may enhance concentration, mental clarity, and overall cognitive performance.
2. **Antioxidant Powerhouse:** Ginkgo contains powerful antioxidants like flavonoids, terpenoids, and bilobalides. These antioxidants help protect the body against oxidative stress and free radical damage, reducing the risk of chronic diseases and supporting overall well-being.
3. **Cardiovascular Health:** Ginkgo's vasodilatory properties are attributed to the active compounds called ginkgolides. By improving blood flow and enhancing circulation, ginkgo may reduce symptoms associated with poor circulation and support cardiovascular health.
4. **Enhances Libido and Sexual Health:** Ginkgo has been traditionally used to support sexual health, and its potential benefits are attributed to improved blood circulation and antioxidant effects. By enhancing blood flow and reducing oxidative stress, ginkgo may help improve libido and sexual function and reduce symptoms of erectile dysfunction.
5. **Memory Support:** Ginkgo's flavonoids and terpenoids, including bilobalides, have been studied for their potential benefits in age-related cognitive decline. These compounds may help slow down cognitive decline, improve memory, and enhance overall brain health in conditions like Alzheimer's disease and dementia.

6. **Anti-inflammatory Effects:** Ginkgo's anti-inflammatory effects are primarily attributed to flavonoids and terpenoids. These compounds help reduce inflammation in the body, providing potential benefits for conditions like arthritis, asthma, and other inflammatory disorders.
7. **Eye Health:** Ginkgo's potential benefits for eye health are linked to its flavonoid content, specifically quercetin and kaempferol. These antioxidants may improve vision, protect against age-related macular degeneration, and reduce the risk of developing cataracts.
8. **Mood Support:** Ginkgo may positively impact mood and mental well-being through its ability to improve blood flow and provide antioxidant support to the brain. The flavonoids and terpenoids in ginkgo are believed to contribute to its mood-stabilizing effects.
9. **Respiratory Health:** Ginkgo's anti-inflammatory properties, primarily due to flavonoids, may help relieve symptoms associated with respiratory conditions like asthma and bronchitis. By reducing inflammation and improving lung function, ginkgo supports respiratory health.
10. **Graceful-aging Effects:** Ginkgo's antioxidant properties, flavonoids, and improved circulation contribute to its potential pro-aging effects. By reducing oxidative stress, improving blood flow, and supporting overall vitality, ginkgo may help reduce the signs of aging, such as wrinkles and age spots.

While ginkgo is generally considered safe to consume, there are certain medical contradictions and precautions to be aware of. Individuals with bleeding disorders or taking blood-thinning medications, such as anticoagulants or antiplatelet drugs, should exercise caution when using ginkgo, as it may increase the risk of bleeding. Ginkgo may also interact with certain medications, including antidepressants, anticonvulsants, and nonsteroidal anti-inflammatory drugs (NSAIDs), potentially affecting their efficacy or increasing the risk of side effects. Allergy warnings include the possibility of hypersensitivity reactions to ginkgo, especially in individuals with known allergies to plants in the Ginkgoaceae family. It is important to note that safety during pregnancy and lactation is not well-established, and it is advisable for pregnant or breastfeeding individuals to consult with their herbalist/practitioner before using ginkgo.

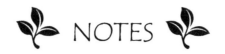

NOTES

GINSENG, AMERICAN

American ginseng, scientifically known as Panax quinquefolius, is a prized herb with a rich history and a plethora of health benefits. Native to North America, specifically the forested regions of the United States and Canada, American ginseng has been treasured for centuries by indigenous tribes and traditional medicine practitioners. The plant's fleshy roots contain bioactive compounds known as ginsenosides, which are responsible for its remarkable medicinal properties. American ginseng has gained worldwide recognition for its adaptogenic properties and its ability to support overall health and well-being.

Now, let's explore ten extensive health and longevity benefits associated with American ginseng:

1. **Adaptogenic Effects:** American ginseng's adaptogenic properties are attributed to the presence of ginsenosides. These active compounds help the body adapt to stress, promote mental clarity, and improve cognitive function by enhancing focus and concentration and reducing anxiety and fatigue.
2. **Energy Boost:** American ginseng's energizing effects are primarily due to the ginsenosides. They can increase stamina, combat fatigue, and improve physical performance, making it beneficial for athletes and those seeking an energy boost.
3. **Cognitive Support:** American ginseng has been studied for its potential to enhance cognitive function and memory. The ginsenosides contribute to improved mental performance, learning, and information processing, supporting overall brain health.
4. **Enhances Libido and Sexual Health:** American ginseng has traditionally been used as an aphrodisiac and for promoting reproductive health. It may improve libido, sexual performance, and fertility in both men and women, although the specific compounds responsible for these effects are not fully understood.
5. **Anti-radiation Effects:** Proponents of using American ginseng as an anti-radiation tool suggest that its bioactive compounds, such as ginsenosides, have antioxidant and immunomodulatory effects. These compounds are believed to support the body's natural defense mechanisms and minimize the harmful effects of radiation. Additionally, ginsenosides are thought to have radioprotective qualities by enhancing DNA repair mechanisms and reducing oxidative stress caused by radiation exposure.

6. **Cardiovascular Health:** American ginseng promotes heart health by reducing cholesterol levels, improving blood flow, and supporting healthy blood pressure. The ginsenosides contribute to these cardiovascular benefits, potentially lowering the risk of heart disease and other cardiovascular conditions.
7. **Antioxidant Powerhouse:** In addition to ginsenosides, American ginseng contains various other antioxidants, such as flavonoids and phenolic compounds. These antioxidants work together with the ginsenosides to neutralize free radicals and protect cells from oxidative stress. By reducing the damage caused by free radicals, American ginseng helps slow down the aging process and may reduce the risk of age-related diseases. The combined antioxidant activity of these compounds supports overall health and promotes longevity.
8. **Immune System Support:** American ginseng stimulates the production of immune cells and enhances the body's defense mechanisms. This immune-enhancing effect is attributed to ginsenosides and polysaccharides, which are known for their immunomodulatory benefits. These active compounds in American ginseng help strengthen the immune system, improve immune cell function, and promote overall immune health.
9. **Anti-inflammatory Effects:** The ginsenosides in American ginseng possess anti-inflammatory properties. These compounds help reduce inflammation in the body, making it potentially beneficial for conditions such as arthritis and inflammatory diseases.
10. **Blood Sugar Regulation:** American ginseng improves insulin sensitivity and enhances glucose metabolism, primarily due to the ginsenosides. This, in turn, helps regulate blood sugar levels, making it beneficial for individuals with diabetes or those at risk of developing the condition.

While American ginseng is generally considered safe to consume, there are certain medical contradictions and precautions to be aware of. American ginseng may interact with certain medications, including immunosuppressants such as cyclosporine and tacrolimus, as it can potentially stimulate the immune system. Additionally, individuals taking anticoagulant or antiplatelet medications like warfarin or aspirin should exercise caution, as American ginseng may increase the risk of bleeding. Individuals with hormone-sensitive conditions, such as breast cancer or endometriosis, should avoid or use American ginseng with caution due to its potential estrogen-like effects. Individuals with known allergies to plants from the Araliaceae family should avoid American ginseng. It is important to note that American ginseng should be avoided during pregnancy unless otherwise advised by your herbalist/practitioner.

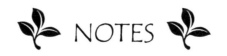

NOTES

GINSENG, KOREAN RED

Korean red ginseng root, derived from the Panax ginseng plant native to the Korean peninsula, is a highly prized herb renowned for its potent medicinal properties and rich cultural heritage. Considered the most potent form of ginseng, Korean red ginseng root has a history that dates back over 2,000 years. The herb undergoes a unique processing method involving steaming and drying, which gives it a distinct reddish color and enhances its bioactive compounds. Korean red ginseng root has gained worldwide recognition for its extensive range of health and longevity benefits, making it a valuable addition to traditional medicine practices.

Now, let's explore ten extensive health and longevity benefits associated with Korean red ginseng root:

1. **Energy Boost:** Korean red ginseng root, rich in active compounds like ginsenosides, polysaccharides, and saponins, is known for its adaptogenic properties. These compounds work together to enhance physical energy, combat fatigue, and improve endurance, making it beneficial for boosting energy levels and overall stamina.
2. **Cognitive Function:** Korean red ginseng root, containing ginsenosides and other active compounds like polyphenols, may improve cognitive function and mental performance. These compounds contribute to enhanced memory, focus, and overall cognitive abilities, supporting optimal brain function.
3. **Immune System Support:** Korean red ginseng root, with its diverse range of active compounds, including ginsenosides, polysaccharides, and peptides, has immune-modulating effects. These compounds help bolster the body's natural defenses, enhance immune cell function, and promote a healthy immune response.
4. **Stress Relief:** Korean red ginseng root, thanks to its adaptogenic properties attributed to ginsenosides, polysaccharides, and phenolic compounds, helps the body adapt to stress and alleviate its negative effects. These active compounds support the body's stress response system and promote overall well-being.
5. **Cardiovascular Health:** Korean red ginseng root, with its active compounds like ginsenosides, flavonoids, and polysaccharides, supports cardiovascular health by regulating blood pressure, improving blood circulation, and reducing the risk of heart disease.

6. **Anti-inflammatory Effects:** Korean red ginseng root's bioactive compounds, such as ginsenosides, polyphenols, and flavonoids, possess anti-inflammatory properties. This synergistic combination helps reduce inflammation in the body, alleviating symptoms associated with inflammatory conditions and promoting overall well-being.
7. **Antioxidant Powerhouse:** Korean red ginseng root, containing a variety of antioxidants, including ginsenosides, polyphenols, flavonoids, and vitamin C, provides strong antioxidant protection. These compounds work together to combat oxidative stress, neutralize free radicals, and protect cells from damage, promoting overall cellular health and longevity.
8. **Enhances Libido and Sexual Health:** Korean red ginseng root, known for its aphrodisiac properties, contains active compounds like ginsenosides, phenolic compounds, and arginine. These compounds may enhance sexual performance, increase libido, and boost overall sexual vitality.
9. **Graceful-aging Effects:** Korean red ginseng root's antioxidant properties attributed to ginsenosides, polyphenols, flavonoids, and other active compounds contribute to its pro-aging effects. Regular consumption may help reduce signs of aging, enhance skin elasticity, and promote a youthful appearance.
10. **Mood Support:** Korean red ginseng root, with its diverse range of active compounds, including ginsenosides, polyphenols, and saponins, has been associated with improvements in mood and mental well-being. These compounds may alleviate symptoms of depression and anxiety, promoting emotional balance and overall psychological health.

While Korean red ginseng root is generally considered safe to consume, it is important to be aware of certain contradictions and potential interactions. Individuals with high blood pressure, diabetes, or bleeding disorders should exercise caution and consult with a healthcare professional before using Korean red ginseng root, as it may affect blood pressure, blood sugar levels, and blood clotting. This herb may interact with certain medications, including blood thinners, antidiabetic drugs, immunosuppressants, and medications metabolized by the liver. Allergy to ginseng is rare but possible, and individuals with known allergies to plants from the Araliaceae family should avoid Korean red ginseng root. Pregnant or breastfeeding women should avoid Korean red ginseng root unless otherwise directed by their herbalist/practitioner.

GOAT'S RUE

Goat's rue, scientifically known as Galega officinalis, is a perennial herb with a long history of medicinal use. Native to Europe and parts of Asia, goat's rue has been valued for centuries for its therapeutic properties. This herb derives its name from its resemblance to the leaves of the rue plant and its attraction to goats. Goat's rue has traditionally been used in herbal medicine for a variety of purposes. It is particularly renowned for its potential health and longevity benefits.

Now, let's explore ten extensive health and longevity benefits associated with goat's rue:

1. **Blood Sugar Regulation:** Goat's rue contains compounds like guanidine derivatives and flavonoids that help regulate blood sugar levels and improve insulin sensitivity, making it potentially beneficial for individuals with diabetes or metabolic conditions.
2. **Liver Health:** Goat's rue contains flavonoids and other compounds that support liver health and assist in detoxification processes, promoting optimal liver function and aiding in the elimination of toxins from the body.
3. **Hormonal Balance:** Goat's rue contains isoflavones and phytoestrogens that may assist in balancing hormones, particularly in women. It may help alleviate symptoms associated with hormonal imbalances, such as irregular periods and menopause.
4. **Digestive Health:** Goat's rue has been traditionally used to support digestive health due to its content of bitter compounds like galegine. It aids in digestion, alleviates gastrointestinal discomfort, and improves nutrient absorption.
5. **Anti-inflammatory Effects:** Goat's rue possesses flavonoids and alkaloids that exhibit anti-inflammatory properties. These compounds help reduce inflammation in the body and alleviate symptoms associated with inflammatory conditions.
6. **Diuretic Effects:** Goat's rue acts as a diuretic due to its content of flavonoids and alkaloids. It promotes increased urine production, aiding in the elimination of toxins from the body and supporting urinary health.
7. **Respiratory Health:** Goat's rue has been used to support respiratory health due to its expectorant properties. It helps alleviate symptoms associated with coughs, bronchitis, and asthma, promoting clearer airways and respiratory comfort.

8. **Lactation Support:** Goat's rue is rich in galactagogue compounds, such as galegine and hydroxyisoleucine, which stimulate the production and flow of breast milk in lactating women.
9. **Antiparasitic Effects:** Goat's rue has been traditionally used as an anthelmintic due to the presence of compounds like galegine. It helps expel intestinal worms and parasites from the body.
10. **Cardiovascular Health:** Goat's rue may have beneficial effects on cardiovascular health due to its content of flavonoids and guanidine derivatives. It may help regulate blood pressure, improve circulation, and reduce the risk of cardiovascular diseases.

While goat's rue is generally considered safe to consume, there are certain medical contradictions and precautions to be aware of. Individuals with hypoglycemia or diabetes should exercise caution when using goat's rue, as it may lower blood sugar levels. It is also important to note that goat's rue may interact with antidiabetic medications, potentially leading to hypoglycemia. Goat's rue may have hormonal effects and should be used with caution in individuals with hormone-sensitive conditions or those taking hormonal medications. Allergy warnings are also important, as goat's rue belongs to the Fabaceae family, which includes other plants like soybeans, peanuts, and lentils. Individuals with known allergies to these plants should avoid goat's rue. Safety during pregnancy and lactation is not well-established, and therefore, pregnant and lactating women should exercise caution and consult with their herbalist/practitioner before using goat's rue.

GOJI BERRY (POWDER)

Goji berries, scientifically known as Lycium barbarum, is a fascinating and revered fruit with a long and storied history dating back thousands of years. Originating from the remote regions of Asia, particularly in China, Tibet, and Mongolia, goji berries have been cherished for centuries for their various uses and esteemed as a symbol of health, longevity, and vitality. Renowned for their vibrant reddish-orange hue, goji berries are often referred to as "red diamonds" due to their precious nature. Traditionally, goji berries were incorporated into Chinese medicine and cuisine, believed to promote well-being and boost overall vitality. Interestingly, goji berries are also associated with a legendary tale of discovery, where ancient Buddhist monks stumbled upon a secret Tibetan valley where goji berries grew in abundance, and those who consumed them were believed to experience increased longevity and vibrant health. Goji berry powder is typically created by freeze drying the goji berries, then pulverizing the berries into a fine powder. This process ensures the preservation of their valuable nutrients. This potent superfood is known for its impressive health and longevity benefits, making it a popular addition to dietary regimes.

Now, let's explore ten extensive health and longevity benefits associated with goji berries.

1. **Antioxidant Powerhouse:** Goji berries are rich in antioxidants such as vitamin C, zeaxanthin, and beta-carotene. These antioxidants help neutralize free radicals, protecting cells from oxidative stress and promoting overall health.
2. **Immune System Support:** Goji berries contain immune-boosting compounds, including polysaccharides and antioxidants, that can enhance the body's natural defense mechanisms, reducing the risk of infections and supporting overall well-being.
3. **Eye Health:** Goji berries are a good source of zeaxanthin and lutein, two antioxidants known for their benefits in promoting eye health. These compounds may help protect against age-related macular degeneration and maintain healthy vision.
4. **Cognitive Support:** Zeaxanthin, a carotenoid found in goji berries, has been linked to improved cognitive function and a positive impact on mental well-being. The B vitamins play a crucial role in brain health, contributing to the production of neurotransmitters and supporting overall cognitive function.

5. **Skin Health:** The antioxidants in goji berries, such as vitamin C and beta-carotene, may help protect the skin from oxidative damage, reduce the signs of aging, improve skin elasticity, and promote a youthful and radiant complexion.
6. **Cardiovascular Health:** Goji berries may contribute to heart health by reducing cholesterol levels, improving blood circulation, and providing a good source of heart-healthy nutrients like antioxidants and fiber.
7. **Energy Boost:** Goji berries contain a compound called polysaccharides, some of which include oligosaccharides and monosaccharides, which are complex carbohydrates that provide a slow and sustained release of energy, helping to prevent energy crashes. Additionally, goji berries are rich in essential nutrients like vitamins B1 (thiamine), B2 (riboflavin), and B6 (pyridoxine), which play crucial roles in energy production and metabolism. These vitamins are involved in converting the food we eat into usable energy for the body. By providing these important nutrients, goji berries can support optimal energy levels and enhance overall vitality.
8. **Mood Support:** The presence of antioxidants, including vitamin C and zeaxanthin, along with other nutrients such as vitamins B1, B2, and B6, in goji berries may help reduce oxidative stress, support brain health, and promote a sense of calmness. Vitamin C acts as an antioxidant, protecting brain cells from damage caused by free radicals and supporting the production of neurotransmitters involved in mood regulation.
9. **Weight Management:** Goji berries are low in calories and high in fiber, which can promote satiety, aid in digestion, and support healthy weight management.
10. **Anti-inflammatory Effects:** Goji berries possess anti-inflammatory properties, such as flavonoids and beta-carotene, which may help reduce inflammation in the body and alleviate symptoms associated with inflammatory conditions such as arthritis, joint pain, and other inflammatory disorders. Flavonoids are plant compounds known for their potent anti-inflammatory effects, helping to inhibit inflammatory pathways and reduce the production of inflammatory molecules. Beta-carotene, a precursor to vitamin A, acts as an antioxidant and may help modulate the immune response to inflammation.

While goji berries are generally considered safe to consume, it is important to be aware of certain medical contradictions and potential interactions with medications. Goji berries may interact with blood thinners, anticoagulant medications, and drugs that lower blood sugar levels. Goji berries are generally considered safe to consume during pregnancy and lactation.

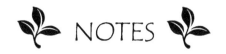

NOTES

GOLDENSEAL

Goldenseal, scientifically known as Hydrastis canadensis, is a perennial herb native to the eastern parts of the United States and Canada. Both the leaf and root of the goldenseal plant hold significance in traditional medicine practices. The goldenseal leaf features deeply lobed leaves and distinctive yellow rhizomes, while the root possesses a bright yellow color and a bitter taste. Each part of the plant offers unique health benefits, and they have been used interchangeably for centuries to address various health concerns.

Now, let's explore ten extensive health and longevity benefits associated with goldenseal:

1. **Immune System Support:** Both goldenseal leaf and root are known for their immune-boosting properties. The active compounds in goldenseal, such as berberine, hydrastine, and canadine, help strengthen the body's natural defense mechanisms during acute illness and infections.
2. **Diaper Rash Support:** Goldenseal can be beneficial in soothing and healing diaper rash in infants when applied topically. Its antimicrobial and anti-inflammatory properties, attributed to compounds like berberine, help reduce irritation and promote healing of the affected area.
3. **Anti-inflammatory Effects:** Both goldenseal leaf and root possess anti-inflammatory properties due to the presence of alkaloids, such as berberine, hydrastine, and canadine, and other bioactive compounds like flavonoids and polyphenols. These compounds help reduce inflammation and alleviate symptoms associated with acute inflammatory conditions.
4. **Antimicrobial Effects:** Goldenseal root contains potent antimicrobial compounds, including berberine, which have broad-spectrum activity against bacteria, fungi, and parasites. These properties make goldenseal useful in combating acute infections.
5. **Skin Health:** The antimicrobial and anti-inflammatory properties of goldenseal, attributed to its bioactive compounds, including berberine and hydrastine, help alleviate skin conditions such as eczema and acne. These properties can combat microbial infections, reduce inflammation, and promote skin healing and balance. Applying goldenseal topically may help soothe irritation, reduce redness, and support overall skin health.

6. **Respiratory Health:** Goldenseal leaf and root have traditionally been used to support respiratory health during acute illness. The antimicrobial and expectorant properties of goldenseal, attributed to its alkaloids, including berberine, can assist in relieving acute respiratory infections such as pneumonia and whooping cough. These properties help combat microbial pathogens and facilitate the removal of excess mucus, promoting respiratory comfort and recovery.
7. **Wound Healing:** Goldenseal contains berberine, a compound with antimicrobial properties that may help prevent infection in minor wounds and promote healing when used topically.
8. **Antifungal Effects:** Goldenseal's antimicrobial properties, primarily attributed to its bioactive compound berberine, make it useful in treating fungal infections topically, such as athlete's foot. Berberine has been shown to have antifungal effects, inhibiting the growth of various fungi and helping to alleviate fungal infections on the skin. Applying goldenseal extract or ointment directly to the affected area may help combat the fungal overgrowth, reduce symptoms, and promote healing.
9. **Eye Infections:** Goldenseal can be used topically as an eyewash to help relieve eye irritation and treat minor eye infections like conjunctivitis (pink eye).
10. **Oral Health:** Goldenseal mouthwashes or gargles may help soothe mouth sores, alleviate gum inflammation, and support oral health by reducing bacteria in the mouth. Goldenseal can also be used as part of a soothing gargle solution for relieving sore throat symptoms. Its antimicrobial properties may help reduce throat inflammation due to an acute infection.

While goldenseal is generally considered safe when used appropriately and for short periods, it's important to note that prolonged internal use may increase the risk of adverse reactions. This can include gastrointestinal distress, allergic reactions, liver toxicity, and changes in blood pressure. Individuals with certain medical conditions, such as high blood pressure, liver disease, or heart conditions, should exercise caution and consult with a healthcare professional before using goldenseal. Goldenseal has been found to inhibit certain enzymes in the liver, particularly the cytochrome P450 enzymes (CYP3A4 and CYP2D6). These enzymes are responsible for metabolizing many medications. Inhibition of these enzymes can lead to higher levels of drugs in the body, potentially increasing the risk of adverse effects. Goldenseal should be used with caution or avoided if you are taking medications metabolized by these enzymes, such as certain antidepressants, antipsychotics, antiarrhythmics, and immunosuppressants. If you are taking medications for high blood pressure, such as beta-blockers, calcium channel blockers, or ACE inhibitors, combining them with goldenseal may further lower blood pressure. Goldenseal contains compounds that may have anticoagulant or antiplatelet effects, which can increase the risk of bleeding. If you are taking medications like warfarin, aspirin, clopidogrel, or other blood thinners, using goldenseal concurrently may enhance their effects and potentially lead to excessive bleeding. Prolonged use of goldenseal can lead to the development of tolerance, where the body becomes less responsive to the herb's active compounds. Prolonged use of goldenseal can also disrupt the natural balance of gut flora. Goldenseal contains antimicrobial compounds, such as berberine, that can affect not only harmful bacteria but also beneficial bacteria in the gut. This disruption may lead to imbalances in the gut microbiota, which can have implications for digestive health. Goldenseal should not be used during pregnancy, as it may have uterine stimulant effects. Consult with your herbalist/practitioner prior to using goldenseal if you are lactating.

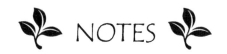

NOTES

GOTU KOLA

Gotu kola, scientifically known as Centella asiatica, is an herbaceous plant with a long history of use in traditional Ayurvedic and Chinese medicine. Native to the wetlands of Asia, particularly in India, Sri Lanka, and other Southeast Asian countries, gotu kola has been revered for centuries for its remarkable health benefits. This herbaceous perennial plant features fan-shaped leaves and small, inconspicuous flowers. Gotu kola is known for its adaptogenic and rejuvenating properties, earning it the title of "herb of longevity" in many ancient cultures.

Now, let's explore ten extensive health and longevity benefits associated with gotu kola:

1. **Cognitive Support:** Gotu kola contains triterpenoid compounds, such as asiaticoside and madecassoside, which have been shown to enhance cognitive function, improve memory, and promote mental clarity and focus.
2. **Anxiety and Stress Relief:** The adaptogenic properties of gotu kola, attributed to compounds like asiaticoside, help regulate the body's response to stress, reducing anxiety and promoting a sense of calm and relaxation.
3. **Skin Health:** Gotu kola contains compounds, including asiaticoside and asiatic acid, that aid in wound healing, stimulate collagen synthesis, and improve the overall health and appearance of the skin.
4. **Wound Healing:** Gotu kola accelerates wound healing by stimulating collagen production, increasing angiogenesis (formation of new blood vessels), and promoting tissue regeneration. Compounds like asiaticoside and asiatic acid support these healing processes.
5. **Cardiovascular Health:** Gotu kola improves cardiovascular health by enhancing blood circulation, reducing cholesterol levels, and supporting the health and functioning of the cardiovascular system. Its active compounds, including asiaticoside, contribute to these effects.
6. **Antioxidant Powerhouse:** The rich antioxidant content in gotu kola, including flavonoids and triterpenoids, helps protect cells from oxidative stress and damage caused by free radicals, promoting overall cellular health.

7. **Graceful-aging Effects:** Gotu kola's ability to promote collagen synthesis, improve skin elasticity, and reduce the appearance of wrinkles is attributed to compounds like asiaticoside and asiatic acid, supporting graceful aging.
8. **Anti-inflammatory Effects:** Gotu kola's anti-inflammatory properties, attributed to triterpenes like asiaticoside and madecassic acid, help reduce inflammation in the body and alleviate symptoms associated with inflammatory conditions.
9. **Venous Health:** Gotu kola supports venous health through its ability to improve circulation, strengthen blood vessels, and reduce venous insufficiency. Compounds like asiaticoside contribute to these benefits.
10. **Hair Health:** Gotu kola's role in promoting hair health and growth is attributed to its ability to improve blood circulation in the scalp, strengthen hair follicles, and nourish the hair strands. Active compounds like asiaticoside contribute to these benefits.

While gotu kola is generally considered safe to consume in mindful quantities, it may have hepatotoxic effects when used in high doses for prolonged periods. Gotu kola may interact with medications such as anticoagulants, antiplatelet drugs, and diuretics, potentially increasing the risk of bleeding or altering the effects of these medications. Allergy warnings for gotu kola are rare, but individuals with a known allergy to plants in the Apiaceae family, such as carrots or celery, may be more prone to an allergic reaction. Safety during pregnancy and lactation is not well-established, and it is recommended to consult your herbalist/practitioner before using gotu kola during these periods.

GRAPEFRUIT PEEL

Grapefruit, scientifically known as Citrus paradisi, is a tropical citrus fruit that has gained global popularity for its refreshing taste and vibrant aroma. While the flesh of the grapefruit is widely enjoyed, the peel of this citrus fruit also holds significant therapeutic properties. Grapefruit peel, derived from the outer layer of the fruit, contains a wealth of bioactive compounds that contribute to its numerous health and longevity benefits. Originating from subtropical regions like the Caribbean and Florida, grapefruit peel has been used in traditional medicine for centuries.

Now, let's explore ten extensive health and longevity benefits associated with grapefruit peel:

1. **Digestive Health:** Grapefruit peel possesses natural enzymes and dietary fiber, such as pectin, that aid in digestion, promote healthy bowel movements, and alleviate digestive issues such as constipation.
2. **Antioxidant Powerhouse:** The peel of grapefruit is rich in antioxidants, including vitamin C and flavonoids like naringin and hesperidin. These antioxidants help combat oxidative stress, neutralize free radicals, and reduce the risk of chronic diseases.
3. **Immune System Support:** Grapefruit peel contains immune-enhancing compounds like vitamin C and various phytochemicals that support the body's natural defense mechanisms, helping to strengthen the immune system and reduce the risk of infections.
4. **Anti-inflammatory Effects:** The phytochemicals present in grapefruit peel, including limonoids and flavonoids, exhibit anti-inflammatory properties. These compounds may help reduce inflammation in the body and alleviate symptoms associated with inflammatory conditions.
5. **Skin Health:** Grapefruit peel is renowned for its skin-enhancing properties, including its rich content of antioxidants and phytochemicals like vitamin C and polyphenols. These compounds promote collagen production, enhance skin elasticity, and combat signs of aging, such as wrinkles and fine lines. The antioxidants in grapefruit peel help protect the skin from free radical damage, while the phytochemicals provide anti-inflammatory benefits, supporting overall skin health and rejuvenation.

6. **Weight Management:** The bioactive compounds in grapefruit peel, such as naringin, contribute to weight management through various mechanisms. Naringin helps suppress appetite by increasing the secretion of hormones that promote feelings of fullness, reducing food intake. It also improves metabolic processes by enhancing the activity of specific enzymes involved in fat metabolism. This leads to increased breakdown and utilization of stored fat for energy. Additionally, naringin stimulates the expression of genes and proteins involved in fat oxidation, increasing the body's fat-burning potential.
7. **Cardiovascular Health:** Grapefruit peel is linked to maintaining a healthy heart due to the presence of flavonoids like naringin and other compounds such as limonoids in the peel. Flavonoids, known for their antioxidant properties, help reduce cholesterol levels, prevent the oxidation of LDL cholesterol, and improve blood vessel function, promoting cardiovascular health. Additionally, the presence of limonoids in grapefruit peel has been associated with reducing blood pressure and inhibiting the formation of blood clots, further supporting overall cardiovascular function.
8. **Detoxification:** The detoxifying compounds found in grapefruit peel, such as naringin and limonoids, support liver health and aid in the elimination of toxins from the body, contributing to liver detoxification.
9. **Respiratory Health:** Consuming grapefruit peel may have beneficial effects on respiratory health. The peel's compounds, including flavonoids and vitamin C, help alleviate congestion, reduce mucus production, and support overall lung function.
10. **Mood Support:** Grapefruit peel is believed to have mood-enhancing properties. The presence of aromatic compounds in the peel, such as limonene, may help reduce stress, anxiety, and symptoms of depression, contributing to overall mental well-being.

While grapefruit peel is generally considered safe to consume as a food ingredient and for its potential health benefits, there are a few medical contradictions and precautions to be aware of. Grapefruit peel contains compounds that can interact with certain medications, specifically those metabolized by the enzyme cytochrome P450 3A4 (CYP3A4). These compounds can inhibit the enzyme, affecting the metabolism and clearance of medications such as statins, calcium channel blockers, and immunosuppressants, which may lead to increased levels of the drugs in the body. It is important to consult with a healthcare professional or pharmacist if you are taking medications that may interact with grapefruit peel. Individuals with known allergies to grapefruit should avoid consuming grapefruit peel. It is worth noting that grapefruit belongs to the Rutaceae family, which includes other citrus fruits such as oranges and lemons. Grapefruit peel is generally considered safe in culinary doses while pregnant or breastfeeding. Consult with your herbalist/practitioner before consuming grapefruit peel in large therapeutic doses during these times. Grapefruit is also a fruit that is more widely being treated with Apeel. Always be sure to source high-quality, organic grapefruit and/or grapefruit peel.

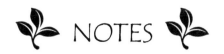
NOTES

GREEK MOUNTAIN TEA

Greek mountain tea, also known as Shepherd's tea or Sideritis tea, is derived from various species of the Sideritis plant, which are found in the mountainous regions of Greece. The specific species used to make Greek mountain tea can vary, but some common species include Sideritis scardica, Sideritis raeseri, Sideritis syriaca, and Sideritis clandestina. These plants share similar characteristics and therapeutic properties, contributing to the following health benefits.
Now, let's explore ten extensive health and longevity benefits associated with Greek mountain tea:

1. **Digestive Health:** Greek mountain tea contains flavonoids such as apigenin and luteolin, known for their anti-inflammatory properties that promote digestive health. These compounds soothe the digestive tract, reduce inflammation, and alleviate symptoms of gastrointestinal disorders.
2. **Anti-inflammatory Effects:** Rich in polyphenols like flavonoids and phenolic acids, Greek mountain tea provides potent anti-inflammatory effects. The presence of antioxidants like verbascoside helps combat chronic inflammation, which is linked to various age-related diseases.
3. **Antioxidant Powerhouse:** Greek mountain tea is a source of antioxidants, including flavonoids, phenolic acids, and terpenoids. Active compounds like luteolin and rosmarinic acid neutralize harmful free radicals, safeguarding cells against oxidative damage and supporting longevity.
4. **Immune System Support:** Greek mountain tea contains compounds like flavonoids, terpenes, and phenolic acids that enhance immune function. These components strengthen the body's defense mechanisms, bolster the immune system, and protect against infections and diseases.
5. **Cognitive Support:** Greek mountain tea's antioxidants and bioactive compounds, such as hydroxycinnamic acids and flavonoids, contribute to cognitive health. These substances protect brain cells from oxidative stress, potentially reducing the risk of neurodegenerative disorders and supporting cognitive function.

6. **Cardiovascular Health:** Flavonoids like apigenin found in Greek mountain tea contribute to cardiovascular health. These compounds lower inflammation, improve blood circulation, and support healthy blood pressure levels, indirectly promoting cardiovascular longevity.
7. **Detoxification:** Greek mountain tea's flavonoids and terpenoids, including quercetin and luteolin, assist in liver detoxification processes. They shield liver cells from oxidative stress and aid in the elimination of toxins from the body.
8. **Respiratory Health:** Essential oils present in Greek mountain tea, such as pinenes and thymol, possess antimicrobial and anti-inflammatory properties. These compounds help reduce inflammation and combat respiratory pathogens, supporting respiratory health.
9. **Graceful-aging Effects:** Greek mountain tea's abundant antioxidants, including phenolic acids and flavonoids, combat oxidative stress and minimize cellular damage, key factors in the aging process. By protecting cells and tissues, Greek mountain tea indirectly promotes graceful aging.
10. **Antimicrobial Effects:** Greek mountain tea exhibits antimicrobial activity attributed to its essential oils and phenolic compounds. These properties help inhibit the growth of bacteria and fungi, bolstering the body's defense against harmful pathogens.

While Greek mountain tea is generally considered safe to consume, there are some medical contradictions and precautions to be aware of. Greek mountain tea may interact with certain medications, especially those metabolized by liver enzymes, such as CYP3A4. The tea contains compounds that can affect the metabolism and clearance of medications, potentially leading to increased or decreased levels in the body. It is important to consult with a healthcare professional or pharmacist if you are taking medications that may interact with Greek mountain tea. Individuals with known allergies to plants in the Lamiaceae family, such as mint, basil, and rosemary, should exercise caution and avoid consumption. Greek mountain tea is generally safe in small quantities during pregnancy and lactation, but it is recommended to consult with your herbalist/practitioner before consuming it in large therapeutic doses during these periods.

GUDUCHI

Guduchi, scientifically known as Tinospora cordifolia, is a versatile medicinal plant deeply rooted in Ayurvedic tradition. Originating from the tropical regions of India, Myanmar, and Sri Lanka, guduchi has been treasured for centuries for its remarkable healing properties. Also known as "Amrita" or the "Divine Nectar" in Sanskrit, guduchi is a climbing shrub with heart-shaped leaves and small yellow flowers. The powdered form of guduchi is derived from the stem of the plant and is highly regarded for its extensive health and longevity benefits. In Ayurveda, guduchi is considered a Rasayana, a category of herbs that promote rejuvenation, vitality, and longevity.

Now, let's explore ten extensive health and longevity benefits associated with guduchi:

1. **Immune System Support:** Guduchi contains active compounds such as tinosporin and berberine that enhance the activity of immune cells, strengthen the immune response, and help prevent infections.
2. **Anti-inflammatory Effects:** Guduchi contains compounds like quercetin and tinosporin that possess potent anti-inflammatory properties. These compounds help reduce inflammation, alleviate pain, and manage inflammatory conditions.
3. **Detoxification:** Guduchi contains antioxidants and bioactive compounds that support the body's detoxification processes. It aids in the elimination of toxins, supports liver function, and promotes overall well-being.
4. **Digestive Health:** Guduchi supports digestive health by improving digestion, reducing indigestion, and alleviating gastrointestinal discomfort. Its active compounds help regulate digestive processes and promote a healthy gut.
5. **Respiratory Health:** Guduchi has been traditionally used to support respiratory health. Its active compounds, including tinosporin and cordifolioside, help manage respiratory infections, allergies, and asthma by reducing inflammation and promoting healthy lung function. These compounds possess anti-inflammatory and immunomodulatory properties that can alleviate respiratory symptoms and enhance lung capacity.

6. **Stress Relief:** Guduchi has adaptogenic properties that help the body cope with stress, anxiety, and mental fatigue. Its active compounds support the adrenal glands, promote a sense of calmness and relaxation, and enhance overall well-being.
7. **Liver Health:** Guduchi contains compounds like tinosporin and berberine that protect the liver from toxins and oxidative damage. It supports liver function, aids in detoxification processes, and contributes to liver health.
8. **Skin Health:** Guduchi's antioxidants and active compounds, including tinosporin and berberine, help purify the blood, reduce skin problems, and improve complexion. These substances combat oxidative stress, reduce inflammation, and promote cellular regeneration, resulting in healthy and radiant skin.
9. **Graceful-aging Effects:** Guduchi powder contains antioxidants like flavonoids and polyphenols that combat oxidative stress, reduce cellular damage, and slow down the aging process, promoting youthful vitality.
10. **Joint Health:** Guduchi's anti-inflammatory properties, attributed to compounds such as tinosporin and berberine, help relieve joint pain, stiffness, and inflammation associated with arthritis and other joint disorders.

While guduchi is generally considered safe to consume, there are certain medical contradictions and precautions to be aware of. Guduchi should be used with caution in individuals with autoimmune disorders or those taking immunosuppressive medications, as it may potentially stimulate the immune system. Additionally, guduchi may lower blood sugar levels, so individuals with diabetes or those taking medications for diabetes should monitor their blood sugar closely when using this herb. Those who are pregnant or lactating should consult with their herbalist/practitioner prior to using guduchi during these times.

GYNOSTEMMA

Gynostemma, scientifically known as Gynostemma pentaphyllum and commonly referred to as "Jiaogulan," is a medicinal herb native to the mountainous regions of China, Japan, and Southeast Asia. With a history dating back thousands of years, gynostemma has been treasured in traditional Chinese medicine for its remarkable health-enhancing properties. This climbing vine belongs to the cucumber family and features delicate leaves and small green flowers. Gynostemma is often referred to as the "Herb of Immortality" due to its association with longevity and vitality. It has gained significant attention worldwide for its numerous health benefits.

Now, let's explore ten extensive health and longevity benefits associated with gynostemma:

1. **Adaptogenic Effects:** Gynostemma contains saponins, including gypenosides, which are responsible for its adaptogenic effects. These compounds help the body adapt to stress, promote resilience, and restore balance.
2. **Energy Boost:** Gynostemma supports enhanced energy levels through its active compounds, particularly gypenosides. Gypenosides have been found to have various bioactive effects, including the stimulation of glucose metabolism and the activation of AMP-activated protein kinase (AMPK), an enzyme involved in cellular energy production and metabolism. By activating AMPK, gypenosides can enhance cellular energy production, promote efficient metabolism of nutrients, and contribute to increased energy and vitality.
3. **Immune System Support:** The immune-boosting effects of gynostemma are attributed to its various bioactive compounds, including saponins and polysaccharides. These compounds stimulate and strengthen the immune system, promoting a robust defense against infections and diseases.
4. **Graceful-aging Effects:** Gynostemma's potent flavonoids, including quercetin and kaempferol, along with gypenosides, contribute to its pro-aging effects. These compounds act as antioxidants, helping to neutralize harmful free radicals and protect cells from oxidative stress, a key factor in the aging process. By reducing oxidative damage, gynostemma supports cellular health, minimizes the appearance of wrinkles and fine lines, and promotes a youthful complexion.

5. **Cardiovascular Health:** Gynostemma helps maintain healthy blood pressure and cholesterol levels due to its saponins and flavonoids. These compounds contribute to cardiovascular health and reduce the risk of heart disease.
6. **Stress Response Modulation:** Gynostemma exerts its adaptogenic properties through its active compounds, such as gypenosides. These compounds interact with the body's stress response system, including the hypothalamic-pituitary-adrenal (HPA) axis, which regulates the production and release of stress hormones like cortisol. Gynostemma helps modulate the HPA axis, promoting a balanced stress response and supporting the body's ability to adapt to various stressors.
7. **Liver Health:** Gynostemma promotes liver health by supporting detoxification processes and protecting against liver damage. Its active compounds, such as saponins and flavonoids, contribute to these liver-protective effects.
8. **Respiratory Health:** Gynostemma has been traditionally used to support respiratory health, including the management of asthma, bronchitis, and other respiratory conditions. The active compounds in gynostemma, such as flavonoids and saponins, contribute to its respiratory health benefits.
9. **Mood Support:** Gynostemma supports mental clarity, focus, and overall cognitive function through its active compounds, including gypenosides. These compounds contribute to improved mental well-being and cognitive performance.
10. **Anti-inflammatory Effects:** The active compounds found in gynostemma, including flavonoids, saponins, and notably gypenosides, play a key role in these anti-inflammatory effects. Gypenosides have been shown to inhibit pro-inflammatory mediators and signaling pathways, thereby suppressing the inflammatory response in the body. By modulating the immune system and reducing inflammation, gynostemma may help manage conditions such as arthritis, joint pain, and other inflammatory disorders.

While gynostemma is generally considered safe for consumption, there are certain drug interactions and medical contradictions to consider. Gynostemma may interact with anticoagulant/antiplatelet drugs (e.g., warfarin, aspirin), antidiabetic medications (e.g., insulin, oral hypoglycemic drugs), and immunosuppressant medications. It is advisable to consult with a healthcare professional before using gynostemma if you are taking any prescription medications. Gynostemma has been reported to have hypotensive (blood pressure-lowering) effects. If you are already taking medications for high blood pressure, combining them with gynostemma may further lower blood pressure, potentially leading to complications. Women who are pregnant or lactating should consult with their herbalist/practitioner prior to using this herb.

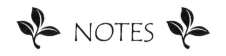

HAWTHORN

Hawthorn, scientifically known as Crataegus, encompasses various species of shrubs and trees. With roots in temperate regions of Europe, Asia, and North America, hawthorn has a rich history woven into diverse cultures. From ancient European herbal practices to traditional Asian medicinal uses, and among indigenous communities in North America, hawthorn has stood the test of time. In Celtic folklore, hawthorn was often associated with magical properties and considered a portal to the fairy realm. It was believed that cutting down a hawthorn tree could bring misfortune, and these trees were sometimes spared even during land development projects. The intertwining of hawthorn with mystical beliefs adds an intriguing layer to its cultural history, showcasing the diverse and captivating ways in which herbs like hawthorn have woven themselves into the fabric of human traditions.

Now, let's explore ten extensive health and longevity benefits associated with hawthorn:

1. **Cardiovascular Health:** Hawthorn leaves and berries contain beneficial compounds that contribute to its cardiovascular support. These include triterpenoids like ursolic acid, as well as flavonoids such as vitexin and hyperoside. These compounds have been studied for their ability to promote healthy blood pressure levels, improve lipid profiles by helping to lower LDL (bad) cholesterol and increase HDL (good) cholesterol, enhance circulation, and support overall heart function.
2. **Antioxidant Powerhouse:** Hawthorn leaves and berries are rich in antioxidants, including procyanidins and flavonoids, which help neutralize free radicals, reduce oxidative stress, and protect cells from damage.
3. **Anti-spasmodic Effects:** Hawthorn leaves and berries contain flavonoids, oligomeric procyanidins, and other compounds that may help dilate blood vessels and improve blood flow. This vasodilatory effect can potentially reduce spasms in blood vessels, leading to enhanced circulation. By preventing or alleviating spasms, hawthorn may contribute to the relaxation of blood vessels and the reduction of blood pressure.
4. **Blood Pressure Regulation:** Both hawthorn leaves and berries exhibit hypotensive properties, thanks to the presence of flavonoids and oligomeric procyanidins. These compounds work together to assist in regulating blood pressure levels.

5. **Digestive Health:** Hawthorn berries are recognized for their digestive benefits, supporting the production of digestive enzymes to aid in food breakdown. This may contribute to easing indigestion and alleviating symptoms of bloating and gas.
6. **Mood Support:** Both hawthorn leaves and berries contribute to the calming effect on the nervous system, attributed to flavonoids like vitexin. This dual combination helps alleviate anxiety, stress, and improves overall mental well-being.
7. **Antimicrobial Effects:** Hawthorn leaves and berries exhibit antimicrobial properties attributed to their active compounds, including flavonoids like vitexin and hyperoside, as well as triterpenic acids. These compounds contribute to the ability of hawthorn to inhibit the growth of certain bacteria and fungi, supporting a healthier immune system and overall well-being.
8. **Cholesterol Management:** Hawthorn leaves and berries have been found to contain compounds like triterpenic acids, which may help lower LDL (bad) cholesterol levels and increase HDL (good) cholesterol levels, promoting a healthier lipid profile.
9. **Anti-inflammatory Effects:** Both hawthorn leaves and berries contain flavonoids and other compounds that possess anti-inflammatory properties, helping to reduce inflammation and alleviate symptoms associated with inflammatory conditions.
10. **Adaptogenic Effects:** The adaptogenic properties of hawthorn are predominantly linked to its vibrant berries. Packed with active compounds like flavonoids, oligomeric proanthocyanidins, and triterpenes, including vitexin, hyperoside, and ursolic acid, hawthorn berries play a key role in modulating stress hormone levels. This, in turn, supports the body's natural ability to cope with stress, fostering a sense of calm and overall well-being.

While hawthorn leaves and berries are generally considered safe to consume, it is important to be aware of certain medical contradictions and precautions. Hawthorn leaves and berries may interact with medications such as beta-blockers, calcium channel blockers, and nitrates, which are commonly prescribed for heart conditions. It is advisable to consult with a healthcare professional before taking hawthorn leaves and berries if you are on any medications or have any underlying medical conditions. Additionally, hawthorn leaves and berries may have hypotensive effects, so caution should be exercised if you have low blood pressure or are already taking medication to lower blood pressure. Individuals with known allergies to plants in the Rosaceae family, such as apples, pears, and cherries, may also be allergic to hawthorn leaves and berries and should avoid its use. Some herbalists suggest that hawthorn leaves and berries may have uterine-stimulating properties, which could potentially lead to contractions. Consult with your herbalist/practitioner prior to incorporating hawthorn leaves and berries into your routine while pregnant or lactating.

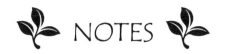
NOTES

HIBISCUS

Hibiscus, scientifically known as Hibiscus rosa-sinensis, is a captivating and vibrant flowering plant with a rich history that spans various cultures and regions. Native to Asia, Africa, and the Pacific Islands, hibiscus has enchanted people with its stunning and distinctive flowers, which come in a wide array of colors, including shades of red, pink, orange, yellow, and white. Notably, it is also the national flower of Malaysia. Throughout history, hibiscus has been esteemed for its diverse uses, from its ornamental beauty in gardens and landscapes to its incorporation in traditional cuisines and beverages in different parts of the world. In various cultures, hibiscus holds special significance, often symbolizing beauty, love, and delicate femininity.

Now, let's explore ten extensive health and longevity benefits associated with hibiscus:

1. **Antioxidant Powerhouse:** Hibiscus flowers are rich in antioxidants, including anthocyanins and flavonoids, which help neutralize free radicals and protect cells from oxidative damage.
2. **Cardiovascular Health:** Flavonoids, such as quercetin and kaempferol, present in hibiscus flowers contribute to their cardiovascular benefits. These compounds help relax blood vessels, lower blood pressure, and reduce LDL cholesterol levels.
3. **Blood Sugar Management:** Hibiscus flowers contain compounds that may help regulate blood sugar levels, including polyphenols and organic acids. These components assist in improving insulin sensitivity and reducing the risk of diabetes.
4. **Digestive Health:** Hibiscus flowers have been traditionally used to support digestive health. Their natural compounds, including mucilage and polyphenols, help soothe the digestive tract, alleviate constipation, and improve overall digestion.
5. **Immune System Support:** The high vitamin C content in hibiscus flowers strengthens the immune system, promoting the production of white blood cells and enhancing immune response against pathogens.
6. **Liver Health:** Hibiscus flowers support liver health by providing antioxidants that protect liver cells from oxidative stress and aid in the detoxification processes of the liver.
7. **Skin Health:** Hibiscus flowers possess natural astringent properties due to their tannin content. This helps tighten pores, improve skin texture, and soothe skin irritations.

8. **Antimicrobial Effects:** The active compounds present in hibiscus flowers, such as organic acids, flavonoids, and polyphenols, contribute to these antimicrobial effects. These compounds can interfere with the growth and reproduction of microorganisms, preventing their proliferation and potentially reducing the risk of infections.
9. **Anxiety Relief:** Hibiscus flowers have calming properties that help reduce anxiety and stress. They promote relaxation by soothing the nervous system and reducing cortisol levels.
10. **Kidney Health:** Hibiscus exhibits diuretic properties due to certain compounds, promoting increased urine production and supporting kidney health. This enhanced urine output aids in efficient waste elimination, benefiting renal function. By promoting fluid balance and urinary flow, hibiscus may reduce the risk of urinary tract infections by flushing out potential pathogens.

While hibiscus is generally considered safe to consume, there are a few medical contradictions and precautions to be aware of. Individuals with low blood pressure should exercise caution when consuming hibiscus, as it may further lower blood pressure levels. Hibiscus can interact with certain medications, particularly antihypertensive drugs, due to its potential hypotensive effects. Additionally, individuals with known allergies to hibiscus or plants in the Malvaceae family, such as marshmallow, okra, and rose of Sharon, should avoid consuming hibiscus. Consult with your herbalist/practitioner prior to using hibiscus during pregnancy and lactation.

HOLY BASIL (KRISHNA TULSI)

Holy basil, also known as Ocimum tenuiflorum or Tulsi, is a sacred herb deeply rooted in the cultural and medicinal traditions of India. Among the various types of holy basil, Krishna Tulsi stands out with its distinct purple or dark green leaves, hence the name "Krishna." Originating from the Indian subcontinent, holy basil has been revered for thousands of years for its spiritual significance and therapeutic properties. Considered a "queen of herbs" in Ayurveda, holy basil offers a myriad of health benefits.

Now, let's explore ten extensive health and longevity benefits associated with holy basil (Krishna):

1. **Adaptogenic Support:** Holy basil (Krishna) contains active compounds such as eugenol and rosmarinic acid, which act as adaptogens, helping the body adapt to stress and enhancing resilience.
2. **Immune System Support:** Holy basil (Krishna) is rich in antioxidants, including flavonoids such as orientin and vicenin, which support a healthy immune system by bolstering the body's defense against infections, viruses, and diseases.
3. **Antioxidant Powerhouse:** The potent antioxidants in holy basil (Krishna), such as eugenol and rosmarinic acid, combat free radicals, reduce oxidative stress, and protect cells from damage, promoting longevity and overall health.
4. **Respiratory Health:** Holy basil (Krishna) contains eugenol, which possesses expectorant and antimicrobial properties that support respiratory health. It helps to alleviate cough, congestion, and respiratory infections.
5. **Anti-inflammatory Effects:** Holy basil (Krishna) contains eugenol and other essential oils with anti-inflammatory properties, assisting in reducing inflammation and alleviating symptoms associated with inflammatory conditions.
6. **Cardiovascular Health:** Eugenol, rosmarinic acid, and flavonoids contribute to its ability to support cardiovascular health. It helps regulate blood pressure, reduce cholesterol levels, and promote healthy blood circulation.
7. **Stress Relief:** Eugenol and other compounds, such as rosmarinic acid and ursolic acid, have calming and stress-reducing effects. These compounds contribute to promoting mental clarity, improving focus, and restoring emotional balance.

8. **Digestive Health:** Eugenol and rosmarinic acid soothe the stomach, reduce bloating, and promote the proper assimilation of nutrients, supporting healthy digestion.
9. **Hormonal Balance:** Holy basil (Krishna) contains compounds like oleanolic acid, ursolic acid, and apigenin that may help regulate hormonal imbalances, particularly in women. These compounds have been found to support menstrual health and alleviate symptoms of menopause, promoting hormonal balance.
10. **Anti-radiation Effects:** This sacred herb is recognized for its potential anti-radiation properties and contains unique bioactive compounds that have been studied for their ability to combat the harmful effects of ionizing radiation in the body. While more research is needed to fully understand the extent of its radioprotective effects, holy basil (Krishna) holds promise as a natural ally in the ongoing efforts to mitigate radiation-related challenges.

> While holy basil (Krishna) is generally considered safe to consume, there are certain medical contradictions and precautions to be aware of. Holy basil (Krishna) may lower blood sugar levels, so individuals with diabetes or those taking medications to regulate blood sugar should exercise caution and monitor their blood sugar levels closely when consuming this herb. Holy basil (Krishna) may have mild blood-thinning effects, so individuals taking blood-thinning medications should consult with their healthcare provider before using this herb. Holy basil (Krishna) belongs to the Lamiaceae family, which includes other plants like mint, rosemary, and sage. Holy basil (Krishna) is generally considered safe during pregnancy and lactation when consumed in small culinary amounts, but it is advisable to consult with your herbalist/practitioner before using it in large therapeutic, supplemental doses, as there may be some potential risk factors to consider. Some herbal traditions suggest that holy basil (Krishna) may have uterine-stimulating properties, which could potentially lead to contractions if used excessively.

HOLY BASIL (RAMA TULSI)

Holy basil, also known as Ocimum tenuiflorum or Tulsi, is a revered herb with a long history rooted in the ancient traditions of India. Among the various types of holy basil, Rama Tulsi stands out with its vibrant green leaves and delightful aroma, making it a prized herb in Ayurvedic medicine. Originating from the Indian subcontinent, holy basil (Rama) has been cherished for centuries for its spiritual significance and therapeutic properties. It is considered a sacred plant and is commonly grown near Hindu temples and households. Holy basil (Rama) offers a plethora of health benefits, making it a valuable addition to any wellness routine.

Now, let's explore ten extensive health and longevity benefits associated with holy basil (Rama):

1. **Stress Relief:** Holy basil (Rama) acts as an adaptogen, helping the body cope with stress and promoting a sense of calm and relaxation. The active compound eugenol contributes to its stress-relieving effects.
2. **Immune System Support:** The presence of flavonoids in holy basil (Rama), such as orientin and vicenin, enhances its immune-boosting properties. These valuable flavonoids are potent antioxidants that play a pivotal role in fortifying the immune system. They not only combat the damaging effects of free radicals but also stimulate the production and activity of vital immune cells, including lymphocytes and macrophages. These immune cells are essential for identifying and eliminating pathogens and foreign invaders within the body, ensuring a robust defense against infections and diseases.
3. **Antioxidant Powerhouse:** Compounds like rosmarinic acid and apigenin contribute to its antioxidant properties. These compounds act as formidable defenders against oxidative stress and free radical damage within the body. Rosmarinic acid, a polyphenol present in holy basil, exhibits exceptional antioxidant capabilities by neutralizing harmful free radicals that can harm cells and DNA. This antioxidant prowess not only promotes overall health but also plays a crucial role in minimizing the risk of chronic illnesses linked to oxidative damage. Additionally, apigenin, a flavonoid found in holy basil, complements its antioxidant effects by further quenching free radicals and enhancing the body's resilience against oxidative stressors.

4. **Respiratory Health:** This herb has expectorant properties that help relieve coughs, and respiratory congestion, promoting clear breathing. The active compound camphene contributes to its expectorant effects.
5. **Anti-inflammatory Effects:** Holy basil (Rama) exhibits potent anti-inflammatory properties attributed to the presence of compounds like ursolic acid and oleanolic acid. These compounds contribute to reducing inflammation in the body and alleviating symptoms associated with inflammatory conditions.
6. **Digestive Health:** Holy basil (Rama) aids in digestion by stimulating the secretion of digestive enzymes, relieving gastrointestinal discomfort, and promoting optimal nutrient absorption. The active compound eugenol contributes to its digestive support.
7. **Cognitive Support:** The presence of compounds like eugenol and ursolic acid contributes to its cognitive-enhancing effects by improving focus, memory, and mental clarity.
8. **Hormonal Balance:** Holy basil (Rama) supports hormonal balance in the body, particularly in women, assisting in regulating menstrual cycles and alleviating symptoms of hormonal imbalances. The active compounds rosmarinic acid and eugenol contribute to its hormonal balancing effects.
9. **Cardiovascular Health:** Holy basil (Rama) offers notable cardiovascular benefits through the presence of compounds such as eugenol and ursolic acid. These active compounds contribute to the regulation of blood pressure, reduction of cholesterol levels, and improvement of blood circulation.
10. **Skin Health:** Holy basil (Rama) purifies the blood and possesses antibacterial properties, contributing to clear and radiant skin. The presence of compounds like eugenol and ursolic acid supports its skin-enhancing effects.

While holy basil (Rama) is generally considered safe to consume, there are a few medical contradictions and precautions to be aware of. Holy basil (Rama) may interact with certain medications, including anticoagulants, antidiabetic drugs, and antihypertensive medications. It is important to consult with a healthcare professional or pharmacist if you are taking any of these medications. Individuals with known allergies to plants in the Lamiaceae family, such as mint or basil, may also be allergic to holy basil (Rama) and should exercise caution. In Ayurveda, some forms of holy basil are traditionally used in limited quantities during pregnancy. Holy basil is considered to have heating properties, and excessive consumption during pregnancy may not be recommended, especially in the early stages when heat can be a concern. Elevated body temperature, especially during the first trimester, may pose certain risks to fetal development. It is recommended to consult with your herbalist/practitioner prior to using holy basil (Rama) during these times.

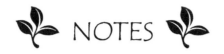

HOLY BASIL (VANA TULSI)

Holy basil, also known as Ocimum tenuiflorum or Tulsi, is a sacred herb with a rich history deeply intertwined with the ancient traditions of India. Among the various types of holy basil, Vana Tulsi stands out with its strong and refreshing fragrance, making it a revered plant in Ayurvedic medicine. Originating from the Indian subcontinent, holy basil (Vana) grows in the wild, flourishing in forests and open fields. This variant of holy basil is cherished for its medicinal properties and spiritual significance. Holy basil (Vana) offers a wide array of health benefits, making it a valuable herb for promoting well-being and longevity.

Now, let's explore ten extensive health and longevity benefits associated with holy basil (Vana):

1. **Stress Relief:** Holy basil (Vana) acts as an adaptogen, supporting the body's ability to cope with stress and promoting a sense of calm and relaxation. The active compounds, including eugenol, contribute to these stress-relieving effects.
2. **Immune System Support:** Holy basil (Vana) strengthens the immune system, helping to ward off infections, viruses, and other diseases. The antioxidants present in holy basil, such as rosmarinic acid, play a role in supporting immune function.
3. **Antioxidant Powerhouse:** The abundant antioxidants in holy basil (Vana) combat free radicals, reducing oxidative stress and promoting cellular health. Compounds like flavonoids and phenols, including apigenin and luteolin, contribute to the antioxidant properties of holy basil (Vana).
4. **Digestive Health:** Eugenol, a compound present in holy basil (Vana), is known for its anti-inflammatory and analgesic properties, which can be particularly beneficial in reducing inflammation and discomfort within the digestive tract. Furthermore, this compound may stimulate the secretion of digestive enzymes, aiding in the efficient breakdown of food and enhancing overall digestive function. In a complementary manner, caryophyllene, a natural component found in holy basil (Vana), has garnered recognition for its gastroprotective attributes, effectively shielding the gastric lining and mitigating the risk of gastric ulcers.
5. **Liver Health:** Holy basil (Vana) supports liver health and aids in detoxification processes, promoting the optimal functioning of this vital organ. Compounds like eugenol and rosmarinic acid may contribute to the liver-supportive properties of this herb.

6. **Respiratory Health:** Camphene and cineole possess expectorant properties that aid in relieving respiratory congestion and coughs, promoting clear breathing.
7. **Anti-inflammatory Effects:** These anti-inflammatory properties are attributed to eugenol, which is said to help reduce inflammation and alleviate various inflammatory conditions. Additionally, compounds like rosmarinic acid and luteolin, present in holy basil (Vana), also contribute significantly to its anti-inflammatory properties. These substances work synergistically to suppress the activity of inflammatory enzymes and pathways, thereby mitigating inflammation and potentially offering relief from various conditions associated with chronic inflammation.
8. **Neuroprotective Support:** Holy Basil (Vana) offers valuable neuroprotective support through its bioactive compounds. Eugenol, one of its key constituents, has demonstrated the ability to safeguard brain cells from damage, promoting optimal cognitive function. Additionally, rosmarinic acid, another component of holy basil, has been linked to enhanced memory and learning capabilities. When combined, these compounds work synergistically to potentially enhance mental clarity and cognitive function.
9. **Hormonal Balance:** Eugenol has been found to have potential estrogenic activity, which may help regulate hormone levels. Apigenin, on the other hand, exhibits anti-estrogenic properties, potentially helping to balance hormone levels by modulating estrogen activity in the body.
10. **Cardiovascular Health:** Holy basil (Vana) promotes heart health by regulating blood pressure, reducing cholesterol levels, and enhancing cardiovascular function. Compounds like eugenol and rosmarinic acid may play a role in supporting cardiovascular health.

While holy basil (Vana) is generally considered safe to consume, there are a few medical contradictions and precautions to be aware of. Holy basil (Vana) may interact with anticoagulant medications, such as warfarin, and medications that affect liver function. Individuals with bleeding disorders or liver conditions should exercise caution and consult with their health care provider prior to using this herb. Some herbal traditions suggest that holy basil (Vana) may have uterine-stimulating properties, which could potentially lead to contractions. It's advisable to consult with your herbalist/practitioner before using this herb during pregnancy and lactation.

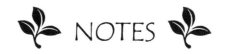

NOTES

HONEYSUCKLE

Honeysuckle, scientifically known as Lonicera, is a beautiful and fragrant flowering plant that has its origins in Asia, Europe, and North America. This climbing vine, with its clusters of vibrant, tubular flowers, has long been appreciated for its aesthetic appeal and enchanting fragrance. In addition to its ornamental value, honeysuckle has a rich history of traditional medicinal use, dating back centuries. This versatile plant is renowned for its numerous health benefits, which can contribute to overall well-being and longevity.

Now, let's explore ten extensive health and longevity benefits associated with honeysuckle:

1. **Anti-inflammatory Effects:** Honeysuckle possesses potent anti-inflammatory compounds such as chlorogenic acid and quercetin. These compounds have been shown to inhibit inflammatory pathways in the body, reducing the production of pro-inflammatory molecules and alleviating inflammation. By doing so, honeysuckle may help alleviate pain and swelling associated with inflammatory conditions.
2. **Immune System Support:** Honeysuckle is rich in antioxidants, including flavonoids and phenolic acids. These antioxidants help neutralize harmful free radicals in the body, which can damage cells and weaken the immune system. Additionally, honeysuckle contains immune-boosting properties, such as polysaccharides, that stimulate the activity of immune cells and enhance the body's defenses against infections and diseases.
3. **Respiratory Health:** Honeysuckle has long been used in traditional medicine for respiratory conditions due to its expectorant and anti-inflammatory effects. The active compound, luteolin, found in honeysuckle, helps loosen mucus and phlegm, making it easier to expel and relieving coughs and congestion. Honeysuckle also contains soothing properties that may help soothe irritated throat tissues, providing relief and aiding in overall respiratory health.
4. **Digestive Health:** Honeysuckle contains compounds such as chlorogenic acid and flavonoids that have been shown to have beneficial effects on the digestive system. These compounds help promote healthy digestion by increasing the production of digestive enzymes, improving nutrient absorption, and reducing digestive discomfort and issues such as bloating and indigestion.

5. **Skin Health:** Honeysuckle possesses antimicrobial properties, primarily due to its active compound, chlorogenic acid. This compound helps inhibit the growth of acne-causing bacteria on the skin, reducing the occurrence of breakouts. Additionally, honeysuckle's anti-inflammatory properties help calm skin inflammation and irritation, promoting a more balanced and youthful complexion.
6. **Antioxidant Powerhouse:** Honeysuckle is packed with antioxidants, including phenolic acids, flavonoids, and carotenoids. These antioxidants help protect cells from oxidative damage caused by free radicals, which can contribute to aging and various diseases. By neutralizing free radicals, honeysuckle's antioxidants reduce oxidative stress, support cellular health, and promote longevity.
7. **Allergy Relief:** Honeysuckle has been traditionally used for its anti-allergic properties. The active compounds, such as chlorogenic acid and quercetin, help inhibit the release of histamine, a compound responsible for allergic reactions. This action may help reduce symptoms associated with allergies, including sneezing, itching, and congestion.
8. **Cardiovascular Health:** Honeysuckle contains active compounds, such as polyphenols and flavonoids, that have been shown to have hypotensive effects. These compounds help relax blood vessels, improve blood flow, and regulate blood pressure. By promoting cardiovascular health and reducing high blood pressure, honeysuckle may lower the risk of heart-related issues.
9. **Antimicrobial Effects:** Honeysuckle possesses antimicrobial properties attributed to compounds like chlorogenic acid and saponins. These compounds have shown effectiveness against various bacteria and viruses, including Staphylococcus aureus and influenza viruses. By inhibiting the growth and spread of harmful microorganisms, honeysuckle supports immune health and helps prevent infections.
10. **Stress Relief:** Honeysuckle has been traditionally used for its calming and soothing properties. The active compound, chlorogenic acid, in honeysuckle has been found to have anxiolytic effects, promoting relaxation and reducing stress. By aiding in stress reduction, honeysuckle contributes to overall mental well-being and helps maintain a balanced state of mind.

While honeysuckle is generally considered safe to consume, there are some medical contradictions and precautions to be aware of. Honeysuckle may interact with certain medications, such as immunosuppressants or anticoagulants, so individuals taking these medications should consult with their healthcare provider before using honeysuckle supplements or products. Additionally, individuals with specific medical conditions such as diabetes, liver disease, or kidney disease should exercise caution and seek medical advice before incorporating honeysuckle into their regimen. Individuals with known allergies to honeysuckle or other plants in the Caprifoliaceae family, such as elderberry or snowberry, should avoid the herb to prevent allergic reactions. It is important to note that honeysuckle berries are toxic and should not be ingested. Women who are pregnant or lactating should consult with their herbalist/practitioner prior to using this herb.

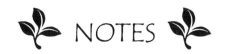

NOTES

HOPS

Hops, scientifically known as Humulus lupulus, is a flowering plant that traces its origins back to ancient civilizations. Native to Europe, hops have been cultivated for centuries and are most famously known for their use in brewing beer. However, beyond their role in the beer-making process, hops have also been recognized for their potential health benefits. These small green flowers, with their distinct aroma and bitter taste, have garnered attention for their therapeutic properties.

Now, let's explore ten extensive health and longevity benefits associated with hops:

1. **Sleep Support:** Hops contain sedative compounds such as xanthohumol and 8-prenylnaringenin that act on GABA receptors in the brain, promoting relaxation and improving sleep quality. These compounds have been shown to have sedative effects, helping to alleviate insomnia symptoms and promote restful sleep.
2. **Anxiety and Stress Relief:** Hops are known to interact with neurotransmitters in the brain, such as GABA and serotonin, which are involved in regulating anxiety and stress.
3. **Anti-inflammatory Effects:** Hops contain potent anti-inflammatory compounds, including humulones and lupulones. These compounds inhibit the activity of pro-inflammatory enzymes, reducing the production of inflammatory molecules and alleviating inflammation in the body. By doing so, hops may benefit conditions such as arthritis by reducing pain and swelling.
4. **Digestive Health:** Hops stimulate gastric secretions, including bile production, which aids in digestion. The bitter acids in hops, such as humulones, have been shown to stimulate the release of digestive enzymes, improving nutrient absorption and reducing gastrointestinal discomfort.
5. **Menopausal Relief:** Hops have been traditionally used to alleviate symptoms associated with menopause. The presence of phytoestrogens in hops, such as 8-prenylnaringenin, may help balance hormone levels and reduce the frequency and intensity of hot flashes, night sweats, and mood swings.
6. **Hormonal Balance:** The phytoestrogens found in hops can interact with estrogen receptors in the body, potentially helping to balance hormone levels, especially in women. This interaction may have a modulating effect on estrogen activity, supporting hormonal balance.

7. **Antioxidant Powerhouse:** Hops are rich in antioxidants, such as flavonoids and phenolic compounds. These antioxidants scavenge free radicals in the body, reducing oxidative stress and protecting cells from damage. By combating free radicals, hops promote overall cellular health and contribute to the body's defense against oxidative damage.
8. **Bone Health:** Hops contain compounds called prenylflavonoids, such as 8-prenylnaringenin, which have shown potential benefits for bone health. These compounds may help enhance bone mineral density and inhibit bone loss, supporting strong and healthy bones.
9. **Anti-cancer Effects:** Studies suggest that hops may have anti-cancer effects due to compounds like xanthohumol. These compounds have demonstrated the ability to inhibit the growth of certain cancer cells and suppress tumor formation.
10. **Respiratory Health:** Hops have been traditionally used to soothe respiratory conditions. The essential oils present in hops, such as humulene and myrcene, possess expectorant and anti-inflammatory properties. These properties help to relieve coughs, congestion, and inflammation in the respiratory tract, promoting respiratory wellness.

While hops are generally considered safe to consume, there are some medical contradictions and precautions to be aware of. Individuals with known allergies to hops or other plants in the Cannabaceae family, such as cannabis or hemp, should avoid the herb to prevent allergic reactions. It is important to note that hops may interact with certain medications, including sedatives, antidepressants, and hormone therapies, so individuals taking these medications should consult with their healthcare provider before using hops supplements or products. Hops may have estrogenic effects, so individuals with hormone-sensitive conditions, such as breast or ovarian cancer, should exercise caution. Consult with your herbalist/practitioner prior to using this herb while pregnant or lactating.

HORSETAIL

Horsetail, scientifically known as Equisetum arvense, is an ancient and unique plant with a history dating back millions of years. Belonging to a family of non-flowering plants, horsetail is a descendant of prehistoric vegetation that once thrived during the Carboniferous period. With its distinctive appearance resembling the tail of a horse, this perennial plant is native to Europe, Asia, and North America. Horsetail has been utilized for centuries due to its potential health benefits and medicinal properties.

Now, let's explore ten extensive health and longevity benefits associated with horsetail:

1. **Bone Health:** Horsetail is rich in silica, a mineral that is essential for the formation and maintenance of strong and healthy bones. Silica plays a crucial role in collagen synthesis, a protein that provides structure and strength to bones. By supplying the body with silica, horsetail supports bone mineralization and may help prevent conditions such as osteoporosis.
2. **Hair and Nail Health:** The high silica content in horsetail contributes to the strength and vitality of hair and nails. Silica helps to strengthen the hair follicles and improve hair thickness, reducing hair brittleness and promoting hair growth. Similarly, silica supports the structure of the nails, reducing nail brittleness and promoting healthier, stronger nails.
3. **Urinary Tract Health:** Horsetail possesses diuretic properties due to its content of compounds like flavonoids and saponins. These diuretic effects help increase urine production and promote the flushing out of toxins from the urinary tract. By assisting in the elimination of waste and supporting urinary tract health, horsetail may be beneficial for individuals with urinary tract infections or kidney stones.
4. **Wound Healing:** Horsetail contains antimicrobial and anti-inflammatory properties attributed to compounds like flavonoids and phenolic acids. These properties may help accelerate wound healing by reducing inflammation and protecting against infections. Additionally, horsetail's high silica content may contribute to tissue repair and regeneration, further supporting the wound healing process.

5. **Skin Health:** Horsetail's antioxidant properties, primarily due to the presence of flavonoids, help protect the skin from free radicals and oxidative stress. By neutralizing free radicals, horsetail promotes a healthy complexion and may reduce the signs of aging. Additionally, its anti-inflammatory effects can soothe skin irritation and inflammation.
6. **Joint and Connective Tissue Support:** Silica, found abundantly in horsetail, supports the health and flexibility of joints and connective tissues. Silica contributes to the formation of collagen, which is a key component of cartilage and other connective tissues. By providing silica, horsetail may benefit individuals with joint conditions like arthritis, as it supports joint health and potentially helps reduce joint pain and stiffness.
7. **Digestive Health:** Horsetail's ability to improve digestion is attributed to its stimulation of digestive enzyme production, primarily due to the presence of plant compounds like flavonoids and saponins. These active compounds in horsetail help increase the secretion of digestive enzymes, such as amylase and lipase, aiding in the breakdown and absorption of nutrients. By enhancing enzymatic activity, horsetail supports efficient digestion and nutrient utilization.
8. **Respiratory Health:** Horsetail has a long history of traditional use for respiratory conditions. Its expectorant properties help to loosen mucus and alleviate coughs, making it useful for respiratory conditions such as bronchitis.
9. **Detoxification:** Horsetail's diuretic properties assist in the elimination of waste products and toxins from the body through increased urine production. This diuretic effect helps support the natural detoxification processes of the body, facilitating the removal of waste materials and promoting overall detoxification.
10. **Antifungal Effects:** Horsetail's antimicrobial properties, primarily attributed to compounds like flavonoids and phenolic acids, can be applied topically to inhibit the growth of fungi that have affected the nails. By doing so, it may promote healthier nail growth and potentially assist in the treatment of nail fungal infections.

While horsetail is generally considered safe to consume, there are some medical contradictions and precautions to be aware of. It is important to note that horsetail contains thiaminase, an enzyme that can break down thiamine (vitamin B1), so excessive and prolonged use of horsetail may lead to thiamine deficiency. Horsetail may interact with certain medications, such as diuretics, lithium, and certain antibiotics, so individuals taking these medications should consult with their healthcare provider before using horsetail. Individuals with specific medical conditions such as kidney disorders, heart conditions, or bleeding disorders should exercise caution and seek medical advice before incorporating horsetail into their regimen. Individuals with known allergies to horsetail or other plants in the Equisetaceae family, such as field horsetail, should avoid the herb to prevent allergic reactions. Women who are pregnant or lactating should consult with their herbalist/practitioner prior to using this herb.

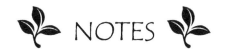

HYSSOP

Hyssop, scientifically known as Hyssopus officinalis, is an ancient and aromatic herb steeped in a fascinating history that dates back to ancient civilizations. Native to the Mediterranean region and parts of Asia, hyssop has been revered for its multitude of uses and symbolic significance. This herb's name likely refers to its associations with purification rituals and religious ceremonies. Throughout history, hyssop has been mentioned in various religious texts, including the Bible, where it symbolizes cleansing and spiritual purification. Renowned for its pleasant and refreshing fragrance, hyssop has been utilized in traditional medicine, culinary arts, and even perfumery. Its delicate blue flowers and slender, woody stems have made it a popular choice for ornamental gardening and attracting pollinators.

Now, let's explore ten extensive health and longevity benefits associated with hyssop:

1. **Respiratory Health:** Hyssop contains compounds such as pinocamphone and myrcene that possess expectorant and bronchodilator properties. These properties help to loosen mucus, clear congestion, and open up the airways, making it beneficial for relieving coughs, congestion, and bronchitis. By promoting clearer breathing, hyssop supports overall respiratory wellness.
2. **Digestive Health:** The essential oils found in hyssop, including pinocamphone and thymol, have carminative properties. These properties help soothe the digestive system, alleviate digestive discomfort, and relieve gas. By promoting healthy digestion and reducing gastrointestinal issues, hyssop supports overall digestive health.
3. **Anti-inflammatory Effects:** Rosmarinic acid and caffeic acid exhibit anti-inflammatory properties. These compounds help reduce inflammation in the body by inhibiting the production of pro-inflammatory molecules. By doing so, hyssop may alleviate symptoms associated with inflammation and promote overall well-being.
4. **Cognative Support:** Hyssop has been traditionally used to enhance mental focus and clarity. The essential oils in hyssop, including pinocamphone and myrcene, possess stimulating properties that can improve concentration and cognitive function. By promoting mental clarity, hyssop may help support cognitive performance and enhance mental well-being.

5. **Immune System Support:** Hyssop is known for its antimicrobial and antioxidant properties. Compounds such as rosmarinic acid and caffeic acid present in hyssop possess antimicrobial effects, helping to inhibit the growth of bacteria and other microbes. Additionally, the antioxidants in hyssop, including flavonoids and phenolic acids, help strengthen the immune system and protect against oxidative stress, supporting overall immune health and defending against microbial infections.
6. **Antioxidant Powerhouse:** Hyssop is rich in antioxidants, such as flavonoids, phenolic acids, and rosmarinic acid. These antioxidants help combat free radicals, reducing oxidative stress and promoting overall cellular health. By neutralizing free radicals, hyssop contributes to the body's defense against oxidative damage and supports overall well-being.
7. **Detoxification:** Hyssop has diuretic properties attributed to compounds like pinocamphone and myrcene. These properties stimulate urine production and promote the elimination of toxins from the body. By supporting the body's detoxification processes, hyssop aids in the removal of waste materials and contributes to overall detoxification.
8. **Skin Health:** Hyssop's antimicrobial and anti-inflammatory properties, primarily due to compounds like rosmarinic acid and thymol, make it beneficial for treating skin conditions such as acne, eczema, and dermatitis. These properties help inhibit the growth of bacteria, reduce inflammation, and promote healthier skin.
9. **Stress Relief:** The soothing aroma of hyssop, attributed to compounds like pinocamphone and myrcene, has calming effects on the mind and body. It helps to alleviate stress, promote relaxation, and enhance a sense of well-being. By reducing stress levels, hyssop contributes to overall mental and emotional balance.
10. **Menstrual Support:** Hyssop has been traditionally used to regulate menstrual cycles and relieve symptoms associated with menstruation. Its compounds, including rosmarinic acid, may help regulate hormone levels and alleviate menstrual discomfort, such as cramps and mood swings.

While hyssop is generally considered safe to consume, there are some medical contradictions and precautions to be aware of. Hyssop should be used with caution or avoided by individuals with epilepsy, asthma, or seizure disorders, as it contains compounds such as pinocamphone and camphor that may potentially trigger seizures or asthma symptoms in susceptible individuals. Additionally, hyssop may interact with certain medications, including anticoagulants and anticonvulsants, so it is important for individuals taking these medications to consult with their healthcare provider before using hyssop. It is crucial to note that individuals with known allergies to hyssop or other plants in the Lamiaceae family, such as mint or basil, should avoid hyssop to prevent allergic reactions. Women who are pregnant or lactating should consult with their herbalist/practitioner prior to using this herb.

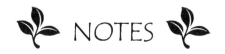

INDIAN SARSAPARILLA

Indian sarsaparilla, scientifically known as Hemidesmus indicus, is a species of medicinal plant native to the Indian subcontinent. With a rich history deeply rooted in Ayurvedic medicine, Indian sarsaparilla has been revered for centuries for its numerous health benefits and contributions to longevity. Extracted from the root of the plant, this versatile herb is renowned for its potent medicinal properties.

Now, let's explore ten extensive health and longevity benefits associated with Indian sarsaparilla:

1. **Blood Cleansing:** Indian sarsaparilla contains compounds such as saponins and flavonoids that promote blood purification. These active compounds help stimulate liver and kidney function, supporting the removal of toxins and impurities from the bloodstream.
2. **Anti-inflammatory Effects:** Indian sarsaparilla has a history of traditional use for its potential anti-inflammatory properties, often attributed to compounds like sarsaponin and pterostilbene. Anecdotal references suggest its effectiveness in alleviating inflammation associated with conditions like arthritis, joint pain, and inflammatory skin disorders.
3. **Digestive Health:** Indian sarsaparilla aids in digestion by stimulating the production of digestive enzymes such as amylase and lipase. These enzymes facilitate the breakdown of carbohydrates and fats, promoting efficient digestion and nutrient absorption. Additionally, Indian sarsaparilla supports gut health by promoting a favorable environment for beneficial gut bacteria. This helps alleviate digestive disorders like indigestion, bloating, and constipation.
4. **Immune System Support:** This herb contains compounds like saponins and flavonoids that help modulate the immune response, supporting the body's defense against infections, allergies, and autoimmune conditions.
5. **Graceful-aging Effects:** Indian sarsaparilla is rich in antioxidants, including polyphenols and flavonoids, which combat free radicals and reduce oxidative stress. By neutralizing free radicals, Indian sarsaparilla helps prevent cellular and tissue damage, thereby slowing down the aging process. The herb's antioxidant properties contribute to maintaining youthful-looking skin and overall cellular health.

6. **Skin Health:** Indian sarsaparilla has been traditionally used for its skin-enhancing benefits. The herb's anti-inflammatory and antioxidant properties help soothe skin inflammation and combat skin conditions such as eczema, psoriasis, and acne. Indian sarsaparilla promotes a healthy complexion and supports overall skin health.
7. **Hormonal Balance:** Indian sarsaparilla is believed to have hormonal balancing properties, particularly in women, due to the presence of compounds such as sarsasapogenin and diosgenin. These compounds are phytoestrogens, plant-based substances that have a similar structure to estrogen. Phytoestrogens can bind to estrogen receptors in the body and modulate estrogen activity. By doing so, Indian sarsaparilla may help regulate hormonal activity and promote hormonal balance. This hormonal balance may alleviate symptoms associated with menstrual irregularities, such as irregular periods and hormonal imbalances, as well as menopausal symptoms, like hot flashes, mood swings, and sleep disturbances.
8. **Respiratory Health:** Indian sarsaparilla aids in respiratory health by soothing respiratory tract inflammation. Its anti-inflammatory properties help alleviate symptoms of cough, bronchitis, and asthma, promoting clear and healthy respiration.
9. **Liver Health:** Indian sarsaparilla exhibits hepatoprotective properties through the presence of compounds like saponins, flavonoids, and phenolic acids. These bioactive compounds help protect the liver from damage caused by toxins and oxidative stress. Indian sarsaparilla supports liver health by enhancing the activity of antioxidant enzymes, such as superoxide dismutase and glutathione peroxidase, which help neutralize harmful free radicals and reduce oxidative stress in the liver. Additionally, the herb supports liver detoxification processes by stimulating the production of phase II detoxification enzymes, such as glutathione-S-transferase, aiding in the elimination of toxins from the body.
10. **Energy and Vitality:** Indian sarsaparilla is known for its energizing properties, which may be attributed to its bioactive compounds, such as saponins, alkaloids, and tannins. These compounds may help stimulate the central nervous system, increase blood circulation, and enhance overall metabolic processes in the body.

While Indian sarsaparilla is generally considered safe to consume, there are some medical contradictions and precautions to be aware of. Indian sarsaparilla should be used with caution or avoided by individuals with a history of hormone-sensitive conditions, such as breast, ovarian, or uterine cancer, as the herb contains phytoestrogens that may potentially affect hormone levels. It is important to note that Indian sarsaparilla may interact with certain medications, including hormonal therapies and anticoagulants, so individuals taking these medications should consult with their healthcare provider before using Indian sarsaparilla. Individuals with known allergies to plants in the Apocynaceae family, such as oleander or periwinkle, should exercise caution when considering the use of Indian sarsaparilla. While cross-reactivity between species in the same family is less common than within closely related species, it's always prudent to be cautious if you have known sensitivities. Women who are pregnant or lactating should consult with their herbalist/practitioner prior to using this herb.

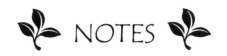

NOTES

JAMAICAN DOGWOOD

Jamaican dogwood, scientifically known as Piscidia piscipula, is a tropical tree native to the Caribbean region, particularly Jamaica. With a history deeply rooted in traditional medicine practices of the indigenous peoples, Jamaican dogwood has gained recognition for its remarkable health benefits and contributions to longevity. The bark, root, and leaves of this tree have been utilized for centuries to alleviate various ailments and promote overall well-being.

Now, let's explore ten extensive health and longevity benefits associated with Jamaican dogwood:

1. **Pain Relief:** Jamaican dogwood contains active compounds like iridoid glycosides and flavonoids that possess analgesic properties. These compounds interact with pain receptors in the body, blocking pain signals and providing relief from migraines, neuralgia, toothaches, and menstrual cramps.
2. **Muscle Relaxant:** Jamaican dogwood acts as a natural muscle relaxant due to the presence of compounds such as isoflavones and tannins. These compounds help relax muscle fibers, reduce spasms, and alleviate muscle-related discomfort, making it valuable for individuals with muscle cramps, spasms, and tension.
3. **Sedative and Sleep Aid:** This herb exhibits sedative effects attributed to compounds like flavonoids and valerianic acid. These compounds interact with neurotransmitters in the brain, such as GABA, promoting relaxation and aiding in sleep. By calming the nervous system, Jamaican dogwood can be beneficial for individuals experiencing insomnia or sleep disturbances.
4. **Anxiety and Stress Relief:** Jamaican dogwood has a long history of use in traditional medicine for alleviating anxiety and stress-related symptoms. The herb contains compounds like tannins and resins that have a calming effect on the nervous system, helping to reduce anxiety and promote a sense of tranquility.
5. **Menstrual Support:** This herb contains compounds such as flavonoids and tannins that exhibit muscle relaxant and antispasmodic properties. These properties help reduce excessive uterine contractions and muscle spasms associated with menstrual cramps. By relaxing the uterine muscles, Jamaican dogwood may help alleviate pain and discomfort during menstruation. Its antispasmodic effects may contribute to regulating irregular menstrual cycles.

6. **Anti-inflammatory Effects:** Jamaican dogwood possesses anti-inflammatory properties due to compounds such as tannins and flavonoids. These compounds help reduce inflammation and swelling in the body by inhibiting pro-inflammatory molecules. By alleviating inflammation, Jamaican dogwood can provide relief from conditions such as arthritis, gout, and joint pain.
7. **Antispasmodic Effects:** Jamaican dogwood has antispasmodic properties attributed to compounds like isoflavones and valerianic acid. These compounds help relax smooth muscles, including those in the digestive tract, reducing spasms and alleviating conditions like irritable bowel syndrome (IBS) and menstrual cramps.
8. **Nervous System Support:** This herb contains compounds like flavonoids and resins that help soothe nervous tension and promote relaxation. Jamaican dogwood's calming properties can be beneficial for individuals experiencing nervousness, restlessness, or mild anxiety.
9. **Respiratory Health:** Jamaican dogwood has been traditionally used to address respiratory issues. Its anti-inflammatory properties help reduce inflammation in the respiratory system, while its relaxant effects promote bronchial relaxation. These actions can be beneficial for conditions such as coughs, bronchitis, and asthma.
10. **Antimicrobial Effects:** Jamaican dogwood exhibits antimicrobial effects due to compounds such as tannins and flavonoids. These compounds may help inhibit the growth of bacteria and fungi, potentially aiding in the treatment of bacterial and fungal infections.

While Jamaican dogwood is generally considered safe to consume, there are some medical contradictions and precautions to be aware of. Jamaican dogwood should be used with caution or avoided by individuals with a history of liver disease or impaired liver function, as the herb may have potential hepatotoxic effects. This caution is due to the presence of compounds such as rotenoids in Jamaican dogwood, which can interact with liver enzymes and potentially lead to liver damage or exacerbation of existing liver conditions if consumed in large doses or for prolonged periods. It is important to note that Jamaican dogwood may interact with certain medications, including sedatives, anticoagulants, and antiplatelet drugs, so individuals taking these medications should consult with their healthcare provider before using Jamaican dogwood. Additionally, individuals with known allergies to plants in the Fabaceae family, such as soybeans, peanuts, or lentils, may have an increased risk of allergic reactions to Jamaican dogwood. Pregnant and lactating women should avoid Jamaican dogwood.

NOTES

JAMAICAN SARSAPARILLA

Jamaican sarsaparilla, also known as Smilax regelii, is a species of vine native to the tropical regions of Jamaica and other parts of the Caribbean. With a history deeply rooted in traditional Jamaican and Ayurvedic medicine, Jamaican sarsaparilla has gained recognition for its extensive health benefits and contributions to longevity. This versatile herb, extracted from the root of the vine, has been valued for centuries for its potent medicinal properties.

Now, let's explore ten extensive health and longevity benefits associated with Jamaican sarsaparilla:

1. **Blood Cleansing:** Jamaican sarsaparilla contains specific saponins known as smilasaponins. These compounds have demonstrated diuretic properties that can assist in eliminating toxins and impurities from the blood, potentially contributing to overall detoxification processes in the body.
2. **Anti-inflammatory Effects:** The powerful anti-inflammatory properties of Jamaican sarsaparilla can be attributed to compounds such as polyphenols and tannins. These compounds help reduce inflammation by inhibiting pro-inflammatory enzymes and cytokines, providing relief from conditions like arthritis and joint pain.
3. **Digestive Health:** Jamaican sarsaparilla stimulates the production of digestive enzymes, including proteases, lipases, and amylases. These enzymes aid in the breakdown of food, improve nutrient absorption, and help to alleviate digestive discomforts such as bloating and indigestion.
4. **Liver Health:** Jamaican sarsaparilla exhibits hepatoprotective qualities that can be attributed to its rich content of flavonoids and terpenes. These bioactive compounds are thought to play a crucial role in bolstering liver health by enhancing liver function, potentially by aiding in the efficient breakdown of toxins and metabolic waste. Moreover, they are believed to promote detoxification processes within the liver, enabling it to more effectively rid the body of harmful substances. Additionally, the presence of these compounds in Jamaican sarsaparilla is believed to act as a shield, guarding the liver against potential damage from oxidative stress and various toxins, contributing to the overall well-being of this vital organ.

5. **Kidney Health:** Jamaican sarsaparilla may support kidney health and promote urinary system health through the presence of active compounds such as saponins and flavonoids. These compounds are believed to have diuretic properties, which can increase urine production and help in the elimination of waste and toxins from the body.
6. **Hormonal Balance:** Jamaican sarsaparilla contains compounds like steroidal saponins that may have hormone-modulating effects. These compounds can potentially help regulate hormonal imbalances, alleviate symptoms of PMS, and promote reproductive health.
7. **Skin Health:** Jamaican sarsaparilla's benefits for skin health are due to its antioxidant and anti-inflammatory properties. These properties help reduce inflammation, soothe skin conditions like acne and eczema, and contribute to a healthier complexion.
8. **Respiratory Health:** The anti-inflammatory and expectorant properties of Jamaican sarsaparilla may help soothe respiratory tract inflammation, ease coughing, and alleviate symptoms of bronchitis and asthma.
9. **Enhances Libido and Sexual Health:** Jamaican sarsaparilla contains saponins, which are phytochemicals that can influence various physiological processes. Some saponins have been associated with potential effects on libido and sexual performance. Saponins may interact with certain receptors in the body, including those involved in the regulation of sex hormones. By modulating hormone levels and promoting hormonal balance, Jamaican sarsaparilla may have a positive impact on libido and sexual desire.
10. **Antioxidant Powerhouse:** Jamaican sarsaparilla boasts an impressive arsenal of antioxidants, including flavonoids, phenolic acids, and various polyphenols. These compounds collectively form a formidable defense against oxidative stress and its detrimental effects. By effectively scavenging harmful free radicals, Jamaican sarsaparilla's antioxidants play a pivotal role in safeguarding the body's cells from oxidative damage, ultimately contributing to the reduction of the risk of premature aging and the development of chronic diseases. These natural protectors not only help maintain cellular integrity but also serve as a shield against the wear and tear of daily life, supporting the body's long-term health and vitality.

While Jamaican sarsaparilla is generally considered safe to consume, there are several medical contradictions and important warnings to be aware of. It is advisable to avoid Jamaican sarsaparilla if you have a history of hormone-sensitive conditions such as breast or ovarian cancer, as the herb may have estrogenic effects. Regarding drug interactions, Jamaican sarsaparilla may interfere with anticoagulant medications, increasing the risk of bleeding. There is limited information available on specific allergy warnings for Jamaican sarsaparilla, but individuals with known allergies to plants in the Smilacaceae family, such as the common greenbrier or carrion flower, should exercise caution when using Jamaican sarsaparilla. Consult with your herbalist/practitioner prior to using this herb while pregnant or lactating.

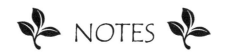

NOTES

JUJUBE SEED

Jujube seed, scientifically known as Ziziphus jujuba, have a rich history and origin that dates back thousands of years. These seeds trace their roots to ancient China, where they were revered for their medicinal properties and were widely used in traditional Chinese medicine. The jujube tree is native to China and has been cultivated for over 4,000 years, making it one of the oldest known fruits. This small, oval-shaped fruit has a sweet and chewy texture, and its seeds have gained recognition for their numerous health and longevity benefits.

Now, let's explore ten extensive health and longevity benefits associated with jujube seed:

1. **Liver Health:** Jujube seeds contain saponins and flavonoids that have been associated with hepatoprotective properties, promoting liver health and function. These compounds contribute to the protective effects on the liver, helping to maintain its well-being and supporting its vital functions.
2. **Digestive Health:** The fiber content in jujube seeds promotes healthy digestion and helps prevent constipation. They also contain polysaccharides that support the growth of beneficial gut bacteria, contributing to a balanced gut microbiome.
3. **Immune System Support:** Jujube seeds are rich in antioxidants, including phenolic compounds like chlorogenic acid, which help neutralize harmful free radicals and strengthen the immune system.
4. **Cardiovascular Health:** The flavonoids and saponins in jujube seeds have been shown to have cardioprotective effects by reducing inflammation, lowering blood pressure, and improving cholesterol levels.
5. **Brain Health:** Jujube seeds contain flavonoids and triterpenes that possess neuroprotective properties. These compounds help protect brain cells from oxidative stress, potentially reducing the risk of neurodegenerative diseases.
6. **Sleep Support:** Jujube seeds contain natural sedatives, such as flavonoids and saponins, that help promote relaxation and improve sleep quality. They also contain compounds that may regulate sleep-wake cycles.
7. **Skin Health:** Jujube seeds are a rich source of vitamin C and various antioxidants, which help protect the skin against oxidative damage, promote collagen synthesis, and maintain skin elasticity.

8. **Respiratory Health:** Jujube seeds contain flavonoids and other bioactive compounds that possess anti-inflammatory properties. These properties contribute to reducing inflammation in the respiratory system, potentially alleviating respiratory discomfort and promoting respiratory health. These compounds work together to support a healthy respiratory system and may provide benefits for individuals dealing with respiratory issues such as inflammation, coughs, or other respiratory conditions.
9. **Anxiety and Stress Relief:** Jujube seeds contain bioactive compounds, including flavonoids and saponins, that have been associated with calming properties and potential anti-anxiety effects. These compounds may help reduce stress levels and promote emotional well-being by modulating neurotransmitters and receptors in the brain. The flavonoids and saponins in jujube seeds have the ability to interact with GABA receptors, which are involved in promoting relaxation and reducing anxiety.
10. **Antimicrobial Effects:** Jujube seeds contain various bioactive compounds, including triterpenoids, flavonoids, and polysaccharides, which have shown potential antiviral, antibacterial, and antifungal activities, contributing to overall immune support and protection against microbial infections.

> While jujube seeds are generally considered safe to consume, there are certain medical contradictions and precautions to be aware of. Individuals with diabetes or hypoglycemia should exercise caution when using jujube seeds, as they may lower blood sugar levels. Jujube seeds may interact with medications that affect blood sugar levels or have sedative effects, so it is important to seek medical advice if taking such medications. It is worth noting that jujube seeds belong to the same family as other fruits in the Rhamnaceae family, which includes buckthorns and jujube trees, so individuals with known allergies to these plants should exercise caution. Pregnant or breastfeeding women should consult with their herbalist/practitioner prior to using jujube seeds.

JUNIPER BERRIES

Juniper berries, scientifically known as Juniperus communis, have a captivating history that stretches back through the ages. These small, dark purple berries come from the juniper shrub, a coniferous plant that is native to regions across the Northern Hemisphere, including Europe, North America, and parts of Asia. Juniper berries have been utilized for a myriad of purposes by various cultures throughout time. In ancient times, they held significant value as a medicinal herb, food source, and even as a flavoring agent for alcoholic beverages. Juniper berries were believed to possess protective qualities and were used in ceremonies and rituals to ward off negative energies.

Now, let's explore ten extensive health and longevity benefits associated with juniper berries:

1. **Digestive Health:** Juniper berries contain terpenes, including alpha-pinene and limonene, which exhibit digestive-stimulating properties. These compounds may help improve digestion, reduce bloating, and alleviate gastrointestinal discomfort.
2. **Detoxification:** The diuretic properties of juniper berries, attributed to the compound terpinen-4-ol, promote increased urine production, aiding in the elimination of toxins and waste products from the body. This can support healthy kidney function and overall detoxification.
3. **Immune System Support:** Juniper berries are rich in antioxidants, such as flavonoids and vitamin C. These compounds help to neutralize harmful free radicals, strengthening the immune system and reducing the risk of oxidative stress-related damage.
4. **Urinary Tract Health:** The diuretic and antimicrobial properties of juniper berries may help prevent and treat urinary tract infections. The active compounds, including terpinen-4-ol and alpha-pinene, assist in flushing out bacteria and reducing inflammation in the urinary system.
5. **Cardiovascular Health:** Juniper berries contain antioxidants that help reduce oxidative stress and prevent the oxidation of LDL cholesterol. This can contribute to improved heart health and a reduced risk of cardiovascular diseases.
6. **Antimicrobial Effects:** The essential oil of juniper berries, containing terpinen-4-ol, has shown antimicrobial activity against certain harmful bacteria, such as H. pylori. This property may be beneficial in managing digestive disorders associated with bacterial overgrowth.

7. **Respiratory Health:** Juniper berries contain compounds like alpha-pinene and limonene, which have expectorant and antimicrobial properties. These properties may help soothe respiratory conditions, support healthy lung function, and relieve coughs and congestion.
8. **Anti-inflammatory Effects:** The essential oil derived from juniper berries contains alpha-pinene, a compound known for its anti-inflammatory properties. This may help reduce inflammation in the body, supporting joint health and potentially reducing the risk of chronic diseases.
9. **Skin Health:** Juniper berries possess antibacterial and antifungal properties, thanks to compounds like terpinen-4-ol and alpha-terpineol. These properties may help cleanse and protect the skin from bacterial or fungal infections, promoting a clear and healthy complexion.
10. **Graceful-aging Effects:** The antioxidants present in juniper berries, including flavonoids and vitamin C, help combat free radicals and protect against premature aging. These compounds may help maintain youthful skin, promote longevity, and support overall cellular health.

While juniper berries are generally considered safe for consumption, there are certain medical contradictions and precautions to be aware of. Juniper berries should be avoided by individuals with gastrointestinal inflammation or ulcers as they may irritate the stomach lining. Juniper berries may also interact with certain medications, including diuretics, lithium, and medications metabolized by the liver. It is important to consult with a healthcare professional if you have any underlying medical conditions or are taking medications to ensure the safe use of juniper berries. Allergy to juniper berries is rare but possible, and individuals with known allergies to other plants in the Cupressaceae family, such as cypress or cedar, may be at a higher risk of developing an allergic reaction. Additionally, juniper berries should not be used during pregnancy due to their potential uterine-stimulating properties, which could lead to complications. Those who are lactating should consult with their herbalist/practitioner prior to using juniper berries.

KAVA KAVA

Kava kava, scientifically known as Piper methysticum, is a plant native to the South Pacific islands, where it has been utilized for centuries in traditional cultural practices. The roots of the kava kava plant are the main part used for their medicinal properties. The roots were traditionally ground and mixed with water to create a beverage that was consumed for its sedative and anxiolytic effects.

Now, let's explore ten extensive health and longevity benefits associated with kava kava:

1. **Anxiety Relief:** Kava kava contains kavalactones, such as kavain, dihydrokavain, and methysticin, which interact with the brain's receptors, promoting relaxation and helping to reduce anxiety.
2. **Sleep Support:** Kavalactones in kava kava have sedative properties that may help promote better sleep quality and support healthy sleep patterns.
3. **Stress Relief:** The active compounds in kava kava may help alleviate stress by acting as an anxiolytic, modulating neurotransmitters in the brain, such as GABA, which promotes a calming effect.
4. **Liver Health:** Kava kava has hepatoprotective properties and contains flavokavains, which may help support liver health by promoting detoxification and protecting against oxidative stress.
5. **Mood Support:** Kavalactones, particularly yangonin and desmethoxyyangonin, can stimulate dopamine receptors in the brain, contributing to an improved mood and overall sense of well-being.
6. **Respiratory Health:** Kava kava's anti-inflammatory properties, attributed to kavalactones, may help reduce inflammation in the respiratory system, supporting lung health and respiratory function.
7. **Muscle Relaxation:** Kavalactones in kava kava exhibit muscle relaxant properties, which may help alleviate muscle tension and support overall musculoskeletal health.
8. **Urinary Tract Health:** Kava kava has diuretic properties attributed to compounds like flavokavains, which may help promote a healthy urinary tract and support proper kidney function.
9. **Digestive Health:** Kava kava has been traditionally used to support digestive health. Compounds like kavalactones may help relax smooth muscles in the digestive system, aiding in digestion and relieving gastrointestinal discomfort.

10. **Immune System Support:** Kava kava contains compounds like yangonin and kavain, which have been shown to possess immunomodulatory properties, potentially supporting a healthy immune response.

> While kava kava is generally considered safe to consume in small quantities, it is important to be aware of certain contradictions and potential interactions. Kava kava may interact with medications that affect the central nervous system, such as sedatives, anxiolytics, and antipsychotics. Individuals with liver disease, a history of liver problems, or those who consume alcohol regularly should avoid the use of kava kava. Allergy to kava kava is rare but possible, and individuals with known allergies to plants in the Piperaceae family, such as black pepper or piperine, may be at an increased risk of allergic reactions. Prolonged and excessive use of kava kava has been associated with adverse effects on the liver, including hepatotoxicity. It is advisable to use kava kava in small quantities and for short durations. If you are pregnant or breastfeeding, it's best to avoid this herb unless otherwise directed by your herbalist/ practitioner.

KELP

Kelp, a type of large brown seaweed, has a fascinating origin rooted in the oceanic depths. It is found in coastal regions across the globe and has been a staple in the diets of various cultures throughout history. From Asia to Europe, kelp has been utilized for its rich nutritional profile and potential health benefits.

Now, let's explore ten extensive health and longevity benefits associated with kelp:

1. **Thyroid Health:** Kelp is a rich source of iodine, a vital nutrient for optimal thyroid function. Iodine is essential for the synthesis of thyroid hormones.
2. **Immune System Support:** Kelp contains various compounds, including fucoidan, which have been shown to exhibit antiviral, antibacterial, and anti-inflammatory properties. These properties help support a healthy immune system and protect against infections.
3. **Detoxification:** The natural compounds present in kelp, such as alginates, bind to heavy metals and other toxins in the body, aiding in their removal. This helps support liver health and overall detoxification processes.
4. **Cardiovascular Health:** Kelp is a good source of omega-3 fatty acids, specifically eicosapentaenoic acid (EPA) and docosahexaenoic acid (DHA). These fatty acids have been linked to a reduced risk of heart disease, improved blood lipid profiles, and decreased inflammation.
5. **Bone Health:** Kelp is rich in minerals like calcium, magnesium, and potassium, which are essential for maintaining strong and healthy bones. These minerals contribute to bone density and help prevent conditions such as osteoporosis.
6. **Digestive Health:** The dietary fiber present in kelp, including alginate, promotes healthy digestion and supports regular bowel movements. It can also help manage cholesterol levels by binding to bile acids in the digestive tract.
7. **Nutrient Dense:** Kelp's rich nutritional profile, including vitamins, minerals, antioxidants, and other bioactive compounds, contributes to overall health and longevity. Its diverse array of nutrients supports various organ systems, such as the thyroid, immune system, cardiovascular system, and brain, helping to promote vitality and well-being.

8. **Brain Function:** Kelp contains essential nutrients like folate, and omega-3 fatty acids, which are important for brain health and cognitive function. These nutrients support neuronal communication and help protect against age-related cognitive decline.
9. **Anti-inflammatory Effects:** Kelp contains fucoxanthin, a carotenoid with potent anti-inflammatory properties. It helps reduce inflammation in the body, supporting joint health and reducing the risk of chronic diseases associated with inflammation.
10. **Skin Health:** The high mineral content in kelp, including zinc and antioxidants like vitamins C and E, promotes healthy skin by nourishing and protecting it from oxidative stress. These nutrients help maintain skin elasticity and support a youthful appearance.

While kelp is generally considered safe to consume, there are certain medical contradictions and precautions to be aware of. Those with bleeding disorders or taking anticoagulant medications should use kelp with caution, as it may have anticoagulant properties and interact with blood-thinning medications. It is important to note that kelp belongs to the seaweed family, which includes other species such as kombu, wakame, and nori. Individuals with allergies to seafood or iodine may also be at risk of allergic reactions to kelp. It is also crucial to source kelp from the Atlantic Ocean to avoid higher levels of contamination from pollutants in the Pacific Ocean. Those who are pregnant or lactating should consult with their herbalist/practitioner prior to consuming kelp in large quantities or for prolonged periods.

KNOTTED WRACK

Knotted wrack, scientifically known as Ascophyllum nodosum, is a brown seaweed with a long history of use and is known for its remarkable health benefits. This seaweed is found in the cold, rocky shores of the North Atlantic Ocean, particularly along the coasts of Europe and North America. Knotted wrack has been revered for centuries for its potent therapeutic properties and has been an integral part of traditional coastal cultures. The health benefits of knotted wrack are attributed to its rich nutritional profile. It is packed with essential vitamins, minerals, antioxidants, and other bioactive compounds that contribute to its medicinal properties. Knotted wrack contains a wide array of minerals, including iodine, potassium, magnesium, calcium, and iron, which are vital for overall health and well-being.

Now, let's explore ten extensive health and longevity benefits associated with knotted wrack:

1. **Thyroid Health:** Knotted wrack is rich in iodine, a crucial nutrient for optimal thyroid function. Adequate iodine intake helps support the production of thyroid hormones, which play a vital role in regulating metabolism, energy levels, and overall growth and development.
2. **Digestive Health:** Knotted wrack contains fucoidan, a unique polysaccharide with prebiotic properties. Fucoidan nourishes beneficial gut bacteria, supporting a healthy gut microbiome and promoting optimal digestion and nutrient absorption.
3. **Anti-inflammatory Effects:** The presence of various antioxidants in knotted wrack, including phlorotannins, fucoxanthin, and fucoidan, contributes to its potent anti-inflammatory effects. These compounds help reduce chronic inflammation, which is associated with various age-related diseases.
4. **Cardiovascular Health:** Knotted wrack provides essential minerals such as magnesium, potassium, and calcium, which are beneficial for cardiovascular health. These minerals help maintain healthy blood pressure levels, support proper heart function, and promote overall cardiovascular longevity.
5. **Immune System Support:** Knotted wrack contains antioxidants, vitamins, and minerals that help strengthen the immune system. These include vitamins C and E, as well as trace elements like zinc and selenium, which support immune function and protect against oxidative stress.

6. **Detoxification:** Knotted wrack contains alginate, a natural compound that binds to heavy metals and toxins in the body, aiding in their removal. This detoxification support helps eliminate harmful substances, contributing to overall health and well-being.
7. **Bone Health:** The rich mineral content of knotted wrack, including calcium and magnesium, supports strong and healthy bones. These minerals, along with other essential nutrients, help maintain bone density and reduce the risk of osteoporosis.
8. **Skin and Hair Health:** Knotted wrack's antioxidants, including vitamins A, C, and E, along with minerals like zinc and selenium, promote healthy skin and hair. These nutrients contribute to collagen production, protect against oxidative damage, and maintain a youthful appearance.
9. **Cognitive Support:** The presence of omega-3 fatty acids, such as docosahexaenoic acid (DHA), in knotted wrack supports cognitive health. DHA is essential for brain development, improving memory, and reducing the risk of neurodegenerative diseases.
10. **Anti-cancer Effects:** Knotted wrack contains bioactive compounds, including phlorotannins and fucoidan, which have shown potential anti-cancer properties in studies. These compounds may help inhibit the growth and spread of cancer cells.

While knotted wrack is generally considered safe to consume, there are certain medical contradictions and precautions to be aware of. Individuals taking medications for thyroid conditions, such as synthetic thyroid hormones, should be cautious as knotted wrack may interact with these medications and affect their efficacy. Individuals with existing kidney conditions or impaired kidney function should exercise caution when consuming foods high in potassium, as knotted wrack is a source of this mineral. People with certain allergies, particularly to seafood or iodine, should avoid or limit their consumption of knotted wrack to prevent allergic reactions. Safety during pregnancy and lactation is an important consideration. While knotted wrack contains beneficial nutrients, excessive iodine intake during pregnancy can be harmful to the developing fetus. Therefore, pregnant or breastfeeding individuals should consult with their herbalist/practitioner to determine safe levels of iodine intake and to ensure the overall safety of consuming knotted wrack during these periods. It is also crucial to source knotted wrack from the Atlantic Ocean to avoid higher levels of contamination from pollutants in the Pacific Ocean.

KOMBU

Kombu, scientifically known as Saccharina japonica or Laminaria japonica, is a type of brown seaweed with a rich history and origin deeply rooted in the coastal regions of East Asia, particularly Japan. For centuries, kombu has been a staple in Japanese cuisine and holds a significant place in their culinary traditions. Its usage can be traced back to ancient times when it was valued not only for its unique umami flavor but also for its nutritional benefits. Kombu was traditionally harvested from the rocky shores and used in various dishes, including soups, stews, and sushi. Over time, its popularity spread beyond Japan, and today it is recognized globally for its versatile culinary applications and potential health-promoting properties. Now, let's explore ten extensive health and longevity benefits associated with kombu:

1. **Immune System Support:** Kombu contains a compound called fucoidan, which exhibits potent antiviral properties. Fucoidan helps support the immune system by inhibiting the replication of viruses and stimulating the activity of immune cells.
2. **Thyroid Health:** Kombu is a rich source of iodine, a crucial mineral for the proper functioning of the thyroid gland. Iodine supports the production of thyroid hormones, which regulate metabolism, energy production, and overall growth and development.
3. **Cardiovascular Health:** The high content of dietary fiber in kombu, along with its unique compound fucoxanthin, helps maintain healthy cholesterol levels. Fucoxanthin has been shown to reduce LDL cholesterol and triglyceride levels, thereby supporting cardiovascular health.
4. **Digestive Health:** Kombu contains a soluble fiber called alginate, which acts as a prebiotic. This fiber supports the growth of beneficial gut bacteria, improving digestion, nutrient absorption, and overall gut health.
5. **Bone Health:** Kombu is a rich source of calcium, magnesium, and other minerals essential for maintaining strong and healthy bones. These minerals, along with the presence of fucoxanthin, contribute to bone density and support skeletal health.
6. **Anti-inflammatory Effects:** Kombu contains phlorotannins, a group of polyphenols with potent anti-inflammatory properties. These compounds help reduce inflammation in the body, which is linked to chronic diseases and supports overall longevity.

7. **Detoxification:** The presence of alginates in kombu has been found to have chelating properties, assisting in the elimination of heavy metals and toxins from the body. This promotes a healthy detoxification process and supports organ function.
8. **Antioxidant Powerhouse:** Kombu is rich in antioxidants, including vitamins C and E, beta-carotene, and various polyphenols. These compounds help neutralize harmful free radicals, protecting cells from oxidative stress and supporting healthy aging.
9. **Cognitive Support:** The omega-3 fatty acids, particularly docosahexaenoic acid (DHA), present in kombu support brain health and cognitive function. DHA is an essential nutrient for brain development and maintenance, contributing to memory, focus, and overall mental well-being.
10. **Skin Health:** The high content of antioxidants, along with the presence of fucoidan, in kombu supports skin health. These compounds help reduce oxidative damage, promote collagen synthesis, and maintain the skin's elasticity and youthful appearance.

While kombu is generally considered safe to consume, there are certain medical contradictions and precautions to consider. Individuals taking medications for thyroid conditions, such as synthetic thyroid hormones, should be cautious as kombu may interact with these medications and affect their efficacy. Individuals with existing kidney conditions or impaired kidney function should exercise caution when consuming foods high in potassium, as kombu is a good source of this mineral. High potassium intake may be problematic for individuals with certain kidney conditions, as their kidneys may have difficulty regulating potassium levels in the body. People with certain allergies, particularly to seafood or iodine, should avoid or limit their consumption of kombu to prevent allergic reactions. Safety during pregnancy and lactation is an important consideration. While kombu contains beneficial nutrients, excessive iodine intake during pregnancy can be harmful to the developing fetus. Therefore, pregnant or breastfeeding individuals should consult with their herbalist/practitioner to determine safe levels of iodine intake and to ensure the overall safety of consuming kombu during these periods. It is also crucial to source kombu from the Atlantic Ocean to avoid higher levels of contamination from pollutants in the Pacific Ocean.

KELPWEED

Kelpweed, scientifically known as Laminaria longicruris, has a rich history and diverse cultural significance across different regions. It is a type of brown seaweed that thrives in cold, nutrient-rich marine environments, particularly along rocky coastlines. Kelpweed has been a staple food source and medicinal plant for coastal communities around the world for centuries. In many Asian countries, such as Japan, China, and Korea, kelpweed has a long-standing culinary tradition and is a key ingredient in various dishes. It is used in soups, salads, and as a flavoring agent due to its unique umami taste. Kelpweed is also an important component of traditional Japanese cuisine, known as "kaiseki," and is used in making dashi, a flavorful stock that forms the basis of many Japanese dishes.

Now, let's explore ten extensive health and longevity benefits associated with kelpweed:

1. **Thyroid Health:** Kelpweed is rich in iodine, a vital nutrient for optimal thyroid function. Iodine supports the production of thyroid hormones, which regulate metabolism, energy levels, and overall growth and development.
2. **Cognitive Support:** The presence of omega-3 fatty acids, such as docosahexaenoic acid (DHA), in kelpweed supports cognitive health. DHA is essential for brain development, improving memory, and reducing the risk of neurodegenerative diseases.
3. **Anti-inflammatory Effects:** Kelpweed contains antioxidants like phlorotannins, fucoxanthin, and fucoidan, which possess anti-inflammatory effects. These compounds help reduce chronic inflammation, a key contributor to various diseases associated with aging.
4. **Cardiovascular Health:** The omega-3 fatty acids in kelpweed, along with its antioxidants, support cardiovascular health. They help lower cholesterol levels, reduce blood pressure, and prevent the formation of blood clots, thereby promoting a healthy heart.
5. **Detoxification:** Kelpweed contains alginate, a natural compound that binds to heavy metals and toxins in the body, facilitating their removal. This detoxification support helps maintain overall health and well-being.
6. **Bone Health:** Kelpweed is a good source of minerals like calcium, magnesium, and potassium, which are essential for strong and healthy bones. These minerals, along with the presence of vitamin K, contribute to bone density and reduce the risk of osteoporosis.

7. **Anti-cancer Effects:** Various active compounds found in kelpweed, including fucoxanthin and fucoidan, have shown potential anti-cancer effects in studies. These compounds may help inhibit the growth and spread of cancer cells.
8. **Digestive Health:** The fiber content in kelpweed promotes healthy digestion and helps regulate bowel movements. It also provides prebiotics that nourish beneficial gut bacteria, supporting overall gut health.
9. **Immune System Support:** Kelpweed's antioxidants, including vitamins A, C, and E, as well as polysaccharides and fucoidan, help strengthen the immune system. They protect against oxidative stress, enhance immune responses, and support overall immune health.
10. **Skin and Hair Health:** Kelpweed mineral content, particularly iodine, iron, and zinc, along with its antioxidants, promotes healthy skin and hair. These nutrients nourish the skin, strengthen hair follicles, and contribute to a youthful appearance.

While kelpweed is generally considered safe to consume, there are certain medical contradictions and precautions to consider. Individuals taking medications for thyroid conditions, such as synthetic thyroid hormones, should be cautious, as kelpweed may interact with these medications and affect their efficacy. Individuals with existing kidney conditions or impaired kidney function should exercise caution when consuming foods high in potassium, as kelp is a good source of this mineral. People with certain allergies, particularly to seafood or iodine, should avoid or limit their consumption of kelpweed to prevent allergic reactions. Regarding pregnancy and lactation, it is important to exercise caution. While kelpweed contains essential nutrients, excessive iodine intake during pregnancy could potentially be harmful to the developing fetus. Therefore, pregnant or breastfeeding individuals should consult with their herbalist/practitioner to determine safe levels of iodine intake and to ensure the overall safety of consuming kelpweed. It is also crucial to source kelp from the Atlantic Ocean to avoid higher levels of contamination from pollutants in the Pacific Ocean.

LAVENDER

Lavender, scientifically known as Lavandula angustifolia, is an herb with a rich and storied history that dates back thousands of years. Native to the Mediterranean region, lavender has been cultivated and cherished by various civilizations, including the ancient Egyptians, Greeks, and Romans. Its name is derived from the Latin word "lavare," meaning "to wash," as the Romans used lavender in their baths and as a fragrance. Lavender's sweet and calming aroma has made it a popular herb for perfumes, soaps, and other scented products throughout history. It has also been highly valued for its medicinal properties, and its essential oil has been used in traditional medicine to soothe aching muscles, promote relaxation, and improve sleep. Lavender has even been associated with superstitions and beliefs in folklore, believed to ward off evil spirits and protect against negative energies.

Now, let's explore ten extensive health and longevity benefits associated with lavender:

1. **Anxiety and Stress Relief:** Lavender contains linalool, a compound known for its anxiolytic and sedative effects. It helps promote relaxation, reduce stress, and improve sleep quality.
2. **Respiratory Health:** The volatile compounds in lavender, including linalool and camphor, possess expectorant properties, aiding in the relief of respiratory conditions such as coughs and congestion.
3. **Skin Health:** Lavender's antimicrobial and anti-inflammatory properties, attributed to compounds like linalool and linalyl acetate, make it beneficial for soothing skin irritations, promoting wound healing, and combating acne-causing bacteria.
4. **Digestive Health:** Lavender's essential oils, including linalool and camphor, may help soothe the digestive system, relieving symptoms such as bloating, indigestion, and abdominal discomfort.
5. **Immune System Support:** Lavender contains various phytochemicals, including terpenes and flavonoids, which exhibit antiviral, antibacterial, and antifungal properties, bolstering the immune system's ability to fend off pathogens.
6. **Cardiovascular Health:** Active compounds like rosmarinic acid and polyphenols found in lavender help protect against oxidative stress and inflammation, supporting cardiovascular health and reducing the risk of heart disease.

7. **Cognitive Support:** Linalool and other aromatic compounds in lavender have been shown to have neuroprotective effects, enhancing cognitive function, memory, and mood regulation.
8. **Pain Relief:** Lavender's analgesic properties, primarily attributed to linalool, may help alleviate headaches, muscle pain, and general discomfort.
9. **Anti-inflammatory Effects:** Lavender's active compounds, such as linalool and rosmarinic acid, possess anti-inflammatory properties, reducing inflammation in the body and potentially protecting against chronic diseases associated with inflammation.
10. **Antioxidant Powerhouse:** Lavender is rich in antioxidants, including polyphenols and terpenes, which help neutralize harmful free radicals, preventing oxidative damage and promoting cellular health.

> While lavender petals are generally considered safe to consume, there are certain medical contradictions and precautions to be aware of. Lavender may have a sedative effect and can enhance the central nervous system depressant effects of medications such as benzodiazepines, barbiturates, and other sedatives. It is important to exercise caution and consult with a healthcare professional if you are taking these medications. Lavender may also have estrogenic effects, so individuals with hormone-sensitive conditions, such as breast cancer, uterine fibroids, or endometriosis, should avoid excessive or prolonged use of lavender. Additionally, lavender may cause skin irritation or allergic reactions in some individuals, particularly those with known allergies to the Lamiaceae family, such as mint, basil, rosemary, and oregano. Women who are pregnant or lactating should consult with their herbalist/practitioner before using this herb, especially if the intention is to consume large quantities for prolonged periods.

LEMON BALM

Lemon balm, scientifically known as Melissa officinalis, is a herb with a fascinating history that dates back centuries. Native to the Mediterranean region, lemon balm has been revered and cultivated by various cultures for its aromatic and uplifting qualities. Its botanical name, "Melissa," is derived from the Greek word for "honeybee," as these buzzing insects have a strong affinity for the fragrant lemon-scented flowers of the plant. In ancient times, lemon balm was believed to have enchanting properties, and it was associated with the Greek goddess of the moon, Artemis. Lemon balm's delightful lemony aroma has also earned it a place as a strewing herb during the Middle Ages, where it was scattered on the floors to release its pleasant scent when walked upon. Furthermore, lemon balm was treasured for its culinary uses, and it was a popular ingredient in medieval European recipes and beverages.

Now, let's explore ten extensive health and longevity benefits associated with lemon balm:

1. **Antiviral Effects:** Lemon balm exhibits antiviral properties against various herpetic viruses because of its active compounds, rosmarinic acid, caffeic acid, and its volatile oils. Lemon balm may help inhibit the replication of the herpes simplex virus (HSV), which is responsible for oral and genital herpes. Lemon balm's antiviral effects are believed to be attributed to various mechanisms, including interference with viral replication, prevention of viral attachment to host cells, and inhibition of viral enzymes.
2. **Anxiety Relief:** Rosmarinic acid has been found to have anxiolytic effects, meaning it may help reduce anxiety and promote relaxation. It acts by modulating neurotransmitters in the brain, such as gamma-aminobutyric acid (GABA), which is known for its calming effects.
3. **Cognitive Support:** Rosmarinic acid, in particular, has been shown to possess neuroprotective properties. It may help protect brain cells from oxidative stress and inflammation, which are known to contribute to cognitive decline. Caffeic acid exhibits antioxidant and anti-inflammatory effects. These properties may help combat oxidative damage and inflammation in the brain and may enhance neuroplasticity, the brain's ability to reorganize and form new neural connections, which is crucial for learning and memory processes.

4. **Immune System Support:** Rosmarinic acid has been shown to possess potent anti-inflammatory and antioxidant properties. These properties help modulate immune responses, reducing inflammation and protecting immune cells from damage caused by harmful free radicals. Caffeic acid exhibits antimicrobial and antiviral properties. It may contribute to strengthening the immune system by combating pathogens and inhibiting their growth. The volatile oils present in lemon balm, such as citral, geraniol, and linalool, have demonstrated antimicrobial and immune-modulating properties.
5. **Respiratory Health:** Lemon balm provides relief from respiratory discomfort, including coughs and congestion, by effectively alleviating such symptoms. This beneficial effect can be attributed to the presence of active compounds like rosmarinic acid, caffeic acid, and volatile oils.
6. **Antioxidant Powerhouse:** Lemon balm offers protection against oxidative stress by demonstrating antioxidant activity, which effectively shields cells from damage caused by oxidative processes. This protective effect can be attributed to the presence of active compounds such as rosmarinic acid, flavonoids, and volatile oils, which are known polyphenols with potent antioxidant properties.
7. **Skin Health:** Lemon balm supports healthy skin by exerting multiple beneficial effects, including reducing inflammation, soothing irritations, and aiding in skin rejuvenation. These effects can be attributed to the active compounds found in lemon balm, such as rosmarinic acid, caffeic acid, and volatile oils.
8. **Sleep Support:** Rosmarinic acid, known for its calming effects, helps to reduce anxiety and promote relaxation, contributing to a more peaceful sleep experience. Flavonoids, on the other hand, possess sedative properties that can aid in promoting a deeper and more restorative sleep. The volatile oils present in lemon balm have soothing effects that may help induce feelings of tranquility, making it easier to drift off into a restful slumber.
9. **Cardiovascular Health:** Lemon balm is linked to supporting heart health by contributing to cardiovascular well-being. It aids in maintaining healthy blood pressure and cholesterol levels, both of which are important factors in overall heart health. These beneficial effects can be attributed to the presence of active compounds, including rosmarinic acid, caffeic acid, and volatile oils.

10. **Menstrual Support:** Rosmarinic acid possesses anti-inflammatory properties that may help reduce inflammation and relieve pain associated with menstrual cramps. By inhibiting the production of inflammatory compounds, it may help to ease uterine contractions and alleviate discomfort. Flavonoids present in lemon balm also play a role, as these compounds have been shown to possess analgesic and antispasmodic properties, which may help relax the uterine muscles and reduce cramping. By modulating pain pathways and reducing muscle contractions, flavonoids contribute to the relief of menstrual discomfort. The volatile oils in lemon balm, including citral and linalool, have soothing and calming effects.

> While lemon balm is generally considered safe to consume, there are some medical contradictions and potential drug interactions to be aware of. Individuals with glaucoma should avoid lemon balm due to its potential to increase eye pressure. Lemon balm has been found to contain compounds that may increase intraocular pressure, which can be problematic for individuals with glaucoma. Lemon balm may interact with sedative medications, such as benzodiazepines and barbiturates, intensifying their effects and causing excessive sedation. It may also interact with thyroid medications, potentially altering their effectiveness. Allergy warnings should be considered, particularly for individuals with known allergies to plants in the Lamiaceae family, such as mint, sage, or basil, as cross-reactivity may occur. Women who are pregnant or lactating should consult with their herbalist/practitioner prior to using this herb.

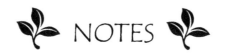

NOTES

LEMON PEEL

Lemon peel has a rich historical origin dating back to the ancient Indus Valley in present-day India, where they were cultivated for their delightful flavor and potential health benefits. As their popularity grew, lemons made their way to the Mediterranean region and eventually spread to various parts of the globe. The aromatic oils and bioactive compounds found in lemon peels make them highly valuable. These peels can be dried and ground to create lemon peel powder, which offers a concentrated form of nutrients and a wide range of potential health benefits.

Now, let's explore ten extensive health and longevity benefits associated with lemon peel:

1. **Liver Health:** Lemon peel contains d-limonene, a naturally occurring compound with potential liver-supportive properties. D-limonene has been studied for its ability to support the liver's detoxification processes and may aid in promoting overall liver health. This compound is found in the essential oil of lemon peel and is believed to have antioxidant and anti-inflammatory effects that can contribute to healthy liver function.
2. **Digestive Health:** The high fiber content in lemon peel, including pectin, supports healthy digestion and may help alleviate constipation.
3. **Immune System Support:** The polyphenols and vitamin C found in lemon peel have immune-enhancing properties, supporting overall immune system function.
4. **Cardiovascular Health:** The flavonoids in lemon peel, such as hesperidin, have been linked to reducing the risk of cardiovascular diseases and promoting heart health.
5. **Skin Health:** The antioxidants in lemon peel, including vitamin C, may help combat oxidative stress and promote healthy, youthful-looking skin.
6. **Respiratory Health:** The essential oils in lemon peel, such as citral and limonene, have expectorant properties that may provide relief from respiratory conditions like coughs and congestion.
7. **Antimicrobial Effects:** The antimicrobial properties of lemon peel, attributed to compounds like limonene and citral, may help inhibit the growth of bacteria and fungi.
8. **Bone Health:** Lemon peel contains calcium and vitamin C, which are essential for maintaining strong and healthy bones.

9. **Cognitive Support:** The antioxidant-rich lemon peel may support brain health and cognitive function, potentially reducing the risk of age-related cognitive decline.
10. **Anti-inflammatory Effects:** Rutin, a flavonoid and bioactive compound in lemon peel, exhibits anti-inflammatory properties that may help reduce inflammation throughout the body.

> While lemon peel is generally considered safe to consume, there are a few medical contradictions and potential drug interactions to be aware of. Lemon peel may interact with certain medications, such as anticoagulants (blood thinners) and antiplatelet drugs, potentially increasing the risk of bleeding. Allergy warnings should be considered, particularly for individuals with citrus fruit allergies, as lemon peel may trigger allergic reactions. Lemon peel belongs to the Rutaceae family, which includes other citrus fruits like oranges and grapefruits. Women who are pregnant or lactating can safely consume culinary amounts of organic lemon peel. Consult with your herbalist/practitioner prior to using lemon peel in high doses in these circumstances. It is advisable to source lemon peel and/or powder from reputable organic sources to ensure its quality and purity.

LEMON VERBENA

Lemon verbena, scientifically known as Aloysia citrodora, is a perennial herb native to South America, particularly Argentina, Chile, and Peru. It has a long history of cultivation and use, dating back to the ancient civilizations of the Inca and the indigenous peoples of South America. Lemon verbena is treasured for its refreshing citrus aroma and its potential health benefits. The herb is typically harvested for its leaves, which are used in various culinary and medicinal preparations. Its origin and cultural significance make it a valuable addition to herbal remedies and culinary creations.

Now, let's explore ten extensive health and longevity benefits associated with lemon verbena:

1. **Digestive Health:** Lemon verbena contains compounds like verbenalin and citral, which exhibit digestive properties, helping to ease indigestion, bloating, and gas.
2. **Anti-inflammatory Effects:** Lemon verbena is rich in flavonoids, such as luteolin and apigenin, which possess anti-inflammatory properties, reducing inflammation and supporting overall health.
3. **Cognitive Support:** Lemon verbena contains rosmarinic acid, which has been shown to support cognitive function, improve memory, and enhance overall brain health.
4. **Antioxidant Powerhouse:** This herb is a potent source of antioxidants, including verbascoside and chlorogenic acid, which help neutralize free radicals, reducing oxidative stress and promoting longevity.
5. **Respiratory Health:** Lemon verbena offers potential relief for respiratory issues by soothing respiratory discomfort and alleviating symptoms such as coughs and congestion. This beneficial effect can be attributed to the presence of specific compounds found in lemon verbena, including verbascoside, cineole, and limonene. These compounds possess properties that help soothe the respiratory system, reduce inflammation, and promote clear airways.
6. **Immune System Support:** Lemon verbena contains immune-boosting compounds, such as verbascoside and eugenol, that help strengthen the immune system, promoting overall health and longevity.

7. **Nervous System Support:** Lemon verbena has soothing effects on the nervous system, thanks to compounds like verbascoside and citral, promoting relaxation, reducing stress, and supporting mental well-being.
8. **Liver Health:** Verbascoside, one of the key compounds found in lemon verbena, has been shown to possess hepatoprotective effects. It helps to shield liver cells from oxidative stress and inflammation, which can contribute to liver damage. By reducing oxidative damage and inflammation, verbascoside aids in preserving liver health and function. Caffeic acid, another important compound present in lemon verbena, exhibits antioxidant and anti-inflammatory properties. These properties are beneficial for liver health, as they help neutralize harmful free radicals and reduce inflammation, which can be damaging to liver cells. Caffeic acid also supports liver detoxification processes by aiding in the elimination of toxins and promoting the breakdown of harmful substances.
9. **Muscle Pain Relief:** Lemon verbena possesses specific compounds that are responsible for its potential analgesic effects, making it a valuable herb for relieving muscle discomfort and alleviating muscle soreness. The active compounds, such as verbascoside and luteolin, have been studied for their ability to reduce pain sensations and provide relief to achy muscles. These compounds work by modulating inflammatory pathways, reducing inflammation associated with muscle soreness and discomfort.
10. **Sleep Support:** Lemon verbena's calming properties, attributed to its verbascoside and citral content, help improve sleep quality, supporting restful sleep, and overall vitality.

Lemon verbena is generally considered safe to consume, but there are certain medical contradictions and precautions to consider. Lemon verbena may have a mild diuretic effect, which can affect fluid balance. Therefore, individuals with kidney or urinary tract disorders should use lemon verbena with caution. Additionally, lemon verbena may lower blood sugar levels, so individuals with diabetes or hypoglycemia should monitor their blood sugar levels closely while using this herb. Lemon verbena may also have a sedative effect, so it should be used cautiously by individuals taking sedatives, sleep aids, or medications that cause drowsiness. Due to its potential impact on blood clotting, individuals with bleeding disorders or those taking anticoagulant medications should consult with a healthcare professional before using lemon verbena. It is important to note that lemon verbena may cause skin sensitization or allergic reactions in some individuals, so it is advisable to perform a patch test before using it topically. Women who are pregnant or breastfeeding should consult with their herbalist/practitioner prior to using this herb.

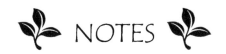

NOTES

LEMONGRASS

Lemongrass, scientifically known as Cymbopogon citratus, is a perennial herb that originated in tropical regions of Asia, particularly India and Sri Lanka. With its distinct citrusy fragrance and culinary versatility, lemongrass has become a cherished herb in many cultures across the globe. Beyond its culinary applications, lemongrass offers a range of extensive health and age-reversal benefits, making it a valuable addition to one's wellness routine.

Now, let's explore ten extensive health and longevity benefits associated with lemongrass:

1. **Immune System Support:** Lemongrass contains citral, a key compound known for its antimicrobial properties. It may help strengthen the immune system and protect against infections.
2. **Digestive Health:** Citronellal possesses antibacterial properties. These properties make lemongrass effective against certain bacteria that can cause gastrointestinal infections. By inhibiting the growth of harmful bacteria, lemongrass may help maintain a healthy balance of gut flora and support optimal digestive function. Lemongrass has been traditionally used to alleviate digestive discomfort and ease digestive disturbances such as bloating, gas, and indigestion. The calming and soothing properties of lemongrass may help relax the muscles of the gastrointestinal tract, promoting smoother digestion and reducing discomfort.
3. **Anti-inflammatory Effects:** The anti-inflammatory properties of lemongrass, particularly geraniol, help to counteract this chronic inflammation. Geraniol has been found to inhibit the production of inflammatory molecules in the body, such as cytokines and prostaglandins. By reducing the levels of these pro-inflammatory substances, lemongrass may help alleviate inflammation and its associated negative effects on health. The anti-inflammatory effects of lemongrass extend beyond its potential impact on specific conditions. By reducing inflammation in the body, lemongrass may contribute to improved overall well-being, support healthy cellular function, and promote longevity.
4. **Antioxidant Powerhouse:** Lemongrass contains phenolic compounds like chlorogenic acid and caffeic acid, which have antioxidant effects. These compounds help neutralize harmful free radicals, promoting cellular health and longevity.

5. **Cardiovascular Health:** Oxidative stress is a key factor in the development and progression of cardiovascular diseases. It occurs when there is an imbalance between the production of harmful free radicals and the body's ability to neutralize them with antioxidants. The antioxidant compounds found in lemongrass, including quercetin and luteolin, play a crucial role in reducing oxidative stress and protecting cardiovascular health. Quercetin, one of the main flavonoids in lemongrass, has been extensively studied for its cardioprotective effects. It helps prevent the oxidation of LDL cholesterol, a key step in the development of atherosclerosis, by scavenging free radicals and inhibiting the inflammatory processes involved in plaque formation.
6. **Nervous System Support:** Lemongrass contains the compound citronellol, which possesses neuroprotective properties. It may help protect against age-related degeneration and support the longevity of the nervous system.
7. **Respiratory Health:** The antifungal and antibacterial properties of lemongrass, attributed to its essential oils like citral and geraniol, may help support respiratory health and protect against respiratory infections.
8. **Skin Health:** Lemongrass is known for its antibacterial and antifungal properties, which may help maintain healthy skin by preventing infections and promoting a clear complexion.
9. **Oral Health:** The antimicrobial properties of lemongrass, particularly its essential oil components like citral and limonene, may help combat oral bacteria and contribute to good oral hygiene.
10. **Stress Relief:** Linalool is a naturally occurring compound found in lemongrass. It has been extensively studied for its potential benefits in reducing anxiety, promoting relaxation, and improving overall mood. By interacting with neurotransmitters in the brain, linalool can have a calming effect and help alleviate stress.

While lemongrass is generally considered safe to consume, there are a few important warnings and contradictions to consider. Lemongrass may interact with certain medications, such as anticoagulants (blood thinners) like warfarin, and increase the risk of bleeding. Individuals taking anticoagulant medications should use lemongrass cautiously and under the guidance of a healthcare professional. Lemongrass may have hypoglycemic effects, potentially lowering blood sugar levels. It is important for individuals with diabetes or those taking antidiabetic medications to monitor their blood sugar levels closely while using lemongrass. Lemongrass, like other plants in the grass family (Poaceae), may potentially trigger allergic reactions in certain individuals, especially those with existing sensitivities to grasses or related plants. Pregnant and breastfeeding women should consult with their herbalist/practitioner before using lemongrass to ensure its safety during these periods.

NOTES

LICORICE ROOT

Licorice root, scientifically known as Glycyrrhiza glabra, has a fascinating history that stretches back to ancient times. Native to the Mediterranean region and parts of Asia, licorice has been cherished and utilized by various cultures for thousands of years. Its botanical name "Glycyrrhiza" is derived from the Greek words "glykys," meaning "sweet," and "rhiza," meaning "root," highlighting its naturally sweet flavor and the part of the plant that is most prized. Interestingly, licorice root has been employed not only for its delightful taste but also for its versatile properties in traditional medicine, culinary arts, and even as a tool for crafting musical instruments. It is said that the ancient Egyptians appreciated licorice for its therapeutic qualities and used it in their recipes. In ancient China, licorice was highly valued for its harmonizing effects in herbal formulations. Throughout history, this remarkable root has found its way into various cultural practices, from Egyptian and Greek medicine to traditional Chinese and Ayurvedic healing systems.

Now, let's explore ten extensive health and longevity benefits associated with licorice root:

1. **Anti-inflammatory Effects:** Licorice root contains glycyrrhizic acid, which exhibits potent anti-inflammatory effects, helping to reduce inflammation in the body and support overall longevity.
2. **Digestive Health:** Licorice root promotes healthy digestion by soothing the stomach lining and reducing discomfort. Its active compound, glycyrrhizin, helps protect against gastric ulcers and supports optimal digestive function.
3. **Cardiovascular Health:** Despite its potential cardioprotective effects, it's essential to note that licorice root has been associated with elevating blood pressure levels. The compound glycyrrhizin, present in licorice root, is believed to contribute to these effects. Therefore, individuals with hypertension should exercise caution.
4. **Antiviral Effects:** Glycyrrhizin and liquiritin have demonstrated antiviral effects against various herpetic viruses, including herpes simplex virus (HSV), respiratory syncytial virus (RSV), and influenza virus.
5. **Skin Health:** Licorice root contains compounds that promote skin health, such as glabridin and liquiritin. These compounds exhibit antioxidant and anti-inflammatory effects, supporting a youthful complexion.

6. **Respiratory Health:** Glycyrrhizin has been studied for its expectorant effects. It helps thin mucus secretions in the respiratory tract, making it easier to expel while promoting productive coughing. By facilitating the removal of excess mucus, licorice root can provide relief from chest congestion and coughs. Flavonoids, such as liquiritin and glabridin, also contribute to the respiratory benefits of licorice root. These compounds possess anti-inflammatory properties that help reduce inflammation in the airways and alleviate bronchial spasms, which are often associated with respiratory conditions. By reducing inflammation and relaxing the airways, licorice root may aid in relieving symptoms of bronchitis and promoting easier breathing.
7. **Immune System Support:** Glycyrrhizin and glycyrrhizic acid are among the key compounds found in licorice root that have been extensively studied for their immunomodulatory properties. These compounds have shown the ability to stimulate the activity of immune cells, such as macrophages and natural killer (NK) cells, which play crucial roles in fighting off infections and maintaining a strong immune response.
8. **Antioxidant Powerhouse:** The antioxidants present in licorice root, including flavonoids, phenolic compounds, and glycyrrhizic acid, act as powerful scavengers of free radicals. Free radicals are highly reactive molecules that can cause damage to cells and tissues, leading to oxidative stress, inflammation, and accelerated aging processes. Licorice root's antioxidants work to neutralize these harmful free radicals, reducing their damaging effects on cellular structures. Licorice root's antioxidant properties extend to protecting against oxidative damage caused by environmental factors such as pollution, UV radiation, and toxins. By shielding cells from this oxidative damage, licorice root helps to maintain cellular integrity and promote healthy aging.
9. **Liver Health:** The active compound glycyrrhizin in licorice root supports liver health by promoting detoxification, reducing inflammation, and protecting liver cells.
10. **Hormonal Balance:** Phytoestrogens are plant compounds that have a similar structure to the hormone estrogen. Licorice root contains phytoestrogens, such as glabridin and liquiritigenin, which can bind to estrogen receptors in the body and exert estrogen-like effects. This allows licorice root to help balance hormone levels and mitigate the symptoms associated with hormonal fluctuations, such as those experienced during menopause.

While licorice root is generally considered safe to consume, there are some medical contradictions and potential drug interactions to be aware of. Individuals with high blood pressure or heart conditions should exercise caution when using licorice root, as it can cause an increase in blood pressure and fluid retention. Licorice root may interact with certain medications, such as blood pressure medications, corticosteroids, and diuretics, potentially altering their effectiveness or increasing the risk of side effects. Allergy warnings should be considered, particularly for individuals with known allergies to plants in the Fabaceae family, such as peas, beans, or soybeans, as cross-reactivity may occur. Women who are pregnant or lactating should consult with their herbalist/practitioner before consuming licorice root, as it contains compounds called glycyrrhizic acid and glycyrrhizin, which can potentially affect hormone levels and blood pressure. High levels of these compounds have been associated with adverse effects during pregnancy, such as increasing the risk of preterm labor and affecting fetal growth.

NOTES

LINDEN LEAF AND FLOWER

Linden leaf and flower, also known as Tilia europaea, have a rich history and origin dating back centuries. This herb is derived from the linden tree, a deciduous tree native to Europe and parts of Asia. The linden tree has long been revered for its beauty, shade, and medicinal properties. The delicate and fragrant linden flowers bloom during the summer months, creating a captivating sight and emitting a sweet aroma. The leaves and flowers of the linden tree have been used in traditional herbal medicine for their numerous health benefits.

Now, let's explore ten extensive health and longevity benefits associated with linden leaf and flower:

1. **Digestive Health:** Linden leaf and flower contain mucilage, a gel-like substance that helps soothe the digestive tract, alleviating indigestion, bloating, and stomach cramps.
2. **Anxiety Relief:** The relaxing effects of linden leaf and flower are attributed to their flavonoids, such as quercetin and kaempferol, which interact with neurotransmitters in the brain to promote relaxation, reduce anxiety, and improve sleep quality.
3. **Respiratory Health:** Linden leaf and flower possess expectorant properties due to their essential oils and tannins, which help loosen mucus and ease coughs. Additionally, their antispasmodic properties, attributed to compounds like farnesol, can relieve respiratory spasms and soothe sore throats.
4. **Antimicrobial Effects:** Linden leaf and flower are known to possess antimicrobial properties, which can contribute to supporting the body's defense against harmful pathogens. Farnesol, which is present in the essential oil of linden exhibits antimicrobial activity against various bacteria and fungi. It works by disrupting the cell membranes of these microorganisms, impairing their growth and survival. Linden leaf and flower contain flavonoids, such as quercetin and kaempferol that exhibit broad-spectrum antimicrobial activity against various bacteria, including both gram-positive and gram-negative strains. They may help inhibit the growth and spread of these bacteria, potentially supporting the body's defense against infections. Tannins found in linden leaf and flower have astringent properties and may help inhibit the growth of certain microorganisms. They can bind to the cell walls of bacteria, interfering with their ability to multiply and causing damage to their structure.

5. **Cardiovascular Health:** Linden leaf and flower contain flavonoids, such as rutin and quercetin, that have antioxidant and anti-inflammatory effects. These compounds help lower blood pressure, reduce inflammation, and support overall cardiovascular health.
6. **Immune System Support:** Linden leaf and flower are rich in antioxidants, including polyphenols and flavonoids, which help strengthen the immune system by neutralizing free radicals, reducing oxidative stress, and supporting the body's defense mechanisms.
7. **Anti-inflammatory Effects:** The anti-inflammatory effects of linden leaf and flower are attributed to their flavonoids and essential oils. These components help reduce inflammation in the body, providing relief from inflammatory conditions.
8. **Skin Health:** Linden leaf and flower's antioxidants, such as quercetin and kaempferol, protect the skin from oxidative stress, enhance skin elasticity, and promote a youthful appearance by reducing the appearance of age-related skin concerns.
9. **Detoxification:** Linden leaf and flower act as diuretics, primarily due to their flavonoids and essential oils. These properties promote kidney function, increase urine production, and support the elimination of toxins from the body.
10. **Menstrual Support:** Linden leaf and flower's antispasmodic properties, attributed to compounds like farnesol and tannins, help relax uterine muscles, alleviate menstrual cramps, and provide relief from discomfort during the menstrual cycle.

While linden leaf and flower are generally considered safe to consume, there are some medical contradictions and potential drug interactions to be aware of. Individuals with low blood pressure should exercise caution when using linden leaf and flower, as it may further lower blood pressure levels. It is also important to note that linden leaf and flower may interact with certain medications, such as anticoagulants and sedatives, potentially enhancing their effects or causing adverse reactions. Individuals with known allergies to plants in the Malvaceae family, including marshmallow, hibiscus, okra, and rose of Sharon, should be cautious as cross-reactivity may occur. Pregnant and breastfeeding women should consult with their herbalist/practitioner before using linden leaf or flower.

LION'S MANE MUSHROOM

Lion's mane is a medicinal mushroom that has gained popularity for its potential health benefits. Originating from various parts of the world, including Asia, North America, and Europe, lion's mane has been used for centuries in traditional medicine practices. It is known for its unique appearance, resembling a lion's mane, which is where it gets its name. Lion's mane powder, derived from the mushroom, offers a range of potential health benefits.

Now, let's explore ten extensive health and longevity benefits associated with lion's mane mushroom:

1. **Brain Health:** Lion's mane contains bioactive compounds called hericenones and erinacines, which have been shown to stimulate the production of nerve growth factor (NGF). NGF promotes the growth, survival, and maintenance of neurons.
2. **Memory Support:** Hericenones and erinacines found in lion's mane play a crucial role in improving memory, concentration, and focus. These compounds support the regeneration and maintenance of brain cells, facilitating better information retention, mental clarity, and cognitive performance.
3. **Nervous System Support:** Hericenones and erinacines are known to support nervous system health. They have demonstrated neuroprotective properties by stimulating the growth and survival of neurons, potentially reducing the risk of neurodegenerative diseases and maintaining overall nervous system well-being.
4. **Mood Support:** Hericenones and erinacines interact with neurotransmitter systems, potentially reducing symptoms of anxiety and depression and promoting a positive emotional state.
5. **Anti-inflammatory Effects:** Hericenones and erinacines modulate inflammatory responses by inhibiting pro-inflammatory molecules and regulating immune cell activity. Triterpenes inhibit inflammation by blocking enzymes and pathways involved in the inflammatory response. Polysaccharides possess immunomodulatory effects, inhibiting pro-inflammatory molecule release and promoting the production of anti-inflammatory substances. Collectively, lion's mane anti-inflammatory properties help alleviate chronic inflammation, reduce tissue damage, alleviate pain, and improve symptoms associated with inflammatory conditions.

6. **Digestive Health:** Hericenones, erinacines, along with triterpenes and polysaccharides in lion's mane contribute to its ability to support digestive health. They help reduce inflammation, promote a healthy gut microbiome, and enhance the function of the digestive system, alleviating issues like indigestion and promoting overall gastrointestinal well-being.
7. **Immune System Support:** Hericenones, erinacines, triterpenes, and polysaccharides possess immune-boosting properties. They can modulate immune responses, enhance the activity of immune cells, and support the body's defense against infections and diseases.
8. **Cardiovascular Health:** Lion's mane is recognized for its potential in supporting cardiovascular health, thanks to the presence of hericenones, erinacines, triterpenes, polysaccharides, and sterols. These bioactive compounds work in synergy to provide cardiovascular benefits. Hericenones and erinacines have shown cholesterol-lowering effects by inhibiting the synthesis and absorption of cholesterol, helping to maintain healthy cholesterol levels. Triterpenes, known for their antioxidant and anti-inflammatory properties, contribute to improved cardiovascular health by reducing oxidative stress and inflammation, which are associated with cardiovascular diseases. Polysaccharides derived from lion's mane exhibit protective effects on the heart and blood vessels, potentially enhancing blood flow and supporting overall cardiovascular function. Additionally, the presence of sterols in lion's mane may help regulate lipid metabolism and reduce the risk of cardiovascular diseases.
9. **Graceful-aging Effects:** Hericenones, erinacines, triterpenes, polysaccharides, and antioxidants provide potential pro-aging effects by protecting against age-related cellular damage caused by oxidative stress. These compounds help maintain cellular health, promote longevity, and contribute to overall healthy aging.
10. **Sleep Support:** Hericenones, erinacines, triterpenes, polysaccharides, and sterols, may help improve sleep quality. By supporting brain health, reducing anxiety and stress, and potentially regulating sleep-wake cycles, lion's mane promotes relaxation, aids in achieving deeper and more restful sleep, and enhances overall sleep quality.

While lion's mane mushrooms are generally considered safe to consume in culinary preparations, using it in concentrated supplement forms should be approached mindfully as there are some medical contradictions and potential drug interactions to be aware of. Individuals with bleeding disorders or those taking anticoagulant medications should exercise caution, as lion's mane may have mild anticoagulant effects. Individuals with low blood pressure or those taking medications for hypertension should monitor their blood pressure closely, as lion's mane may have hypotensive effects in high doses. Individuals with known allergies to mushrooms should be cautious when consuming lion's mane as cross-reactivity can occur, leading to allergic symptoms. Women who are pregnant or lactating can safely consume lion's mane mushroom in culinary preparations, however it's advisable to consult with your herbalist/practitioner before using large doses of supplemental lion's mane mushroom during these times.

NOTES

LOBELIA

Lobelia, scientifically known as Lobelia inflata, boasts a rich and intriguing history that dates back centuries. Indigenous to North America, particularly the eastern regions, lobelia has been an integral part of Native American traditional medicine. The plant was held in high regard for its various uses, and it was often referred to as "Indian tobacco" due to its resemblance to tobacco plants and its historical use as a smoking herb. However, it's essential to note that lobelia is not related to true tobacco and does not contain nicotine. The name "Lobelia" is a tribute to Matthias de Lobel, a Flemish botanist who significantly contributed to the field of botany during the Renaissance period.

Now, let's explore ten extensive health and longevity benefits associated with lobelia:

1. **Respiratory Health:** Lobelia contains alkaloids such as lobeline, lobelanidine, lobelanine, and isolobelanine, which promote healthy lung function, ease congestion, and act as bronchodilators, opening up the airways for improved respiratory support.
2. **Anxiety and Stress Relief:** Lobelia's calming properties can be attributed to lobeline, lobelanidine, and lobelanine, which act as natural relaxants and sedatives, helping to alleviate stress, anxiety, and tension, promoting relaxation and mental well-being.
3. **Smoking Cessation:** Lobelia has been traditionally included in smoking cessation formulations due to its constituents, believed to have properties that may support individuals trying to quit smoking. Lobelia contains alkaloids, including lobeline, which bears a structural resemblance to nicotine. This similarity has led to the belief that lobelia might help ease withdrawal symptoms associated with nicotine addiction. The lobeline content in lobelia is often considered the key component thought to interact with the same receptors in the brain that respond to nicotine.
4. **Digestive Health:** Lobelia's digestive benefits can be attributed to the alkaloids lobeline and lobelanidine. These compounds stimulate digestion, improve gastric secretions, relieve indigestion, and reduce stomach discomfort, promoting digestive health.
5. **Muscle Relaxation:** Lobelia's muscle relaxant properties are due to lobeline, lobelanidine, and lobelanine, as well as flavonoids such as apigenin. These compounds help relax smooth muscles, providing relief from muscle tension, spasms, and cramps.

6. **Pain Relief:** Lobeline, lobelanidine, and lobelanine possess analgesic properties, helping to alleviate various types of pain, including headaches, migraines, and menstrual cramps.
7. **Cardiovascular Health:** Lobeline is believed to have vasodilatory properties, meaning it helps to widen blood vessels and improve blood circulation. By promoting better blood flow, lobeline may support overall cardiovascular health. Additionally, lobeline has been studied for its potential ability to help reduce blood pressure. By helping to relax blood vessel walls and reducing resistance to blood flow, lobeline may contribute to maintaining healthy blood pressure levels.
8. **Antispasmodic Effects:** Alkaloids such as lobeline, lobelanidine, and lobelanine work synergistically to relax smooth muscles, making lobelia an effective natural remedy for relieving bronchial spasms, asthma, and other respiratory conditions characterized by constricted airways. These alkaloids in lobelia act as bronchodilators, helping to open up and widen the air passages, thus facilitating easier breathing. They work by relaxing the smooth muscles of the bronchial tubes, reducing their constriction, and alleviating symptoms associated with respiratory spasms.
9. **Anti-inflammatory Effects:** Lobelia possesses anti-inflammatory properties due to the presence of lobeline and lobelanidine. These compounds help reduce inflammation in the body, providing relief from conditions like arthritis and joint pain.
10. **Mood Support:** Lobelia's mood-enhancing effects can be attributed to lobeline, lobelanidine, and lobelanine, which interact with neurotransmitters in the brain. These compounds interact with neurotransmitters in the brain, such as dopamine and serotonin, which play vital roles in regulating mood and emotional well-being. Lobeline, in particular, has been found to act as a dopamine reuptake inhibitor, meaning it helps increase dopamine levels by blocking its reabsorption in the brain.

While lobelia is generally considered safe to consume, there are certain medical contradictions and important considerations to be aware of. Individuals with cardiovascular conditions, including hypertension, heart disease, or arrhythmias, should avoid using lobelia as it may affect heart rate and blood pressure. Individuals with gastrointestinal conditions such as ulcers, inflammatory bowel disease, or diverticulitis should exercise caution due to lobelia's potential to irritate the digestive tract. Lobelia may also interact with medications that affect the cardiovascular system, such as beta-blockers, calcium channel blockers, and antiarrhythmics, leading to potential complications. It is crucial to be aware of the potential side effects of lobelia, which can include nausea, vomiting, and dizziness, especially if consumed in excessive amounts. Lobelia should not be used by individuals with a history of seizures as it may lower the seizure threshold. Allergy warnings should also be noted, particularly for individuals allergic to plants in the Campanulaceae family, such as Bellflower and Canterbury bells, as cross-reactivity may occur. Women who are pregnant or lactating should consult with their herbalist/practitioner prior to using this herb.

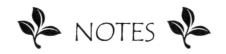
NOTES

LOMATIUM ROOT

Lomatium root, scientifically known as Lomatium dissectum, is a perennial herb indigenous to the Western regions of North America. In addition to its rich Native American traditional use, Lomatium root has an intriguing historical connection to the Spanish flu pandemic that occurred in the early 1900s. During this devastating global health crisis, Native American medicine practitioners shared their knowledge of Lomatium root with other communities. Lomatium root gained attention for its potential antiviral and immune-boosting properties, making it a valuable resource during the Spanish flu outbreak. Native American healers recommended using Lomatium root to support respiratory health and strengthen the immune system against the influenza virus. The herb's traditional use focused on addressing respiratory symptoms and alleviating congestion, which made it a sought-after remedy when effective flu treatments were limited.

Now, let's explore ten extensive health and longevity benefits associated with Lomatium root:

1. **Immune System Support:** Lomatium root contains potent compounds such as coumarins, furanocoumarins, and polysaccharides that enhance the immune system's function. These compounds stimulate immune cell activity, increase the production of immune-enhancing cytokines, and help fortify the body's defense against infections, viruses, and harmful bacteria.
2. **Digestive Health:** Lomatium root supports digestive health through its active compounds, including coumarins and polysaccharides. These constituents help soothe digestive discomfort, improve digestion, and alleviate symptoms associated with conditions like bloating, indigestion, and gastritis. Lomatium root's anti-inflammatory properties also contribute to a healthy digestive system.
3. **Anti-Allergic Effects:** Lomatium root's traditional use for allergies and hay fever suggests its potential anti-allergic effects. Allergic reactions involve an immune response to substances such as pollen, dust, or pet dander, resulting in symptoms like sneezing, runny nose, and itchy eyes. Lomatium root may help alleviate these symptoms by modulating the immune system's response and reducing inflammation. It is believed to have a calming effect on the body's hypersensitivity to allergens, potentially making it an herbal remedy for individuals seeking natural relief from seasonal allergies and hay fever.

4. **Urinary Tract Support:** Lomatium root possesses diuretic properties attributed to its coumarins and other active compounds. These constituents increase urine production and promote urine flow, aiding in flushing out harmful bacteria from the urinary system. This can provide support for urinary tract health and help relieve symptoms of urinary tract infections (UTIs).
5. **Respiratory Health:** Lomatium root's respiratory benefits can be attributed to its active compounds, including coumarins, alkaloids, and polysaccharides. These constituents act as expectorants, promoting the expulsion of mucus and relieving congestion. By soothing the respiratory tract, they help alleviate coughs and bronchial discomfort and promote overall lung health.
6. **Antiviral Effects:** Lomatium root's antiviral properties stem from its rich composition of potent compounds, including coumarins, furanocoumarins, and alkaloids. These constituents exhibit remarkable broad-spectrum antiviral activity, demonstrating the ability to inhibit the replication of various types of viruses. Lomatium root has shown efficacy against herpetic viruses, including herpes simplex virus (HSV), mumps virus, measles virus, and the Epstein-Barr virus (EBV). The active compounds interfere with the viral replication process by disrupting the synthesis of viral DNA or RNA, thereby hindering the virus's ability to proliferate and spread. Additionally, these compounds modulate the immune response, enhancing the body's defense mechanisms against viral infections.
7. **Antioxidant Powerhouse:** Lomatium root is rich in antioxidants (coumarins, flavonoids, and phenolic compounds). These antioxidants help neutralize free radicals, preventing oxidative stress and cellular damage. By protecting cells from oxidative damage, Lomatium root contributes to overall cellular health, supports graceful aging, and promotes optimal well-being.
8. **Skin Health:** Lomatium root's anti-inflammatory and antioxidant effects extend to the skin. Its active compounds, including coumarins and flavonoids, help reduce skin inflammation, soothe irritations, and support overall skin health and radiance. They may help address skin conditions and promote a healthy complexion.
9. **Stress Relief:** Lomatium root is believed to possess adaptogenic properties, thanks to its active compounds like coumarins. These constituents may help the body cope with stress, promote a sense of calmness, and support emotional well-being. Lomatium root is often used as a natural remedy for anxiety, nervousness, and emotional imbalances.

10. **Anti-inflammatory Effects:** The anti-inflammatory effects of Lomatium root are attributed to its coumarins, flavonoids, and other active compounds. These constituents help reduce inflammation by inhibiting inflammatory pathways and suppressing the production of pro-inflammatory molecules. This makes Lomatium root valuable in alleviating symptoms associated with inflammatory conditions like arthritis, joint pain, and skin irritations.

> While Lomatium root is generally considered safe to consume, there are certain medical contradictions and precautions to be aware of. Lomatium root may interact with immunosuppressant medications, such as corticosteroids or drugs used after organ transplantation, as it may interfere with their efficacy. Allergy warnings should be noted, especially for individuals sensitive to plants in the Apiaceae family, which includes celery, carrots, and parsley, as cross-reactivity may occur. Women who are pregnant or lactating should consult with their herbalist/practitioner prior to using this root.

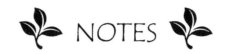
NOTES

MANGOSTEEN PEEL (POWDER)

Mangosteen, scientifically known as Garcinia mangostana, is a captivating and exotic fruit with a rich history rooted in Southeast Asia. Native to countries such as Indonesia, Malaysia, Thailand, and the Philippines, mangosteen holds a special place in the hearts and cultures of these regions. Revered for its delectable taste and unique appearance, it has earned the nickname "queen of fruits" in some parts of the world. Despite its name, mangosteen is not related to the mango; instead, it belongs to the Garcinia family. The fruit's exterior is dark purple and thick, while the interior reveals juicy, sweet, and tangy segments that are often described as a blend of flavors like peach, strawberry, and citrus. Mangosteen has been cultivated and cherished for centuries, with its significance extending beyond its culinary uses. In traditional medicine practices, the mangosteen peel and even parts of the tree have been utilized for their potential health benefits.

Now, let's explore ten extensive health and longevity benefits associated with mangosteen peel:

1. **Anti-inflammatory Effects:** Mangosteen peel contains xanthones, such as alpha-mangostin and gamma-mangostin, which possess strong anti-inflammatory properties. These compounds help reduce inflammation in the body, supporting joint health and overall well-being.
2. **Immune System Support:** The high vitamin C content in mangosteen peel enhances immune function by stimulating the production of immune cells and protecting against oxidative stress. Vitamin C acts as a powerful antioxidant, promoting a strong immune system and defending against pathogens.
3. **Cardiovascular Health:** Mangosteen peel's antioxidants, including xanthones and flavonoids, contribute to cardiovascular health. These compounds help reduce oxidative stress, support healthy blood vessels, and promote optimal heart function.
4. **Antimicrobial Effects:** Mangosteen peel exhibits antimicrobial activity due to its xanthones. These compounds possess antibacterial and antifungal properties, aiding in the body's defense against harmful pathogens.
5. **Detoxification:** Mangosteen peel contains compounds like xanthones that aid in detoxification processes. These compounds support liver function, promoting the elimination of toxins from the body.

6. **Anti-cancer Effects:** The xanthones found in mangosteen peel, such as alpha-mangostin and gamma-mangostin, have shown potential anti-cancer effects. These compounds inhibit the growth of cancer cells and may help prevent the development and spread of tumors.
7. **Digestive Health:** Mangosteen peel has been traditionally used to support digestive health and promote a healthy digestive system. It contains natural compounds, including xanthones and other antioxidants, which contribute to its potential digestive benefits. These substances have been found to possess anti-inflammatory properties, which may help soothe inflammation in the digestive tract and alleviate digestive discomfort.
8. **Skin Health:** The antioxidants present in mangosteen peel, including xanthones and vitamin C, contribute to vibrant and healthy skin. These compounds protect against oxidative stress, reduce inflammation, and promote collagen production.
9. **Cognitive Support:** Mangosteen peel contains a variety of antioxidants, including xanthones, that play a crucial role in supporting brain health and cognitive function. These antioxidants have been found to possess neuroprotective properties, helping to protect brain cells from oxidative stress and damage caused by harmful free radicals. By reducing oxidative stress in the brain, mangosteen peel may contribute to the maintenance of healthy brain function and potentially lower the risk of cognitive decline and age-related neurological disorders. The antioxidant activity of mangosteen peel helps to promote overall brain health by combating inflammation and supporting proper blood flow to the brain.
10. **Graceful-aging Effects:** Mangosteen peel's antioxidant activity combats oxidative stress, a key factor in aging. Xanthones and other antioxidants in mangosteen peel help minimize cellular damage, reduce inflammation, and indirectly support healthy aging.

While mangosteen peel is generally considered safe to consume, there are certain medical contradictions to consider. Individuals with existing kidney conditions or impaired kidney function should exercise caution when consuming mangosteen peel due to its naturally occurring potassium content. Additionally, individuals taking medications that affect potassium levels, such as certain diuretics or potassium-sparing medications, should be mindful of their mangosteen peel consumption to avoid excessive potassium levels in the body. Allergy warnings should be noted, especially for individuals sensitive to plants in the Clusiaceae family, which includes Garcinia cambogia, kokum, and bacupari. They should avoid its consumption to prevent allergic reactions. While mangosteen peel is generally considered safe during pregnancy and lactation in small quantities, it's recommended to consult with your herbalist/practitioner prior to using mangosteen peel in large therapeutic quantities.

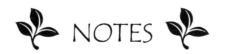

NOTES

MAQUI BERRY (POWDER)

Maqui berries, scientifically known as Aristotelia chilensis, holds a rich history deeply rooted in the Patagonia region of South America. For centuries, the indigenous Mapuche people revered the maqui berry for its exceptional health benefits and regarded it as a sacred fruit. Traditionally, the Mapuche would consume the fresh berries or prepare herbal infusions using dried maqui berries to harness its therapeutic properties. Maqui berry powder is derived by a meticulous process of dehydration and grinding. After thorough cleaning and sorting, the berries are dehydrated using methods like freeze-drying to remove moisture while retaining their nutrients. This powder encapsulates the concentrated goodness of the fruit, preserving its unique flavor and nutritional properties.

Now, let's explore ten extensive health and longevity benefits associated with maqui berries:

1. **Antioxidant Powerhouse:** Maqui berries boasts an exceptional antioxidant profile, attributed to its abundant anthocyanins, delphinidins, and flavonoids. These potent antioxidants help combat oxidative stress, safeguarding cells from damage and promoting healthy aging.
2. **Cardiovascular Health:** The wealth of antioxidants in maqui berries, particularly anthocyanins, contributes to cardiovascular well-being. These compounds help reduce inflammation, support healthy blood vessels, and aid in maintaining optimal heart function.
3. **Immune System Support:** Maqui berries offer essential vitamins and minerals, such as vitamin C and manganese, which bolster immune function. Vitamin C enhances immune responses, while manganese supports the production of immune cells.
4. **Anti-inflammatory Effects:** The anthocyanins and other antioxidants found in maqui berries exhibit potent anti-inflammatory properties, diminishing chronic inflammation within the body. This contributes to overall well-being and may assist in preventing age-related diseases.
5. **Digestive Health:** Maqui berries contain natural compounds, including polyphenols, known to promote digestive health. These compounds help soothe gastrointestinal inflammation, fostering a healthy digestive system.

6. **Detoxification:** The antioxidants present in maqui berries assist in detoxification processes, aiding the body in eliminating harmful toxins and promoting optimal liver health, the primary organ responsible for detoxification.
7. **Eye Health:** Maqui berries' anthocyanins, notably delphinidins, play a crucial role in supporting eye health. These antioxidants safeguard the retina from oxidative damage, reducing the risk of age-related macular degeneration and maintaining healthy vision.
8. **Anti-cancer Effects:** Maqui berries contain compounds, including anthocyanins and delphinidins, that exhibit promising anti-cancer effects. These compounds may impede the growth of cancer cells and provide protection against certain types of cancer.
9. **Energy Boost:** Maqui berries are a source of essential nutrients that may help boost energy levels and enhance stamina. They offer a remarkable antioxidant content and a nutrient profile that includes vitamins B2 and B6, iron, magnesium, and manganese, which collectively contribute to supporting optimal energy production and reducing fatigue.
10. **Skin Health:** These berries are abundant in essential vitamins and minerals, including vitamin C, vitamin E, vitamin A, zinc, and manganese. Vitamin C acts as a potent antioxidant, shielding the skin from oxidative stress, promoting collagen synthesis, and reducing the appearance of wrinkles and fine lines. Vitamin E contributes to maintaining the skin's moisture balance, preventing dryness, and ensuring a smooth and supple complexion. Vitamin A supports cell turnover, rejuvenating the skin and improving its texture while also regulating sebum production. Zinc helps regulate oil production, aids in wound healing, and possesses anti-inflammatory properties, reducing redness and irritation. Manganese plays a crucial role in collagen synthesis, supporting skin elasticity and firmness.

While maqui berries are generally considered safe to consume, there are certain medical contradictions and precautions to be aware of. Maqui berry may interact with certain medications, such as anticoagulants or antiplatelet drugs, due to its antioxidant properties, potentially increasing the risk of bleeding. It is advisable to consult with a healthcare professional if you are taking such medications. Maqui berry is generally considered safe to consume in culinary amounts during pregnancy and lactation, however individuals should consult with their herbalist/practitioner prior to consuming maqui berry in large therapeutic quantities.

NOTES

MARJORAM

Marjoram, scientifically known as Origanum majorana, is an aromatic and versatile herb with a fascinating history dating back to ancient times. Believed to have originated in the Mediterranean region, marjoram has been cherished by various civilizations for its culinary and medicinal properties. Its name, "marjoram," is thought to have come from the Greek word "mármaros," which means "joy of the mountains," highlighting its prevalence in mountainous areas. This herb has been a beloved addition to traditional dishes, imparting a warm and slightly citrusy flavor to culinary creations. In ancient Egypt, marjoram was revered for its aromatic qualities and was used in religious rituals and burial practices. Greeks and Romans valued marjoram for its potential medicinal benefits and associated it with love, happiness, and peace.

Now, let's explore ten extensive health and longevity benefits associated with marjoram:

1. **Digestive Health:** Marjoram contains compounds like carvacrol and terpinene, which have been shown to possess digestive properties, promoting healthy digestion and reducing gastrointestinal discomfort.
2. **Anti-inflammatory Effects:** The flavonoids and phenolic acids found in marjoram, such as rosmarinic acid and apigenin, exhibit anti-inflammatory activity, potentially reducing inflammation in the body and supporting overall health.
3. **Cardiovascular Health:** Marjoram contains antioxidants like quercetin and kaempferol, which help protect against oxidative stress and support cardiovascular health by reducing the risk of heart disease and improving blood vessel function.
4. **Immune System Support:** Marjoram is rich in vitamin C, an essential nutrient for a healthy immune system. Vitamin C helps boost immunity, fight against pathogens, and protect cells from oxidative damage.
5. **Respiratory Health:** Compounds like thymol and linalool found in marjoram possess antimicrobial and expectorant properties, supporting respiratory health and aiding in the management of coughs, colds, and congestion.
6. **Cognitive Support:** The antioxidant-rich profile of marjoram, including phenolic acids and flavonoids, may help protect against age-related cognitive decline and support brain health.

7. **Sleep Support:** Marjoram contains compounds such as terpinen-4-ol and linalool, which have been shown to have calming and sedative effects, promoting relaxation, reducing anxiety, and supporting restful sleep.
8. **Liver Health:** Marjoram contains caffeic acid, which may exhibit hepatoprotective properties and support liver health by promoting detoxification processes and protecting against oxidative damage.
9. **Antimicrobial Effects:** The essential oils present in marjoram, including thymol and carvacrol, exhibit antimicrobial properties, potentially inhibiting the growth of harmful bacteria, fungi, and other microorganisms.
10. **Anti-cancer Effects:** Marjoram contains antioxidants such as rosmarinic acid and apigenin, which have been studied for their potential anti-cancer effects by inhibiting the growth of cancer cells and reducing oxidative stress.

> While marjoram is generally considered safe to consume, there are certain medical contradictions and precautions to be aware of. Individuals with bleeding disorders or scheduled surgeries should exercise caution, as marjoram may have mild anticoagulant properties. Marjoram may interact with certain medications, such as anticoagulants, antidiabetic drugs, and sedatives. It is advised to avoid marjoram if you have a known allergy to other plants in the Lamiaceae family, which includes basil, mint, and oregano, as cross-reactivity may occur. As for safety during pregnancy and lactation, it's generally considered safe to consume this herb in culinary amounts. Consult with your herbalist/practitioner before using marjoram in large therapeutic quantities during these times.

MARSHMALLOW ROOT

Marshmallow root, scientifically known as Althaea officinalis, is a perennial plant native to Europe, Western Asia, and North Africa. It holds cultural significance and symbolism in ancient civilizations, ranging from ancient Egypt, where it was revered for its medicinal properties, to Greek mythology associating it with protection under Hera's watchful gaze. Romans, influenced by Greek traditions, documented its healing benefits, and in Arabic, Middle Eastern, and European folklore, it emerged as a symbol of protection and well-being.

Now, let's explore 10 extensive health and longevity benefits associated with marshmallow root:

1. **Respiratory Health:** Marshmallow root, enriched with mucilage and anti-inflammatory compounds, plays a pivotal role in supporting respiratory health. Its mucilaginous properties, characterized by a gel-like substance that becomes viscous when mixed with water, form a protective layer along the respiratory tract. This layer soothes irritations and effectively reduces inflammation, offering significant relief for individuals experiencing bronchial irritation, asthma symptoms, or bronchitis.
2. **Skin Health:** The flavonoids and phenolic acids in marshmallow root exhibit potent anti-inflammatory effects, effectively soothing the skin. Additionally, the root boasts a considerable presence of antioxidants that contribute to shielding the skin from oxidative stress. One noteworthy component is ceramides, which are lipids crucial for maintaining the skin's protective barrier. Ceramides play a vital role in preventing moisture loss and safeguarding the skin from external irritants. Marshmallow root's ceramide-rich content enhances its moisturizing properties, working in conjunction with mucilage. This makes marshmallow root a valuable asset for alleviating conditions such as eczema, psoriasis, and minor wounds, promoting skin hydration, suppleness, and resilience.
3. **Urinary Tract Health:** The synergistic properties of marshmallow root, enriched with mucilage, flavonoids, and tannins, comprehensively support urinary tract health. Mucilage forms a protective layer, alleviating irritation and inflammation along the urinary tract, while flavonoids and tannins contribute anti-intlammatory properties. This holistic approach aids in managing symptoms related to urinary tract infections and bladder inflammations.

4. **Anti-inflammatory Effects:** The synergistic action of anti-inflammatory compounds, such as flavonoids and phenolic acids, within marshmallow root works harmoniously to alleviate discomfort associated with respiratory issues. Whether triggered by environmental factors like pollution or allergens, these compounds demonstrate the root's potent soothing effects. By modulating inflammatory responses, they contribute to a profound sense of relief and play a pivotal role in promoting optimal respiratory function.
5. **Oral Health:** Marshmallow root emerges as a champion for oral health, leveraging its demulcent and anti-inflammatory properties. When used as a mouthwash or gargle, it promotes oral well-being by soothing mouth sores, gum inflammations, and sore throats. The root's mucilage and beneficial compounds contribute to reducing inflammation and fostering healing within the oral cavity.
6. **Digestive Health:** Marshmallow root, with its abundance of mucilage and anti-inflammatory properties, plays a crucial role in promoting digestive well-being. It addresses concerns such as indigestion, acid reflux, and gastritis by soothing the digestive tract. Its effective relief from discomfort supports a healthier digestive environment.
7. **Immune System Support:** Marshmallow root, rich in antioxidants, fortifies the immune system by combating oxidative stress and reducing inflammation. Its immune-supporting qualities contribute to overall well-being, providing a natural defense against external stressors.
8. **Joint Health:** With its anti-inflammatory compounds, marshmallow root plays a crucial role in supporting joint health. By reducing inflammation, it contributes to alleviating joint pain, stiffness, and swelling associated with conditions like arthritis, promoting increased comfort and mobility.
9. **Throat Support:** Marshmallow root, when consumed with water, transforms into a gel-like substance that gently coats the throat. This soothing effect proves beneficial for persistent coughing or throat irritation. The mucilage not only alleviates discomfort but also acts as a natural cough suppressant, reducing irritation and inflammation in the respiratory passages and aiding in mucus clearance.

10. **Nervous System Support:** The calming and soothing properties of marshmallow root, attributed to flavonoids like quercetin and kaempferol, contribute to nervous system support. These compounds interact with neurotransmitters and receptors in the brain, fostering a sense of relaxation and tranquility, thereby promoting overall nervous system well-being.

> While marshmallow root is generally considered safe to consume, it's crucial to be mindful of potential medical contradictions and drug interactions. Individuals with diabetes or blood sugar imbalances should exercise caution when using marshmallow root, as it may impact blood sugar levels. The root may interact with medications that lower blood sugar, such as insulin and oral antidiabetic drugs. Additionally, individuals with a history of gastrointestinal obstruction should avoid marshmallow root due to its mucilage content, which can potentially exacerbate the condition. Allergy to plants in the Malvaceae family, such as hibiscus, okra, and rose of Sharon, may occur in some individuals, particularly those with known sensitivities. For individuals who are pregnant or lactating, it is advisable to consult with your herbalist/practitioner prior to using marshmallow root during these times.

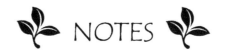

NOTES

MEADOWSWEET

Meadowsweet, scientifically known as Filipendula ulmaria, is a perennial herb native to Europe and Western Asia. This herb has a long history of traditional use dating back to ancient times when it was highly valued for its medicinal properties. Meadowsweet is commonly found in damp meadows, riverbanks, and wetlands, and its delicate white flowers and pleasant fragrance make it a popular ornamental plant as well.

Now, let's explore ten extensive health and longevity benefits associated with meadowsweet:

1. **Pain Relief:** Meadowsweet contains salicylates, including salicin and other salicylic acid derivatives, which provide analgesic and anti-inflammatory effects. These compounds function similarly to aspirin by inhibiting the production of inflammatory substances and relieving pain associated with conditions such as headaches, menstrual cramps, and joint discomfort.
2. **Digestive Health:** Meadowsweet contains tannins, including ellagitannins and hydrolysable tannins, which have astringent properties that help soothe stomach irritation and reduce acidity. Additionally, flavonoids like quercetin and kaempferol found in meadowsweet contribute to its anti-inflammatory effects, supporting digestive health and relieving symptoms of gastritis, peptic ulcers, and indigestion.
3. **Anti-inflammatory Effects:** Meadowsweet's anti-inflammatory effects are primarily attributed to its salicylates, which help reduce inflammation throughout the body. These compounds inhibit the activity of cyclooxygenase enzymes involved in the production of inflammatory mediators, making meadowsweet beneficial for conditions like arthritis, gout, and inflammatory bowel diseases.
4. **Fever Reduction:** Meadowsweet contains salicylates that possess cooling and diaphoretic properties, promoting sweating and aiding in fever reduction. These compounds help regulate body temperature and alleviate febrile conditions.
5. **Skin Health:** When used topically, meadowsweet's astringent properties, attributed to its tannins, play a role in tightening pores and reducing excess oiliness. These tannins have a mild drying effect on the skin, which may help reduce the appearance of enlarged pores and control oil production. By tightening the skin, meadowsweet can contribute to a smoother complexion and help improve the appearance of acne-prone skin.

6. **Respiratory Health:** Meadowsweet acts as an expectorant due to the presence of tannins and mucilage. These compounds help loosen mucus and facilitate its expulsion, providing relief from respiratory conditions such as coughs, bronchitis, and congestion.
7. **Urinary Tract Health:** Meadowsweet's diuretic properties, in part due to its tannins and flavonoids, promote urine flow and assist in flushing out toxins from the urinary tract. This may help support urinary tract health and reduce the risk of urinary tract infections.
8. **Headache Relief:** The analgesic properties of meadowsweet's salicylates, including salicin, make it effective in relieving headaches, including tension headaches and migraines. These compounds help reduce pain and inflammation associated with headaches.
9. **Cardiovascular Health:** Meadowsweet's flavonoids, including quercetin, kaempferol, and rutin, contribute to its potential cardiovascular benefits. These antioxidants help reduce oxidative stress, improve blood flow, and lower the risk of heart-related conditions by promoting healthy blood vessels and reducing inflammation.
10. **Anxiety and Stress Relief:** The flavonoids found in meadowsweet, such as quercetin and rutin, have been studied for their calming effects on the nervous system. These compounds interact with neurotransmitters in the brain, including gamma-aminobutyric acid (GABA), which is known for its calming and relaxing effects. By modulating GABA receptors, meadowsweet's flavonoids may help reduce anxiety and promote a sense of calmness.

While meadowsweet is generally considered safe to consume, there are certain medical contradictions and precautions to be aware of. Individuals with kidney or liver diseases should use meadowsweet with caution, as the herb may potentially affect kidney function and require additional liver processing. Meadowsweet may interact with certain medications, such as blood thinners, antiplatelet drugs, and nonsteroidal anti-inflammatory drugs (NSAIDs), leading to an increased risk of bleeding or adverse effects. It is important to consult with a healthcare professional before using meadowsweet if you have any underlying medical conditions or are taking medications. Individuals who have a known allergy or sensitivity to aspirin or salicylates should exercise caution when considering the use of meadowsweet, as it contains salicylates that are similar to those found in aspirin. This can potentially trigger an allergic reaction in susceptible individuals. It is also worth noting that meadowsweet belongs to the Rosaceae family, which includes various other plants such as roses, strawberries, and raspberries. People who have known allergies to plants within this family may have an increased risk of developing an allergic reaction to meadowsweet as well. Women who are pregnant or lactating should consult with their herbalist/practitioner prior to using this herb.

NOTES

MILK THISTLE SEED

Milk thistle, scientifically known as Silybum marianum, is a flowering plant that has been used for centuries due to its numerous health benefits. Native to the Mediterranean region, milk thistle has a long history of traditional use in herbal medicine. The plant gets its name from the milky white veins that run through its leaves. The seeds of milk thistle are particularly valued for their medicinal properties and are commonly used in herbal preparations.

Now, let's explore ten extensive health and longevity benefits of milk thistle seed:

1. **Liver Health:** The active compound in milk thistle, silymarin, found primarily in the seeds, plays a key role in liver protection and regeneration. It helps promote the growth of new liver cells, supports detoxification processes by enhancing liver function, and protects the liver against damage caused by toxins, alcohol, and certain medications.
2. **Antioxidant Powerhouse:** Milk thistle, particularly in its seeds, is a rich source of antioxidants, including silymarin—a complex of flavonoids. These antioxidants, such as silibinin, silychristin, and silydianin, help combat oxidative stress by neutralizing harmful free radicals in the body, promoting overall well-being, and supporting the body's natural aging processes.
3. **Digestive Health:** Milk thistle, particularly in its seeds, supports a healthy digestive system by stimulating bile production. Bile plays a crucial role in the breakdown and absorption of dietary fats, promoting efficient digestion. Additionally, milk thistle's anti-inflammatory properties may help alleviate digestive issues such as indigestion and bloating, supporting optimal digestive health.
4. **Anti-radiation Effects:** Milk thistle seeds, rich in active compounds, particularly silymarin, have gained attention for their potential as a natural anti-radiation tool. The seeds have been studied for their ability to mitigate the harmful effects of ionizing radiation on the body's cells and tissues. While more research is needed to fully understand the extent of milk thistle's radioprotective properties, it holds promise as a natural remedy in efforts to counteract radiation-related challenges and support overall well-being.
5. **Anti-cancer Effects:** Milk thistle's potent antioxidant activity and anti-inflammatory effects, particularly in its seeds, have shown potential in protecting against certain types of cancer.

6. **Blood Sugar Regulation:** Milk thistle, specifically its seeds, may assist in regulating blood sugar levels. Silymarin, the key component found in the seeds, helps improve insulin sensitivity and promotes balanced glucose metabolism, contributing to better blood sugar control.
7. **Anti-inflammatory Effects:** Silymarin, mainly found in the seeds, possesses potent anti-inflammatory effects by inhibiting various inflammatory pathways and reducing the production of inflammatory mediators. These properties may help alleviate symptoms associated with chronic inflammatory conditions, such as arthritis, rheumatoid arthritis, and inflammatory bowel diseases, promoting improved joint health and mobility.
8. **Skin Health:** The antioxidants present in milk thistle, particularly in its seeds, including the flavonoid complex silymarin, help protect the skin from oxidative damage. By neutralizing free radicals, milk thistle supports skin health and prevents premature aging signs. In addition to its antioxidant activity, milk thistle's anti-inflammatory properties contribute to skin health, improving conditions such as acne, rosacea, and eczema.
9. **Immune System Support:** The antioxidants found in milk thistle, such as silymarin and other phenolic compounds, help protect immune cells from oxidative stress. Milk thistle aids in reducing cellular damage and supports the optimal functioning of immune cells. Its anti-inflammatory properties contribute to immune system support, creating an environment that supports a robust immune system.
10. **Cognitive Support:** Milk thistle, primarily in its seeds, may have neuroprotective effects, benefiting cognitive function and memory. The antioxidant properties of milk thistle, particularly silymarin, help protect brain cells from oxidative damage, potentially reducing the risk of age-related cognitive decline and supporting overall brain health.

While milk thistle seed is generally considered safe for consumption, it's crucial to be mindful of specific medical contradictions and potential interactions. Milk thistle seeds may interact with certain medications, including anticoagulants (blood thinners), antidiabetic drugs, and medications metabolized by the liver. Individuals taking these medications should exercise caution and seek guidance from a healthcare professional before incorporating any form of milk thistle into their regimen. Additionally, individuals with specific medical conditions, such as hormone-sensitive cancers or allergies to the Asteraceae/Compositae family (which includes daisies, ragweed, and chrysanthemums), should approach milk thistle seeds with caution. Pregnant or breastfeeding women should consult their herbalist or healthcare practitioner before considering the use of any form of milk thistle.

NOTES

MIMOSA ROOT

Mimosa root, scientifically known as Albizia julibrissin, is an herb that has a fascinating origin and a long history deeply rooted in Asian cultures. Native to Asia, particularly China and Korea, it has been an integral part of traditional medicine systems in these regions for centuries. The use of mimosa root can be traced back to ancient times when it was highly valued for its therapeutic properties and wide-ranging health benefits. In traditional Chinese medicine, mimosa root is known as "He Huan Pi" and is revered for its ability to calm the spirit, soothe the heart, and uplift the mood. It is considered a Shen tonic, which means it nourishes the spirit and enhances emotional well-being. Mimosa root has been traditionally used to address conditions related to stress, anxiety, and mood imbalances, promoting a sense of inner peace and tranquility.

Now, let's explore ten extensive health and longevity benefits associated with mimosa root:

1. **Anxiety Relief:** Mimosa root contains active compounds such as saponins, flavonoids (including rutin and quercetin), and alkaloids. These compounds interact with neurotransmitters in the brain, potentially promoting relaxation, reducing anxiety and stress, and uplifting mood.
2. **Sleep Support:** Mimosa root's ability to support healthy sleep patterns can be attributed to its compounds, including flavonoids and alkaloids. These constituents may have calming effects on the nervous system, promoting relaxation and aiding in achieving restful sleep.
3. **Respiratory Health:** The expectorant properties of mimosa root can be attributed to its active compounds, including saponins. These compounds help alleviate coughs and chest congestion and promote healthy respiratory function by facilitating the expulsion of mucus from the respiratory tract.
4. **Skin Health:** Mimosa root's antioxidant activity, attributed to its flavonoids and other phenolic compounds, helps protect the skin against oxidative stress and damage caused by free radicals. This antioxidant effect contributes to maintaining a youthful and radiant complexion.
5. **Digestive Health:** Mimosa root's potential to support digestive health is linked to its anti-inflammatory properties, attributed to compounds like flavonoids and saponins. These constituents may help reduce inflammation in the gastrointestinal tract, soothe digestive discomfort, and alleviate symptoms of indigestion.

6. **Cognitive Support:** Flavonoids, such as rutin and quercetin, possess antioxidant properties that help protect brain cells from oxidative stress and damage caused by free radicals. These antioxidants contribute to the overall health of brain cells and may help maintain cognitive function. The alkaloids found in mimosa root, like mimosine and tetrahydroharman, are believed by some to have positive effects on the brain. People who use mimosa root often claim that these alkaloids contribute to better cognitive function by possibly enhancing communication between neurons. Many individuals share their experiences of feeling more mentally alert and focused after using mimosa root.
7. **Cardiovascular Health:** Mimosa root's ability to support cardiovascular health may be due to its flavonoids and other active compounds. These constituents may help maintain healthy cholesterol levels, promote blood circulation, and support overall cardiovascular well-being.
8. **Immune System Support:** The immune-boosting properties of mimosa root can be attributed to its active compounds, particularly saponins and flavonoids. Saponins are natural compounds known for their immunomodulatory effects, meaning they can enhance the activity of the immune system. These compounds have been shown to stimulate the production of immune cells, such as lymphocytes and natural killer cells, which play vital roles in defending the body against infections and diseases. Flavonoids, on the other hand, possess antioxidant and anti-inflammatory properties that contribute to immune system support. These compounds help reduce oxidative stress and inflammation, which can weaken the immune response.
9. **Liver Health:** Mimosa root contains a range of bioactive substances that contribute to its hepatoprotective properties. Among these, flavonoids such as quercetin and rutin provide antioxidant and anti-inflammatory effects, protecting liver cells from oxidative stress and reducing inflammation. The presence of alkaloids, including mimosine, adds to its hepatoprotective benefits. Saponins found in mimosa root exhibit diverse biological activities and may support liver function and promote detoxification processes. Phenolic compounds, including phenolic acids and phenolic glycosides, contribute antioxidant and anti-inflammatory properties, further supporting the liver's health.

10. **Anti-inflammatory Effects:** The anti-inflammatory effects of mimosa root are attributed to its active compounds, including flavonoids and alkaloids. These constituents help reduce inflammation in the body, potentially alleviating symptoms associated with inflammatory conditions like arthritis.

While mimosa root is generally considered safe to consume, there are several medical contradictions and precautions to consider. Mimosa root may have sedative effects and can potentiate the effects of sedative medications or central nervous system depressants. Caution should be exercised when using mimosa root in conjunction with medications that have sedative properties, such as benzodiazepines or opioids. Additionally, individuals with low blood pressure or hypotension should use mimosa root cautiously, as it may further lower blood pressure levels. Those with known allergies to plants in the Fabaceae family (legume family), including peanuts and soybeans, may also be at risk of experiencing allergic reactions to mimosa root. Consult with your herbalist/practitioner prior to using mimosa root if you are pregnant or breastfeeding.

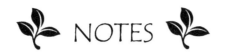

NOTES

MISTLETOE (EUROPEAN)

European mistletoe, scientifically known as Viscum album, is a fascinating parasitic plant with a long history and cultural significance in various civilizations. This unique plant grows on and derives nutrients from other host plants, making it a true parasite. Often associated with holiday traditions and folklore, mistletoe can be found growing on trees and shrubs. It has been valued for centuries for its medicinal properties and its ability to adapt and thrive in diverse environments. It's important to note that while European mistletoe (Viscum album) has been traditionally used for its therapeutic benefits, it does contain a certain degree of toxic compounds. However, the level of toxicity is generally lower compared to the American mistletoe (Phoradendron spp.), which should be strictly avoided as it contains higher concentrations of toxic compounds.

Now, let's explore ten extensive health and longevity benefits associated with European mistletoe:

1. **Immune System Support:** European mistletoe may help support the immune system. Advocates of this herb often express a feeling of increased resilience. This suggested effect is believed to be linked to certain active substances like lectins and viscotoxins, which are thought to work synergistically. There are even anecdotal reports of a potential positive connection with natural killer (NK) cells, important defenders of the immune system, which target irregular cells linked to infections and diseases.
2. **Cardiovascular Health:** Specific flavonoids present in European mistletoe, such as quercetin and kaempferol, contribute to cardiovascular health. They help reduce inflammation, lower blood pressure, improve blood flow, and protect against oxidative stress, supporting heart health.
3. **Anti-cancer Effects:** European mistletoe extracts have been examined for their potential anti-cancer properties. These extracts demonstrate cytotoxic effects against cancer cells, boost the immune system's anti-cancer response, and could potentially alleviate the side effects associated with conventional cancer treatments.
4. **Anti-inflammatory Effects:** European mistletoe contains phenolic compounds, such as caffeic acid derivatives, that possess anti-inflammatory effects. These compounds help reduce chronic inflammation, a major contributor to age-related diseases, and promote overall well-being.

5. **Liver Health:** European mistletoe extracts contain antioxidants, including flavonoids and phenolic acids, that protect the liver from oxidative stress and damage. They support liver detoxification processes and promote healthy liver function.
6. **Antimicrobial Effects:** European mistletoe exhibits antimicrobial, antiviral, and antifungal properties attributed to its various bioactive compounds. These properties help combat pathogens, protect against infections, and boost overall immune function.
7. **Nervous System Support:** Certain compounds found in European mistletoe, such as alkaloids and flavonoids, have neuroprotective effects. They help protect nerve cells from oxidative damage, promote cognitive function, and may potentially contribute to age reversal of the nervous system.
8. **Skin Health:** European mistletoe extracts contain antioxidants and polyphenols that protect the skin from free radicals and oxidative stress. They help promote skin elasticity, reduce signs of aging, and support a youthful complexion.
9. **Detoxification:** European mistletoe plays a significant role in stimulating liver function and facilitating the elimination of toxins from the body. European mistletoe's bioactive compounds, such as phenolic acids and flavonoids, actively participate in the body's detoxification processes, promoting a thorough cleansing and purification of various systems. European mistletoe promotes the production and activity of specific enzymes involved in the detoxification pathways, such as phase I and phase II liver enzymes. These enzymes facilitate the breakdown and conversion of toxins into less harmful substances, enabling their safe elimination.
10. **Respiratory Health:** European mistletoe has traditionally been used to support respiratory health. Its expectorant properties help relieve coughs, soothe the respiratory tract, and promote healthy lung function.

While some parts of European mistletoe (leaves, stems) are generally considered safe to consume when under the guidance of your herbalist, there are several medical contradictions and considerations to keep in mind. It is advised to avoid European mistletoe if you are taking medications that affect the immune system, such as immunosuppressants or corticosteroids, as European mistletoe may interact with these drugs. Individuals with known allergies to other plants in the Santalaceae family, such as sandalwood or boxwood, may be at higher risk of allergy. The berries of European mistletoe plants are known to be toxic and should never be consumed. They contain toxic compounds, including lectins and phoratoxins, which can cause serious health risks if ingested in any quantity for prolonged periods. European mistletoe should only be used under the supervision of your herbalist. Safety during pregnancy and lactation is a significant concern, and it is crucial to avoid all mistletoe use during these periods due to potential adverse effects on the developing fetus or nursing infant. American mistletoe (Phoradendron spp.) should be strictly avoided as it contains higher concentrations of toxic compounds.

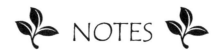

NOTES

MORINGA

Moringa, scientifically known as Moringa oleifera, is a tree native to the sub-Himalayan regions of India, Pakistan, and Afghanistan. It has a rich history dating back thousands of years and has been revered for its remarkable health benefits. This versatile plant, often referred to as the "Miracle Tree" or "Tree of Life," is valued for its leaves, seeds, flowers, and roots, all of which possess potent medicinal properties. Moringa leaves are highly nutritious, containing a wide array of essential vitamins, minerals, and antioxidants. These nutritional powerhouses provide numerous health and longevity benefits, promoting overall well-being.

Now, let's explore ten extensive health and longevity benefits associated with moringa:

1. **Immune System Support:** Moringa contains potent antioxidants such as vitamin C, beta-carotene, and quercetin, which help strengthen the immune system and protect against oxidative stress.
2. **Cardiovascular Health:** The presence of compounds like quercetin, kaempferol, and polyphenols in moringa supports cardiovascular health by reducing oxidative stress, improving blood lipid profiles, and promoting healthy blood pressure levels.
3. **Digestive Health:** Moringa aids in digestion and promotes a healthy gastrointestinal system. Additionally, compounds like isothiocyanates help combat harmful bacteria such as Helicobacter pylori, supporting a balanced gut environment.
4. **Respiratory Health:** Moringa's anti-inflammatory and antimicrobial properties, including compounds like quercetin and isothiocyanates, help reduce respiratory inflammation, promote healthy lung function, and support respiratory health.
5. **Skin Health:** Moringa contains vitamin E, vitamin C, and other antioxidants that nourish the skin, protect against oxidative stress, and promote a healthy complexion. The plant's antimicrobial properties also help combat skin infections.
6. **Joint Health:** The anti-inflammatory properties of moringa, attributed to compounds like quercetin and kaempferol, help alleviate joint discomfort and promote healthy joint function.
7. **Bone Health:** Moringa is a good source of calcium, phosphorus, and other minerals essential for maintaining strong and healthy bones. These nutrients, along with anti-inflammatory properties, support bone density and overall bone health.

8. **Liver Health:** Moringa is known to support liver health and function through the presence of antioxidants and phytochemicals. Compounds such as quercetin, kaempferol, and chlorogenic acid, have been shown to have hepatoprotective properties. These antioxidants help neutralize harmful free radicals, reducing oxidative stress and preventing damage to liver cells. Additionally, these phytochemicals aid in the detoxification processes of the liver, promoting the elimination of toxins and harmful substances from the body.
9. **Cognitive Support:** Moringa is a rich source of antioxidants and essential nutrients like vitamin E, vitamin C, and flavonoids, which help protect the brain against oxidative stress and support cognitive function.
10. **Anti-inflammatory Effects:** Moringa is well-known for its potent anti-inflammatory effects, attributed to its bioactive compounds such as isothiocyanates and quercetin. These compounds have been found to modulate the inflammatory response in the body, inhibiting the production of pro-inflammatory molecules and reducing inflammation. Isothiocyanates, in particular, have been shown to inhibit the activity of inflammatory enzymes and cytokines, contributing to the suppression of inflammation. Quercetin, on the other hand, acts as a powerful antioxidant and anti-inflammatory agent, scavenging free radicals and reducing oxidative stress, which can trigger inflammation.

> While moringa is generally considered safe to consume, there are certain medical contradictions and precautions to consider. Moringa may interact with medications such as anticoagulants (blood thinners) and antihypertensive drugs, potentially affecting their effectiveness. Individuals with bleeding disorders or low blood pressure should exercise caution and consult with a healthcare professional before using moringa. Additionally, moringa has been shown to have potential hypoglycemic effects, which may lower blood sugar levels. Therefore, individuals with diabetes or those taking medications for diabetes should monitor their blood sugar levels closely. Moringa leaves contain various bioactive compounds, including alkaloids, that have been found to possess uterine-stimulant properties in animal studies. It is recommended that pregnant women exercise caution and consult with their herbalist/practitioner prior to using moringa.

MOTHERWORT

Motherwort, scientifically known as Leonurus cardiaca, has a rich history and fascinating origin. Its name, "Motherwort," reflects its traditional use for women, especially mothers. This herb has been cherished and cultivated for centuries in various cultures for its diverse properties. In ancient Greek and Roman civilizations, motherwort was valued for its medicinal attributes and believed to support heart health. The Latin name "Leonurus" refers to the plant's leaves' jagged edges resembling a lion's tail. Motherwort's reputation as a nurturing herb for women dates back to traditional herbal practices in Europe and Asia. In Chinese traditional medicine, it was called "Yi Mu Cao," emphasizing its use during pregnancy, childbirth, and postpartum care. Ancient herbalists like Nicholas Culpeper praised its beneficial properties, earning it the name "Mother's Wort." Motherwort's significance extended beyond medicine; it was believed to offer protection to women against evil spirits and bad luck.

Now, let's explore ten extensive health and longevity benefits associated with motherwort:

1. **Hormonal Balance:** Motherwort is known for its ability to support hormonal balance, particularly in women, due to its active compounds like alkaloids, flavonoids, and phenolic acids. These constituents, including leonurine, rutin, quercetin, and phenolic acids, help alleviate menstrual cramps, regulate menstrual cycles, and ease symptoms associated with menopause, such as hot flashes and mood swings.
2. **Digestive Health:** The essential oils present in motherwort contribute to its digestive properties by promoting the secretion of digestive enzymes and enhancing the breakdown of food. This aids in relieving digestive discomfort such as bloating, gas, and indigestion. The tannins found in motherwort have astringent properties that help tone and tighten the digestive tract, reducing excessive secretion and supporting healthy bowel movements. The bitter compounds in motherwort stimulate the production of digestive juices and enhance appetite, making it useful for individuals with poor appetite or sluggish digestion.
3. **Uterine Tonic:** Motherwort's uterine tonic properties are attributed to its alkaloids, flavonoids, and phenolic acids. These compounds, including leonurine, rutin, and other phenolic acids, help tone and strengthen the uterus. They regulate menstrual flow, reduce excessive bleeding, and support overall uterine health.

4. **Cardiovascular Health:** Motherwort's cardiovascular benefits are attributed to its constituents, including alkaloids, flavonoids like rutin, and tannins. These compounds promote healthy blood circulation, regulate blood pressure, reduce palpitations, and strengthen the cardiovascular system, supporting heart health.
5. **Stress Relief:** Motherwort's calming effect on the nervous system is attributed to its alkaloids, flavonoids like rutin, and essential oils. These constituents help reduce anxiety, nervousness, and stress by promoting relaxation, improving sleep quality, and easing tension.
6. **Anti-inflammatory Effects:** Motherwort exhibits anti-inflammatory effects due to its flavonoids, including rutin and quercetin, and phenolic acids. These compounds help reduce inflammation in the body, making motherwort beneficial for managing conditions associated with inflammation, such as arthritis and joint pain.
7. **Liver Health:** Motherwort supports liver health through its bitter compounds, flavonoids, including rutin, and essential oils. These constituents aid in detoxification processes, promote liver function, and assist in the elimination of toxins from the body.
8. **Immune System Support:** Motherwort contains immune-supporting compounds, including alkaloids like leonurine and flavonoids such as rutin. These constituents help strengthen the immune system, promoting overall wellness and aids in graceful aging.
9. **Nervous System Support:** Motherwort acts as a tonic for the nervous system due to its alkaloids, such as leonurine and essential oils. These constituents help restore balance and strengthen nerve function, making motherwort beneficial for conditions such as nervous exhaustion, irritability, and tension headaches.
10. **Respiratory Health:** Motherwort's respiratory benefits are attributed to compounds like leonurine and stachydrine. These constituents exhibit anti-inflammatory and bronchodilatory properties, reducing inflammation, relaxing bronchial muscles, and supporting respiratory health. Motherwort may alleviate coughs, ease breathing difficulties, and promote overall respiratory well-being.

While motherwort is generally considered safe to consume, there are certain medical contradictions and precautions to consider. Motherwort may interact with anticoagulant or antiplatelet medications, increasing the risk of bleeding. Individuals with bleeding disorders or those scheduled for surgery should exercise caution and consult with a healthcare professional before using motherwort. Due to its potential to lower blood pressure, individuals with hypotension or those taking medications to manage blood pressure should also use motherwort with caution. Individuals with hormone-sensitive conditions or those taking hormone medications should consult their healthcare provider, as motherwort may have hormonal effects. Individuals taking medications that affect the liver should use motherwort with caution, as it may interact with liver function. Pregnant women should avoid motherwort due to its potential to stimulate uterine contractions. Those who are lactating should consult with their herbalist/practitioner prior to using this herb.

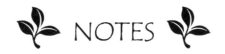

NOTES

MUGWORT

Mugwort, scientifically known as Artemisia vulgaris, is a herb with a rich historical and cultural significance that spans various regions and traditions. Belonging to the Asteraceae family, mugwort is native to Europe, Asia, and North Africa, and it has since spread to other parts of the world. Known for its unique aroma and distinctive feathery leaves, mugwort has been utilized for centuries for its medicinal properties, culinary uses, and ceremonial practices.

Now, let's explore ten extensive health and longevity benefits associated with mugwort:

1. **Brain Health:** Mugwort provides notable support for brain health by virtue of its vitamin E content, an antioxidant that safeguards the brain against oxidative stress, preserving cognitive function and overall brain health. It also contains flavonoids and coumarins, which further contribute to the promotion of optimal brain function and well-being. These bioactive constituents work synergistically to bolster brain health, offering protective effects and supporting healthy aging of cognitive abilities.
2. **Digestive Health:** Essential oils found in mugwort, including cineole and camphor, possess antibacterial and antifungal properties that support a healthy gut microbiome. Mugwort can also aid digestion by promoting bile production and enhancing gastrointestinal motility.
3. **Respiratory Health:** Cineole and camphor have been found to have anti-inflammatory properties. These compounds help soothe respiratory tissues, reducing inflammation and irritation. Mugwort's anti-inflammatory effects may help relieve congestion, open up the airways, and support healthy lung function. Mugwort also contains flavonoids, such as quercetin and rutin, which have antioxidant properties. These antioxidants may help protect respiratory cells from oxidative damage, promoting overall respiratory well-being.
4. **Skin Health:** Phenolic compounds like coumarins, along with flavonoids such as quercetin and rutin, play a vital role in protecting the skin from oxidative stress. By neutralizing harmful free radicals, these compounds help prevent cellular damage and premature aging. This antioxidant defense supports skin health, preserving its integrity, and promoting a resilient and youthful appearance.

5. **Impact on Dreams:** One of the key compounds in mugwort is thujone (both alpha-thujone and beta-thujone), which is believed to play a role in altering dream patterns. Thujone is a neuroactive compound that can interact with certain receptors in the brain, including GABA receptors. GABA (gamma-aminobutyric acid) is an inhibitory neurotransmitter associated with relaxation and sleep. By modulating GABA receptors, thujone may potentially promote relaxation and lucid dreaming and enhance dream recall.
6. **Liver Health:** Bitter compounds present in mugwort, including sesquiterpene lactones, stimulate liver function and assist in the detoxification process. Mugwort supports the liver's ability to metabolize toxins and promotes overall liver health.
7. **Antiparasitic Effects:** Mugwort's potential antiparasitic effects are attributed to bioactive compounds, such as sesquiterpene lactones and flavonoids. These compounds have shown activity against certain parasites, including intestinal worms.
8. **Anti-inflammatory Effects:** Mugwort contains various anti-inflammatory compounds, along with terpenes such as beta-thujone, camphor, and cineole which may help reduce inflammation throughout the body.
9. **Immune System Support:** Mugwort's bioactive compounds, including polysaccharides and flavonoids, enhance immune function. They stimulate immune responses and support the body's defense against pathogens.
10. **Sleep Support:** Mugwort possesses calming properties that can promote relaxation, relieve anxiety, and improve sleep quality. Its sedative effects are attributed to compounds like coumarins and volatile oils.

While mugwort is generally considered safe to consume, there are important medical contradictions to consider. Mugwort may interact with certain medications, particularly those that increase the risk of bleeding or affect blood clotting. Examples include anticoagulants (warfarin) and antiplatelet drugs (aspirin). Although significant interactions are not well-documented, it is advisable to consult with a healthcare professional if you are taking such medications to ensure there are no potential risks or interactions. Mugwort belongs to the Asteraceae family, which includes plants that may cause allergic reactions in sensitive individuals, such as ragweed, daisies, and marigolds. Individuals with known allergies to these plants may also experience cross-reactivity or allergic responses to mugwort. Safety during pregnancy is a concern with mugwort due to its potential effects on uterine stimulation. It is recommended to avoid mugwort during pregnancy as it may increase the risk of uterine contractions. Consult with your herbalist/practitioner before using this herb while breastfeeding.

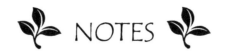

MULLEIN LEAF

Mullein leaf, scientifically known as Verbascum thapsus, is an intriguing and ancient herb with a rich history that spans continents and cultures. Native to Europe and Asia, mullein leaf has also made its home in North America, where it was introduced by early settlers. This herb's unique appearance is characterized by its tall, erect stem adorned with soft, fuzzy leaves, earning it the nickname "velvet plant" or "flannel leaf." Mullein has been valued by various civilizations for its versatile properties. In traditional folk medicine, the fuzzy leaves were used as natural torches or lamp wicks, giving rise to the name "candlewick plant." The ancient Greeks and Romans also admired mullein for its potential medicinal benefits and called it "Jupiter's staff" due to its towering stem. Native American tribes recognized mullein's significance and incorporated it into their herbal practices, utilizing it for various remedies. Throughout history, mullein leaf has been woven into folklore and cultural traditions, symbolizing resilience and protection.

Now, let's explore ten extensive health and longevity benefits associated with mullein leaf:

1. **Respiratory Health:** Mullein leaf is highly regarded for its ability to support respiratory health. It contains active compounds such as saponins, flavonoids, and mucilage, which help alleviate coughs, congestion, and respiratory discomfort. These constituents have expectorant properties, promoting the clearance of mucus from the respiratory system and supporting conditions such as bronchitis and asthma.
2. **Lung and Throat Support:** Mullein leaf's soothing properties are attributed to its mucilage content. Mucilage forms a protective coating that helps relieve irritation and inflammation in the throat and respiratory tract. This makes mullein leaf beneficial for soothing sore throats and irritated lungs.
3. **Expectorant Effects:** Mullein leaf acts as an expectorant, primarily due to its saponins and flavonoids. These compounds stimulate the production and clearance of mucus, helping to clear congestion and promote healthy respiratory function. By supporting the removal of mucus, mullein leaf aids in respiratory comfort.
4. **Ear Health:** Mullein leaf oil, derived from the flowers, has been traditionally used for ear health. Its antibacterial and anti-inflammatory properties may help alleviate earaches, ear infections, and inflammation in the ear canal.

5. **Anti-inflammatory Effects:** Mullein leaf's anti-inflammatory properties can be attributed to its flavonoids and other bioactive compounds. These constituents help reduce inflammation throughout the body, making mullein leaf potentially beneficial for managing conditions such as arthritis and inflammatory skin conditions.
6. **Immune System Support:** Mullein leaf contains compounds like flavonoids and polysaccharides that support immune system function. These constituents enhance immune response, strengthen the body's defense against infections, and promote overall immune health and resilience.
7. **Sleep Support:** Flavonoids found in mullein leaf, such as apigenin and luteolin, have been shown to possess anxiolytic and sedative properties. These compounds interact with neurotransmitters in the brain, promoting a sense of calmness and relaxation. Saponins present in mullein leaf have adaptogenic properties, which help the body adapt to stress and promote overall relaxation. These saponins have a regulatory effect on the nervous system, helping to balance its response to stressors and promoting a state of calmness.
8. **Digestive Health:** Mullein leaf has been used to support gastrointestinal health. Its anti-inflammatory properties and mucilage content may help relieve digestive discomfort, soothe inflammation in the digestive tract, and promote healthy digestion. Mullein leaf may assist in alleviating symptoms such as bloating, gas, and indigestion.
9. **Skin Health:** Mullein leaf's soothing and anti-inflammatory properties benefit various skin conditions. The herb's active compounds, including flavonoids and saponins, help alleviate skin irritations, rashes, and inflammation. Mullein leaf promotes healthier skin by soothing and supporting its natural balance.
10. **Urinary Tract Health:** Mullein leaf's diuretic properties may support urinary tract health. It promotes urine production, which can aid in flushing out toxins, reducing inflammation, and supporting proper urinary function. Mullein leaf's diuretic effects may be attributed to its saponins and flavonoids.

While mullein leaf is generally considered safe to consume, there are several medical contradictions and precautions to be aware of. Mullein may interact with certain medications, particularly anticoagulants, antiplatelet drugs, and immunosuppressants, leading to potential adverse effects. Individuals with bleeding disorders or those scheduled for surgery should avoid mullein leaf. Individuals with known allergies to mullein or related plants in the Plantaginaceae family, such as figwort or snapdragons, should avoid its use. Mullein leaf may cause skin irritation in some individuals, so a patch test is recommended prior to topical use. Pregnant or breastfeeding women should exercise caution and consult with their herbalist/practitioner before using mullein leaf.

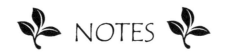

MUSTARD SEED

Mustard seed, derived from the mustard plant of the Brassicaceae family, have a rich history and wide-ranging culinary and medicinal applications. Believed to have originated in the Mediterranean region, mustard seeds have been cultivated and used for thousands of years, making them one of the oldest known spices. Mustard plants are known for their vibrant yellow flowers and pungent taste. The seeds are small and round, with a distinctive flavor and aroma that adds depth and zest to various dishes. Now, let's explore ten extensive health and longevity benefits associated with mustard seed:

1. **Brain Health:** Mustard seeds are rich in nutrients like folate, niacin, and vitamin B6, which play essential roles in brain health and cognitive function. These nutrients support the production and regulation of neurotransmitters, helping to maintain optimal brain function.
2. **Cardiovascular Health:** Mustard seeds, containing alpha-linolenic acid (ALA) and phytosterols, contribute to heart health. Although not as abundant in omega-3 fatty acids as some sources, the ALA in mustard seeds may still play a role in reducing inflammation and supporting overall cardiovascular well-being. Additionally, the presence of phytosterols in mustard seeds is associated with potential benefits for lowering cholesterol levels.
3. **Anti-inflammatory Effects:** Mustard seeds possess anti-inflammatory properties due to the presence of compounds such as isothiocyanates and selenium. These compounds help reduce inflammation in the body, which may contribute to various chronic conditions and support healthy aging.
4. **Digestive Health:** Mustard seeds can aid digestion and promote a healthy digestive system. They contain enzymes like myrosinase, which helps break down food components and enhance nutrient absorption. Additionally, mustard seeds may help alleviate symptoms of indigestion and improve bowel movements.
5. **Antimicrobial Effects:** Mustard seeds have antimicrobial properties, including antibacterial and antifungal effects. Compounds like allyl isothiocyanate and glucosinolates contribute to these properties, helping to combat harmful pathogens and promote a healthy immune system.

6. **Skin Health:** Mustard seeds are a source of essential minerals like zinc and selenium, as well as antioxidants such as vitamin E. These nutrients and antioxidants help protect the skin from damage caused by free radicals, promoting healthy skin and supporting a youthful appearance.
7. **Detoxification:** Mustard seeds contain compounds that support the body's detoxification processes. Glucosinolates, in particular, are metabolized into isothiocyanates, which aid in detoxification and help eliminate toxins from the body.
8. **Bone Health:** Mustard seeds are rich in minerals essential for bone health, including calcium, magnesium, and phosphorus. These minerals contribute to maintaining strong and healthy bones, reducing the risk of age-related bone disorders such as osteoporosis.
9. **Respiratory Health:** Mustard seeds have been used traditionally to support respiratory health. They possess expectorant properties that may help relieve congestion and promote clear airways, making them beneficial for individuals with respiratory conditions.
10. **Anti-cancer Effects:** Mustard seeds contain compounds with potential anti-cancer properties, such as glucosinolates and isothiocyanates. These compounds have been studied for their ability to inhibit the growth of cancer cells and reduce the risk of certain types of cancer.

While mustard seeds are generally considered safe to consume, there are certain medical contradictions and precautions to be aware of. Mustard seeds may interact with specific medications, particularly those that affect blood clotting or have anticoagulant properties, such as warfarin or aspirin. Individuals taking these medications should consult with a healthcare professional before incorporating mustard seeds into their diet. Individuals with a known allergy to mustard or other members of the Brassicaceae family, including cabbage, broccoli, or radishes, should avoid mustard seeds due to the risk of allergic reactions. Mustard seeds are generally recognized as safe during pregnancy and lactation when consumed as a spice or food ingredient in normal culinary amounts. However, pregnant or lactating individuals should consult with their herbalist/practitioner before consuming mustard seeds in high doses for prolonged periods during these times.

MYRRH GUM

Myrrh gum, scientifically known as Commiphora myrrha, is derived from the resin of the Commiphora myrrha tree. With its rich history in ancient civilizations, particularly in the Middle East and North Africa, this aromatic resin holds a significant place in traditional medicine. Revered for its medicinal properties, myrrh gum has been used for centuries and is even mentioned in ancient texts like the Bible, highlighting its value and significance. Its enduring popularity can be attributed to the extensive range of health benefits it offers, making myrrh gum a treasured natural remedy throughout the ages.

Now, let's explore ten extensive health and longevity benefits associated with myrrh gum:

1. **Oral Health:** Myrrh gum contains active compounds such as terpenoids and tannins that contribute to its oral health benefits. These compounds possess antimicrobial properties, helping to promote healthy gums, alleviate gum inflammation, and inhibit the growth of oral bacteria responsible for plaque formation and bad breath.
2. **Wound Healing:** The antiseptic and wound-healing properties of myrrh gum are attributed to its terpenoids and sesquiterpenes. These compounds have antimicrobial effects, cleansing wounds and preventing infection. They also support tissue regeneration and promote the formation of healthy granulation tissue, accelerating the healing process.
3. **Anti-inflammatory Effects:** Myrrh gum's anti-inflammatory properties are primarily due to its active compounds, including terpenoids, sesquiterpenes, and flavonoids. These compounds help reduce inflammation by inhibiting inflammatory enzymes and mediators, making myrrh gum beneficial for alleviating inflammation in the joints, muscles, and gastrointestinal system.
4. **Skin Health:** Myrrh gum's skincare benefits are due to its terpenoids, flavonoids, and resins. These compounds possess antioxidant and anti-inflammatory properties, promoting a more youthful and radiant complexion. Myrrh gum aids in soothing dry and irritated skin, providing hydration and enhancing skin elasticity.
5. **Anxiety Relief:** Myrrh gum has been used in aromatherapy for its calming and grounding effects on emotions. The aromatic compounds in myrrh gum, such as sesquiterpenes and terpenoids, promote relaxation, reduce stress, anxiety, and promote emotional balance.

6. **Digestive Health:** Myrrh gum supports digestive health through its terpenoids and resins. These compounds stimulate digestive enzymes, enhance bile secretion, and promote healthy gut function. Myrrh gum may aid in improving digestion, alleviating indigestion and stomach discomfort, and supporting a healthy gastrointestinal system.
7. **Respiratory Health:** Myrrh gum's beneficial effects on the respiratory system are attributed to its antimicrobial and anti-inflammatory properties. These properties help soothe inflammation, reduce coughs, and alleviate congestion. Myrrh gum also supports healthy mucus production, assisting in clearing the respiratory passages and combating respiratory infections.
8. **Immune System Support:** Myrrh gum contains immune-supporting compounds, including terpenoids and flavonoids. These constituents help strengthen the immune system by enhancing immune cell activity and protecting against microbial infections. Myrrh gum promotes overall wellness and aids in maintaining a robust immune response.
9. **Antioxidant Powerhouse:** Myrrh gum's antioxidant activity is attributed to its flavonoids, terpenoids, and phenolic compounds. These antioxidants protect cells from oxidative damage caused by free radicals, supporting graceful aging and preserving cellular integrity. Myrrh gum's antioxidant properties contribute to the maintenance of healthy cells.
10. **Menstruation Support:** Myrrh gum has been traditionally used to support women's health during menstruation. Its beneficial effects are attributed to its terpenoids and flavonoids, which may help regulate menstrual cycles, reduce menstrual pain, and alleviate symptoms associated with premenstrual syndrome (PMS).

While myrrh gum is generally considered safe to consume, there are certain medical contradictions and precautions to consider. Myrrh gum may interact with anticoagulant or antiplatelet medications, such as warfarin or aspirin, due to its potential blood-thinning properties. People with bleeding disorders or scheduled surgeries should consult with their healthcare provider prior to using myrrh gum. Individuals with hormone-sensitive conditions, such as breast cancer or uterine fibroids, should exercise caution and consult with their herbalist/practitioner before using myrrh gum, as it may have hormonal effects. It is important to note that myrrh gum should not be ingested in large quantities for extended periods of time due to the potential for toxic effects. This is primarily due to the presence of certain compounds, such as furanosesquiterpenes and sesquiterpene lactones, which can have adverse effects on the liver and kidneys if myrrh gum is abused. Individuals with a history of allergic reactions or sensitivity to plants in the Burseraceae family, such as frankincense, should avoid its use. Pregnant and breastfeeding women should consult with their herbalist/practitioner prior to using myrrh gum.

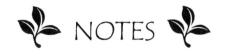

NOTES

NEEM LEAF

Neem, scientifically known as Azadirachta indica, has a rich cultural and historical significance in India and neighboring regions. It has been revered for thousands of years and is often referred to as the "divine tree" or "miracle tree" due to its exceptional properties and wide range of applications. In ancient Indian texts, such as the Vedas and Ayurvedic scriptures, the neem tree is mentioned as a sacred plant with profound healing abilities. It is believed to have been used for medicinal purposes since ancient times, with Ayurvedic practitioners recognizing its remarkable therapeutic potential. The neem tree's significance goes beyond its medicinal properties. It has been an integral part of cultural practices and rituals, symbolizing purity, protection, and well-being. Neem leaves are often used in religious ceremonies and festivals to purify the environment and ward off negative energies.

Now, let's explore ten extensive health and longevity benefits associated with neem leaf:

1. **Skin Health:** Neem leaf is renowned for its skincare properties thanks to its active compounds, such as nimbin, nimbidin, and quercetin. These compounds help cleanse and purify the skin, reducing the appearance of blemishes and promoting a healthy complexion. Neem leaf's antimicrobial properties also aid in combating skin infections, while its antioxidant content supports graceful aging by protecting the skin from free radical damage.
2. **Oral Health:** Neem leaf supports oral health through its active compounds like gedunin and nimbidin. These compounds possess antibacterial properties that help maintain healthy gums, reduce plaque buildup, and alleviate gum inflammation. Neem leaf's natural astringent properties also contribute to freshening breath and promoting overall oral hygiene.
3. **Digestive Health:** Neem leaf's digestive benefits are attributed to compounds like nimbin and nimbidin. These compounds help alleviate digestive discomfort, support healthy bowel movements, and maintain the balance of beneficial gut bacteria. Neem leaf's anti-inflammatory properties also aid in soothing the digestive tract.
4. **Blood Cleansing:** Neem leaf acts as a blood purifier due to its active compounds, including nimbin, nimbidin, and azadirachtin. These compounds help cleanse the blood, support liver function, and aid in the body's detoxification processes.

5. **Immune System Support:** Neem leaf's immune-boosting effects can be attributed to its rich content of catechin and quercetin. Polysaccharides are complex carbohydrates that play a crucial role in modulating the immune system. They stimulate immune cell activity and enhance the production of immune-regulating molecules, such as cytokines, which help coordinate immune responses. Catechin, a type of flavonoid, exhibits potent antioxidant and anti-inflammatory properties. It helps neutralize harmful free radicals and reduce inflammation, thus supporting immune health. Quercetin, another flavonoid present in neem leaf, has been shown to have immunomodulatory effects. It helps regulate immune responses, enhances the activity of immune cells, and promotes the production of antibodies, which are essential for immune defense.
6. **Respiratory Health:** Neem leaf's respiratory benefits are attributed to its active compounds like nimbidin and gedunin. These compounds help alleviate respiratory congestion, support clear breathing, and maintain a healthy respiratory tract. Neem leaf's anti-inflammatory properties also aid in reducing respiratory inflammation.
7. **Joint and Muscle Health:** Neem leaf's anti-inflammatory properties, including compounds like nimbidin and nimbin, help soothe joint and muscle discomfort. These compounds support joint health, maintain flexibility, and promote overall mobility. Neem leaf's analgesic properties also contribute to pain relief.
8. **Hair and Scalp Health:** Neem leaf's nourishing properties for hair and scalp are attributed to compounds like nimbidin and quercetin. These compounds help promote healthy hair growth, reduce dandruff, and soothe an itchy scalp. Neem leaf's antimicrobial properties also aid in maintaining a healthy scalp environment.
9. **Antioxidant Powerhouse:** Neem leaf exhibits potent antioxidant effects due to its active compounds, such as flavonoids and phenolic acids. These compounds help protect cells from oxidative damage caused by free radicals, promoting overall cellular health and reducing the risk of chronic diseases.
10. **Pest Control:** Neem leaf's natural insect-repelling properties are attributed to compounds like azadirachtin. These compounds help deter pests such as mosquitoes, fleas, and lice, making neem leaf useful for personal and environmental pest control.

While neem leaf is generally considered safe to consume, there are certain medical contradictions and precautions to be aware of. Neem leaf may interact with certain medications, including antidiabetic drugs, immunosuppressants, and medications processed by the liver. It may potentially lower blood sugar levels, so individuals with diabetes or hypoglycemia should exercise caution and monitor their blood sugar levels closely. Neem leaf may also have immunomodulatory effects, which can be problematic for individuals taking immunosuppressant medications. Individuals taking medications metabolized by the liver should consult with a healthcare professional before using neem leaf, as it may affect liver function. Pregnant or breastfeeding women should exercise caution and consult with their herbalist/practitioner prior to consuming neem leaf.

NOTES

NETTLE LEAF

Nettle leaf, scientifically known as Urtica dioica, is an ancient and versatile herb with a fascinating history that spans civilizations and continents. Native to Europe, Asia, and parts of North America, nettle leaf has been esteemed for its numerous uses by various cultures. This herb's name, "nettle," is believed to have originated from the Old English word "netel," which means "needle," referring to the stinging sensation caused by the tiny hairs on its leaves and stems upon contact. Despite its initial sting, nettle leaf has found a place in folk traditions and herbal practices for its potential benefits. The ancient Greeks and Romans admired nettle for its various properties and used it as a food source, herbal remedy, and even a textile fiber. In medieval Europe, nettle was woven into fabric, providing clothing and bedding. Additionally, nettle leaf was used in traditional Native American medicine, where it was valued for its potential therapeutic effects.

Now, let's explore ten extensive health and longevity benefits associated with nettle leaf:

1. **Joint and Muscle Support:** The anti-inflammatory properties of nettle leaf are attributed to its active compounds, including flavonoids, phenolic acids, and lignans. These bioactive constituents work synergistically to help reduce inflammation in the joints and muscles, which may contribute to alleviating pain and discomfort associated with conditions like arthritis and muscle strain. By inhibiting pro-inflammatory enzymes and cytokines, nettle leaf helps modulate the inflammatory response, promoting a more balanced and comfortable state for the joints and muscles.
2. **Blood Sugar Balance:** One of the key ways in which nettle leaf may contribute to blood sugar regulation is through its effects on glucose metabolism. Certain compounds found in nettle leaf, including flavonoids, lectins, and polysaccharides, may play a role in modulating glucose absorption and utilization in the body. These constituents may help regulate enzymes involved in carbohydrate metabolism, which can aid in maintaining balanced blood sugar levels. Nettle leaf's active compounds, such as flavonoids and phenolic acids, may have the potential to enhance insulin sensitivity and improve insulin signaling, promoting a more balanced response to glucose.

3. **Allergy Relief:** This remarkable herb offers support for individuals dealing with respiratory conditions, such as seasonal allergies, COPD (Chronic Obstructive Pulmonary Disease), chronic coughs, and tuberculosis. One of the key ways in which nettle leaf promotes respiratory wellness is by addressing the symptoms associated with seasonal allergies. It contains active compounds, including flavonoids, quercetin, and histamine receptors. These constituents work together to help reduce the release of histamine and other inflammatory mediators that contribute to allergy symptoms. By mitigating the allergic response, nettle leaf may help alleviate symptoms such as sneezing, itching, runny nose, and congestion, promoting clearer breathing and a greater sense of comfort.
4. **Detoxification:** One way in which nettle leaf contributes to detoxification is by assisting in the removal of toxic antigens, such as xenoestrogens. Xenoestrogens are synthetic chemicals that mimic the effects of estrogen in the body and can disrupt hormonal balance. Nettle leaf's active compounds, including flavonoids and lignans, have been shown to exhibit estrogen-modulating effects, helping to counteract the impact of xenoestrogens and support hormone balance. Another aspect of nettle leaf's detoxification support lies in its ability to promote liver health. Nettle leaf contains various compounds, including polyphenols and antioxidants, that help protect liver cells from damage caused by oxidative stress and promote optimal liver function. Anecdotally, nettle leaf has been suggested to provide support against radiation exposure, through its detoxifying and antioxidant properties.
5. **Urinary Tract Health:** Nettle leaf is rich in vitamins and minerals that contribute to its beneficial effects on urinary tract health. It contains vitamins A, C, and K, which support the integrity and function of the urinary tract epithelial cells, protect against oxidative damage, and aid in blood clotting. The leaf is also a good source of calcium, magnesium, and potassium, essential for proper muscle function, relaxation, and maintaining fluid and electrolyte balance in the body. Nettle leaf's bioactive compounds, including flavonoids like quercetin and kaempferol, provide antioxidant and anti-inflammatory properties that reduce inflammation and protect against oxidative stress in the urinary tract. By providing these essential nutrients and bioactive compounds, nettle leaf promotes optimal urine flow, maintains urinary system integrity, and supports overall urinary tract health.

6. **Skin Health:** Nettle leaf, enriched with silica, flavonoids, and a host of other active compounds, is renowned for its exceptional skincare properties. Silica, a trace mineral found in nettle leaf, plays a crucial role in maintaining healthy skin, hair, and nails. It supports the production of collagen, a protein that provides structure and elasticity to the skin, promoting a clear and youthful complexion. The flavonoids present in nettle leaf, such as quercetin and kaempferol, possess antioxidant and anti-inflammatory properties. These compounds help soothe irritated skin, reduce redness, and protect against environmental damage.
7. **Reproductive Health:** Nettle leaf is packed with essential vitamins, minerals, and antioxidants, including vitamins A, C, and K, iron, calcium, magnesium, and zinc. These nutrients play a vital role in supporting reproductive health. This herb is also a natural remedy to balance hormones which helps to support the endocrine system.
8. **Lymphatic Support:** Nettle leaf can contribute to a healthy lymphatic system, which plays a crucial role in eliminating waste and toxins from tissues. The lymphatic system acts as a drainage system, helping to remove cellular debris, toxins, and pathogens. Nettle leaf's active compounds, such as flavonoids and terpenoids, have been shown to possess lymphatic-supportive properties, aiding in the proper flow and function of the lymphatic system.
9. **Immune System Support:** One of the key components of nettle leaf's immune-boosting properties is its high content of flavonoids, including quercetin, rutin, and kaempferol. These flavonoids exhibit strong antioxidant and anti-inflammatory effects, which help reduce oxidative stress and inflammation in the body. By mitigating these harmful processes, nettle leaf supports the immune system by preserving the integrity of immune cells and preventing excessive immune responses. Nettle leaf also contains a rich source of vitamin C, a potent antioxidant that enhances immune cell activity and supports the production of antibodies. Additionally, nettle leaf provides essential minerals such as iron, zinc, and selenium, which are vital for optimal immune system functioning. Nettle leaf also contains bioactive compounds, including polysaccharides, lectins, and lignans, which have been shown to modulate immune responses. These compounds interact with immune cells and promote their activation, helping to strengthen the body's defense mechanisms against pathogens and foreign invaders.

10. **Adaptogenic Effects:** Nettle leaf is renowned for its ability to provide a natural energy boost and support overall vitality. This herb possesses adaptogenic properties, meaning it helps the body adapt to stress and promotes balance in various physiological processes. Nettle leaf's energy-enhancing effects can be attributed to its ability to support adrenal health. The adrenal glands are responsible for producing hormones, including cortisol, which play a crucial role in regulating energy levels and managing stress. This herb also contains bioactive compounds such as sterols and polyphenols that support adrenal function, helping to optimize hormone production and maintain balanced energy levels.

> While nettle leaf is generally considered safe to consume, there are certain medical contradictions and precautions to be aware of. Nettle leaf may interact with anticoagulant or antiplatelet medications, such as warfarin or aspirin, due to its potential blood-thinning effects. Individuals with bleeding disorders or scheduled surgeries should consult with their healthcare provider before using nettle leaf. Individuals with diabetes or hypoglycemia should monitor their blood sugar levels closely when using nettle leaf, as it may lower blood sugar levels. Nettle leaf may also have diuretic effects and interact with medications that have a diuretic effect, or affect blood pressure. Allergy to nettle is rare but possible, especially in individuals sensitive to plants in the Urticaceae family, which includes other nettles and related species. Safety during pregnancy and lactation is generally safe in small quantities. Consult with your herbalist/practitioner before using nettle leaf in large therapeutic doses for prolonged periods during these times.

OATSTRAW

Oatstraw, scientifically known as Avena sativa, has a remarkable history that spans centuries. Derived from the green stem and leaves of the oat plant, oatstraw has been widely used and revered in traditional herbal medicine practices. Recognized for its nourishing and rejuvenating properties, oatstraw was highly regarded in ancient civilizations for its ability to promote vitality and well-being. It holds a prominent place in ancient texts and folklore, where its potential to support various aspects of health has been documented. Oatstraw's benefits extend across different cultures, with its use valued for its calming effects on the nervous system, support for cognitive function, promotion of a healthy stress response, and positive impact on skin health, digestive well-being, and overall vitality. Now, let's explore ten extensive health and longevity benefits associated with oatstraw:

1. **Nervous System Support:** Oatstraw is rich in active compounds such as flavonoids and saponins and minerals like magnesium and calcium. These constituents contribute to its ability to support the nervous system by promoting relaxation, alleviating anxiety, and calming the mind.
2. **Cognitive Support:** Oatstraw's positive impact on cognitive function can be attributed to its rich content of essential nutrients. It is a valuable source of vitamins, including B vitamins such as thiamine (B1), riboflavin (B2), niacin (B3), and folate (B9), which play a crucial role in supporting brain health and cognitive function. Oatstraw is also abundant in minerals like magnesium and calcium, which support neurotransmitter function and communication between brain cells.
3. **Hormonal Balance:** Oatstraw's support for hormonal balance is attributed to its phytoestrogen content, essential nutrients like vitamins (including B vitamins) and minerals (such as magnesium and zinc), and adaptogenic properties. Phytoestrogens in oatstraw interact with estrogen receptors, helping to regulate hormonal fluctuations and alleviate symptoms associated with imbalances. The essential nutrients present in oatstraw play a vital role in hormone production, metabolism, and regulation, contributing to overall hormonal well-being. Oatstraw's adaptogenic properties support the adrenal glands, which are involved in hormone production and stress response, aiding in maintaining hormonal equilibrium.

4. **Stress Relief:** Oatstraw's adaptogenic properties are attributed to compounds like avenacosides and saponins. These compounds help the body adapt to stress, support adrenal function, and reduce the negative effects of stress on the body and mind.
5. **Digestive Health:** Oatstraw's soothing effect on the digestive system is attributed to its mucilaginous fibers, which help alleviate digestive discomfort and support healthy bowel movements. The presence of phenolic compounds also contributes to its positive impact on digestive health.
6. **Bone Health:** Oatstraw's benefits for bone health are due to its high silica content, as well as calcium and magnesium. Silica is essential for collagen formation, which is crucial for maintaining strong bones. Calcium and magnesium support bone density and prevent age-related bone loss.
7. **Cardiovascular Health:** Oatstraw's cardiovascular benefits are attributed to its antioxidant compounds, such as avenanthramides and flavonoids. These antioxidants help maintain healthy cholesterol levels, promote optimal blood circulation, and support heart health.
8. **Sleep Support:** Oatstraw's sleep-inducing properties can be attributed to its rich content of bioactive compounds, including flavonoids and alkaloids. Flavonoids, such as rutin and quercetin, possess sedative effects and help modulate neurotransmitters in the brain, promoting relaxation and preparing the body for sleep. These compounds interact with GABA receptors, known for their calming effects, reducing neuronal excitability and promoting tranquility. Oatstraw also contains alkaloids like gramine and trigonelline, which exhibit mild sedative properties, alleviating restlessness and promoting a restful sleep cycle. The combined actions of flavonoids and alkaloids in oatstraw create a calming effect on the nervous system, facilitating a restful and rejuvenating sleep.
9. **Adaptogenic Support:** Oatstraw's remarkable ability to enhance energy and vitality can be attributed to its adaptogenic properties. As an adaptogen, oatstraw works to support the body's response to stress and restore balance. It specifically targets the adrenal glands, which play a crucial role in regulating stress hormones like cortisol. By promoting adrenal health and optimizing the body's stress response, oatstraw helps combat fatigue and improve overall energy levels.

10. **Skin Health:** Oatstraw's exceptional skin benefits can be attributed to its rich array of antioxidants, including avenanthramides, phenolic acids, and vitamins E and C. These antioxidants work together to protect the skin from oxidative stress caused by environmental factors and free radicals. Avenanthramides, unique to oats, have anti-inflammatory properties that help soothe irritated skin, reducing redness and inflammation. Phenolic acids, such as ferulic acid and caffeic acid, contribute to the antioxidant activity of oatstraw, neutralizing harmful free radicals and preventing damage to the skin cells. Vitamins E and C are essential for skin health, with vitamin E providing deep moisturization and vitamin C promoting collagen synthesis for a youthful appearance. Oatstraw is particularly rich in silica, a trace mineral known for its role in collagen formation, which supports skin elasticity and strength. Silica helps maintain a firm and plump complexion, reducing the appearance of fine lines and wrinkles.

> While oatstraw is generally considered safe to consume, there are certain medical contradictions and precautions to consider. Oatstraw may interact with certain medications, such as anticoagulants, antiplatelet drugs, and sedatives. It may enhance the effects of these medications, increasing the risk of bleeding or excessive sedation. Individuals with bleeding disorders or those scheduled for surgery should exercise caution. Oatstraw may also lower blood sugar levels, so individuals with diabetes or hypoglycemia should monitor their blood sugar closely. Individuals with hormone-sensitive conditions, such as breast or uterine cancer, should consult with their herbalist/practitioner prior to using oatstraw, as it may have estrogenic effects. Individuals allergic to oats should avoid oatstraw. Pregnant or breastfeeding women should consult with their herbalist/practitioner before using this herb.

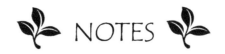

NOTES

ORANGE PEEL

Orange peel, scientifically known as Citrus sinensis pericarpium, constitutes the outer layer of the orange fruit. Originating from the Citrus species, orange peel is often discarded but is actually a rich source of beneficial compounds. Centuries ago, oranges were not just a tasty treat; they symbolized prestige and opulence. In medieval Europe, where oranges were considered rare luxuries, the peel became a status symbol. Adorning banquet tables of the elite, the vibrant orange peel showcased wealth and sophistication.

Now, let's explore ten extensive health and longevity benefits associated with orange peel:

1. **Digestive Health:** Orange peel contains flavonoids, such as nobiletin and tangeretin, which have been found to support digestive health by promoting proper digestion and reducing the risk of gastrointestinal disorders.
2. **Cardiovascular Health:** The peel contains polymethoxyflavones, including hesperidin and polymethoxylated flavones, which have shown potential in improving heart health by reducing cholesterol levels, lowering blood pressure, and supporting healthy blood vessel function.
3. **Anti-inflammatory Effects:** Orange peel contains powerful antioxidants, including hesperidin, naringin, and limonene, which have demonstrated anti-inflammatory properties, supporting the reduction of chronic inflammation and associated health issues.
4. **Liver Health:** The compounds in orange peel, such as nobiletin and polymethoxylated flavones, exhibit hepatoprotective effects by supporting liver function, enhancing detoxification processes, and reducing oxidative stress in the liver.
5. **Bone Health:** Orange peel provides minerals like calcium and magnesium, which are crucial for maintaining strong bones and preventing conditions such as osteoporosis. Additionally, the presence of hesperidin and other flavonoids may contribute to bone health by reducing inflammation and supporting bone density.
6. **Skin Health:** The antioxidants, vitamins C and E, and polymethoxyflavones found in orange peel contribute to its potential benefits for the skin. They may help protect against oxidative damage, promote collagen synthesis, and improve skin elasticity, indirectly supporting graceful aging and longevity.

7. **Respiratory Health:** The essential oil derived from orange peel contains compounds like limonene and citral, which possess expectorant properties, aiding in the relief of respiratory symptoms and supporting respiratory health.
8. **Immune System Support:** Orange peel contains vitamin C and antioxidants like hesperidin, which can support a healthy immune system by strengthening immune responses and protecting against oxidative stress.
9. **Anti-cancer Effects:** The presence of d-limonene, a natural compound in orange peel, has been associated with anti-cancer effects, particularly against breast, lung, and colon cancer cells, by inducing apoptosis (cell death) and inhibiting tumor growth.
10. **Graceful-aging Effects:** The combination of antioxidants, vitamins, and flavonoids found in orange peel contributes to its potential pro-aging effects by protecting against oxidative stress, supporting cellular health, and promoting overall longevity.

> While organic orange peel is generally considered safe to consume and offers various health benefits, there are certain medical contradictions and warnings to consider. Orange peel contains compounds that can interact with specific medications. For instance, the furanocoumarins in orange peel can inhibit the activity of liver enzymes responsible for metabolizing certain drugs, potentially leading to increased drug concentrations in the body. Therefore, individuals taking medications metabolized by these enzymes, such as statins, calcium channel blockers, or immunosuppressants, should exercise caution and consult with a healthcare professional before consuming orange peel. Individuals with known citrus allergies should avoid consuming orange peel, as it may trigger allergic reactions. It is worth noting that orange peel may also contain pesticide residues, so it is advisable to opt for organic or pesticide-free sources whenever possible and always wash the fruit to remove any potential contaminants. Organic orange peel is generally safe to use during pregnancy and lactation in culinary amounts.

OLIVE LEAF

Olive leaf, scientifically known as Olea europaea, is derived from the olive tree and has a rich history dating back thousands of years and is renowned for its numerous health benefits. Originating in the Mediterranean region, the olive tree has been a symbol of peace and prosperity, and its leaves have been used in traditional medicine for centuries.

Now, let's explore ten extensive health and longevity benefits associated with olive leaf:

1. **Immune System Support:** Verbascoside, a phenolic compound found in olive leaf, has been studied for its immunomodulatory properties. It can enhance the activity of immune cells, such as natural killer cells and lymphocytes, which play a crucial role in recognizing and eliminating harmful pathogens. Verbascoside also exhibits antioxidant effects, protecting immune cells from oxidative damage and supporting their optimal functioning. Luteolin, another important compound in olive leaf, has been shown to possess potent immunomodulatory effects. It helps regulate the immune response by modulating various immune cells and their signaling pathways. Luteolin exhibits anti-inflammatory properties, reducing excessive immune responses that can lead to tissue damage. Apigenin, a flavonoid present in olive leaf, has been recognized for its immunomodulatory and antimicrobial properties. It can modulate the activity of immune cells, such as macrophages and lymphocytes, and enhance their ability to fight against pathogens. Apigenin also exhibits antimicrobial effects, directly targeting and inhibiting the growth of various microorganisms, including bacteria and viruses.
2. **Antioxidant Powerhouse:** Olive leaf is rich in a variety of antioxidants, including compounds such as oleuropein, hydroxytyrosol, and tyrosol, as well as other beneficial antioxidants like verbascoside, rutin, and quercetin. These antioxidants play a vital role in neutralizing free radicals and reducing oxidative stress within the body. By scavenging free radicals, these compounds help prevent cellular damage and support overall health and graceful aging. Additionally, verbascoside, rutin, and quercetin further enhance the antioxidant capacity of olive leaf by inhibiting oxidative processes and synergistically working with other antioxidants.

3. **Cardiovascular Health:** Along with oleuropein, hydroxytyrosol, and tyrosol, olive leaf contains secoiridoids such as ligstroside and oleocanthal, which contribute to its cardiovascular benefits. These compounds have anti-inflammatory and vasodilatory effects, helping to improve blood pressure, cholesterol levels, and overall heart health.
4. **Anti-inflammatory Effects:** Olive leaf's remarkable anti-inflammatory effects can be attributed not only to the presence of oleuropein, hydroxytyrosol, and tyrosol but also to other beneficial compounds such as verbascoside, luteolin, and maslinic acid. These compounds work synergistically to combat inflammation and promote overall well-being. By inhibiting inflammatory pathways and reducing the production of pro-inflammatory molecules, olive leaf helps alleviate inflammation in the body.
5. **Blood Sugar Regulation:** Building on the foundation of well-known constituents like oleuropein, hydroxytyrosol, and tyrosol, olive leaf further incorporates compounds such as maslinic acid and oleanolic acid. These specific constituents have garnered attention in scientific studies for their potential in regulating blood sugar levels. Maslinic acid and oleanolic acid play a role in improving insulin sensitivity and enhancing glucose metabolism, ultimately contributing to the promotion of balanced blood sugar levels.
6. **Digestive Health:** Maslinic acid and oleanolic acid found in olive leaf possess anti-inflammatory properties that help soothe digestive discomfort and reduce inflammation in the gastrointestinal tract. They also contribute to maintaining a healthy gut environment by supporting the growth of beneficial gut bacteria and inhibiting the proliferation of harmful pathogens. Verbascoside, a potent antioxidant, aids in maintaining a balanced digestive system by neutralizing free radicals and protecting the integrity of the digestive tissues.
7. **Respiratory Health:** The health benefits of olive leaf for respiratory health are primarily attributed to its key compounds, oleuropein, hydroxytyrosol, and tyrosol. These compounds exhibit remarkable anti-inflammatory properties, which play a crucial role in reducing inflammation in the respiratory system. By reducing inflammation, they help alleviate respiratory symptoms and promote clearer airways, facilitating easier breathing. These compounds also possess antioxidant properties that help protect respiratory cells from oxidative stress and damage caused by free radicals.

8. **Bone Health:** Expanding on the well-established components like calcium and magnesium found in olive leaf, the presence of compounds such as verbascoside and oleuropein further enriches its impact on bone health. These specific constituents are recognized for their contributions to supporting bone density, preventing age-related bone loss, and promoting overall bone health.
9. **Cognitive Support:** Olive leaf's impact on cognitive function extends beyond oleuropein, hydroxytyrosol, and tyrosol. It also contains other notable compounds, such as verbascoside and oleocanthal, which contribute to its cognitive benefits. Verbascoside, a phenolic compound, helps protect brain cells from oxidative stress and reduces the risk of cognitive decline. It also has neuroprotective effects, promoting the growth and survival of neurons. Oleocanthal has been shown to exhibit anti-inflammatory properties and may help reduce the inflammation that can negatively impact brain function. By reducing neuroinflammation, oleocanthal may support cognitive health and improve memory and learning abilities.
10. **Skin Health:** Olive leaf's skin benefits extend beyond the widely recognized compounds of oleuropein, hydroxytyrosol, and tyrosol. Additional compounds present in olive leaf, such as verbascoside and rutin, also contribute to its remarkable effects on the skin as they possess potent antioxidant properties, helping to protect the skin from oxidative damage caused by free radicals. By neutralizing these harmful molecules, they support a youthful complexion by reducing the appearance of fine lines and wrinkles. Verbascoside and rutin exhibit anti-inflammatory properties, which help soothe and calm the skin, reducing redness, irritation, and inflammation.

While olive leaf is generally considered safe to consume, there are certain medical contradictions and precautions to be aware of. Individuals with low blood pressure should exercise caution when using olive leaf, as it has hypotensive effects and may further lower blood pressure. Individuals taking medications for blood pressure management should consult with a healthcare professional before using olive leaf. Additionally, individuals with diabetes or those taking antidiabetic medications should use olive leaf with caution, as it may lower blood sugar levels. If you have scheduled surgery, it is important to inform your healthcare provider about your olive leaf use, as it may interfere with blood clotting and blood sugar control during the perioperative period. Individuals with allergies to olive tree pollen or related plants may be at an increased risk of developing allergic reactions to olive leaf. Women who are pregnant or lactating should consult with their herbalist/practitioner prior to using this herb.

OREGANO LEAF

Oregano leaf, scientifically known as Origanum vulgare, has a fascinating history deeply rooted in the Mediterranean region. For centuries, it has been an integral part of Mediterranean cuisine, prized for its distinct aroma and flavor that adds depth and complexity to various dishes. However, its significance extends far beyond culinary uses, as oregano leaf has been valued for its remarkable medicinal properties as well. Throughout ancient civilizations, from the Greeks and Romans to the Egyptians, oregano leaf has been revered for its therapeutic benefits. It was used as an herbal remedy to address a wide range of health issues, ranging from digestive complaints to respiratory ailments. The ancient Greeks even considered oregano leaf to be a symbol of joy and happiness. Oregano leaf's popularity and widespread use continued to flourish over the centuries, with its medicinal properties being passed down through generations. Its reputation as a potent natural remedy made it a staple in traditional herbal medicine practices.

Now, let's explore ten extensive health and longevity benefits associated with oregano leaf:

1. **Immune System Support:** Oregano leaf contains carvacrol, rosmarinic acid, and other compounds known for their immune-boosting properties. These compounds help support a healthy immune system by enhancing immune responses and providing defense against harmful pathogens.
2. **Digestive Health:** The beneficial effects of oregano leaf on the digestive system can be attributed to its unique combination of active compounds, including carvacrol, thymol, and rosmarinic acid. These compounds possess antimicrobial properties that help combat harmful bacteria and parasites in the digestive tract, promoting a healthy microbial balance and supporting optimal digestive function. Oregano leaf contains volatile oils that stimulate the production of digestive enzymes, which play a crucial role in breaking down food and facilitating nutrient absorption. By enhancing the efficiency of digestion, oregano leaf may help alleviate common digestive symptoms such as bloating, indigestion, and gas. It aids in the proper breakdown of food, allowing nutrients to be absorbed more effectively by the body.

3. **Antimicrobial Effects:** Oregano leaf possesses potent antimicrobial properties attributed to its active compounds. Carvacrol, in particular, has been shown to combat harmful bacteria, fungi, and parasites, promoting a healthy microbial balance in the body.
4. **Respiratory Health:** The therapeutic benefits of oregano leaf can be attributed to its unique combination of active compounds, including carvacrol, thymol, and rosmarinic acid, which possess antimicrobial, anti-inflammatory, and expectorant properties. The antimicrobial properties of oregano leaf help combat harmful microorganisms that can contribute to respiratory infections and discomfort. It may help inhibit the growth of bacteria, viruses, and fungi that may cause respiratory symptoms. By reducing the presence of these pathogens, oregano leaf supports a healthy respiratory system and aids in alleviating coughs and congestion.
5. **Anti-inflammatory Effects:** Rosmarinic acid acts as a powerful anti-inflammatory agent by inhibiting the production of inflammatory compounds in the body, such as prostaglandins and leukotrienes. Inflammation is a natural response of the immune system to protect the body from infection or injury. However, chronic inflammation can contribute to the development of various health conditions, including cardiovascular disease, arthritis, and chronic inflammatory disorders. By reducing inflammation, oregano leaf helps to maintain a balanced inflammatory response, promoting overall well-being.
6. **Antioxidant Powerhouse:** The abundant presence of antioxidants in oregano leaf helps safeguard cells from the harmful effects of free radicals and unstable molecules that can cause cellular damage and contribute to various health issues. The antioxidants found in oregano leaf, such as rosmarinic acid, thymol, and carvacrol, act as scavengers, neutralizing free radicals and preventing them from causing oxidative damage to cells and tissues. By donating an electron to the free radicals, antioxidants help stabilize them, reducing their ability to initiate harmful chain reactions in the body. Oxidative stress occurs when there is an imbalance between the production of free radicals and the body's ability to neutralize them with antioxidants. This imbalance can lead to cellular damage, inflammation, and the progression of chronic diseases. Oregano leaf's rich antioxidant content helps combat oxidative stress by effectively neutralizing free radicals and minimizing their detrimental effects on cellular structures and DNA.

7. **Cardiovascular Health:** Rosmarinic acid and carvacrol have been shown to support healthy blood pressure regulation. These compounds may help relax and dilate blood vessels, promoting optimal blood flow and reducing the strain on the heart. Oxidative stress and inflammation can contribute to the development of cardiovascular diseases, including atherosclerosis and heart disease. The antioxidants in oregano leaf help protect against oxidative damage and reduce inflammation, which may help maintain the health of blood vessels and prevent the formation of plaques. Cholesterol management is another essential aspect of cardiovascular health, and oregano leaf may offer support in this area as well.
8. **Bone Health:** Oregano leaf contains essential minerals like calcium, iron, and manganese, which are vital for maintaining healthy bones and supporting bone density.
9. **Cognitive Support:** Oregano leaf contains compounds like rosmarinic acid and carvacrol, which have been linked to potential cognitive benefits. These compounds may contribute to improved cognitive function by protecting brain cells from oxidative stress, promoting neuronal health, and potentially enhancing memory and learning abilities. While more research might be needed in this area, the neuroprotective and anti-inflammatory properties of oregano leaf's active compounds suggest a possible role in supporting brain health and cognitive function.
10. **Skin Health:** Oregano leaf offers potential benefits for skin health, making it a valuable ingredient in topical applications and skincare products. Its soothing properties and rich composition of bioactive compounds contribute to its ability to promote a clear complexion, soothe skin irritations, and provide age-reversal effects. The soothing properties of oregano leaf may help calm various skin irritations, such as redness, itching, and inflammation. Oregano leaf possesses potent antimicrobial and anti-inflammatory properties, making it beneficial for healing the skin. When applied topically, oregano leaf may help combat skin infections, soothe inflammation, and support the skin's natural healing process.

While oregano leaf is generally considered safe to consume, there are certain medical contradictions and precautions to consider. Oregano leaf may interact with anticoagulant medications, such as warfarin, increasing the risk of bleeding. Individuals with bleeding disorders or scheduled for surgery should exercise caution. Oregano leaf may also interfere with the absorption of iron due to its high content of tannins. Individuals with iron deficiency or anemia should consider spacing out the consumption of oregano leaf from iron-rich foods or supplements. Individuals with known allergies to plants in the Lamiaceae family, including basil, mint, or lavender, may be at risk of allergic reactions to oregano leaf. Oregano leaf has been reported to have potential uterine-stimulating effects, so pregnant women should avoid consuming it in large amounts to minimize the risk of contractions. Those who are lactating can safely consume culinary amounts of oregano. Consult with your herbalist/practitioner before consuming large therapeutic doses of this herb during lactation.

OREGON GRAPE ROOT

Oregon grape root, scientifically known as Mahonia aquifolium, is a flowering plant that thrives in the western regions of North America. This perennial plant is notable for its striking yellow flowers and clusters of small purple berries. Oregon grape root has been valued for centuries by various Native American tribes for its diverse range of medicinal properties and is an important herb in traditional herbal medicine. The historical use of Oregon grape root by Native American tribes reflects its significance as a medicinal plant. It has been employed to address various health concerns, including digestive issues, skin conditions, and infections. The roots of the plant contain numerous bioactive compounds that contribute to its therapeutic effects.

Now, let's explore ten extensive health and longevity benefits associated with Oregon grape root:

1. **Digestive Health:** Oregon grape root is known for its ability to support digestive health through various mechanisms. One of its primary actions is the stimulation of bile production. Bile is essential for the digestion and absorption of fats, and adequate bile flow helps in emulsifying fats and enhancing their breakdown. By promoting bile production, Oregon grape root aids in the efficient digestion of fats, preventing symptoms such as bloating and indigestion that can occur due to impaired fat metabolism. Oregon grape root contains berberine, a bioactive compound known for its beneficial effects on digestion. Berberine has been found to enhance digestive enzyme activity, including amylase and lipase, which are responsible for the breakdown of carbohydrates and fats, respectively. By increasing the activity of these enzymes, Oregon grape root supports the proper digestion and utilization of nutrients, leading to improved digestive function. Oregon grape root exhibits mild laxative properties, helping to promote regular bowel movements and prevent constipation.
2. **Liver Health:** The beneficial effects of Oregon grape root on liver function are attributed to compounds like berberine, which help protect and support the liver's detoxification processes, contributing to overall liver health.
3. **Antioxidant Powerhouse:** Oregon grape root is rich in antioxidants that protect cells from damage caused by free radicals. These antioxidants contribute to overall health and longevity by neutralizing harmful free radicals.

4. **Immune System Support:** Berberine's ability to combat harmful microorganisms, including bacteria, viruses, and fungi, not only helps the body ward off infections but also assists in maintaining a balanced microbial environment within the body. By supporting the immune system's ability to recognize and eliminate harmful pathogens, berberine aids in promoting overall immune health, making it a valuable ally in bolstering the body's natural defense mechanisms. Additionally, berberine's anti-inflammatory properties may further contribute to its immune-boosting capabilities by reducing excessive inflammation that can weaken the immune response.
5. **Skin Health:** The anti-inflammatory compounds present in Oregon grape root, including berberine, may help reduce inflammation of the skin, soothing these conditions and promoting a calmer, more balanced complexion. In addition to its anti-inflammatory properties, Oregon grape root also exhibits antimicrobial activity. Certain skin conditions, such as acne, can be exacerbated by the presence of harmful bacteria on the skin's surface. The antimicrobial compounds in Oregon grape root, including berberine, may help combat these bacteria, reducing the risk of infection and promoting a healthier skin environment. Oregon grape root is rich in antioxidants, which play a vital role in maintaining skin health. Antioxidants help protect the skin cells from oxidative damage caused by free radicals, which can contribute to premature aging and skin damage. By neutralizing these free radicals, Oregon grape root's antioxidants contribute to a healthier complexion and support the skin's natural defenses against environmental stressors.
6. **Anti-cancer Effects:** Berberine has garnered attention for its potential anti-cancer properties. It may play a role in inhibiting the growth and proliferation of specific cancer cells. This anti-cancer effect is thought to be multifaceted, as berberine influences various cellular processes that are critical to cancer development and progression. It has been shown to interfere with the signaling pathways involved in uncontrolled cell growth, trigger apoptosis (programmed cell death) in cancer cells, and impede angiogenesis, which is the formation of new blood vessels that tumors rely on for nutrients and oxygen. Furthermore, berberine's ability to modulate inflammation and oxidative stress, which are known contributors to cancer development, adds to its potential as a natural anti-cancer agent.

7. **Anti-inflammatory Effects:** Berberine inhibits the production of pro-inflammatory molecules, such as cytokines and prostaglandins, which are responsible for triggering and sustaining inflammation in the body. By reducing the production of these inflammatory mediators, Oregon grape root helps to dampen the inflammatory response and alleviate symptoms like pain, swelling, and redness. The anti-inflammatory effects of Oregon grape root extend beyond its action on specific inflammatory mediators. It also supports the overall health of tissues and organs affected by inflammation. By reducing inflammation, Oregon grape root may help promote tissue repair, enhance the body's healing processes, and support overall well-being.
8. **Urinary Tract Health:** Berberine is a natural alkaloid that exhibits antimicrobial properties, making it effective against certain bacteria, fungi, and parasites that can cause urinary tract infections (UTIs) and other urinary tract issues. When consumed, berberine may help inhibit the growth and activity of harmful microorganisms that may infect the urinary tract. It works by interfering with the microbial cell walls, preventing their adherence to the urinary tract walls and reducing their ability to cause infection. This antimicrobial action helps to promote a healthy microbial balance in the urinary system. In addition to its antimicrobial effects, Oregon grape root may also support urinary tract health by soothing the tissues of the urinary tract. It is believed to have a calming and toning effect on the urinary system, helping to maintain proper functioning and promoting comfort.
9. **Cardiovascular Health:** The berberine in Oregon grape root may help regulate cholesterol metabolism by reducing the production of cholesterol in the liver and enhancing the clearance of LDL (bad) cholesterol from the bloodstream. By promoting healthy cholesterol levels, Oregon grape root may contribute to the prevention of plaque buildup in the arteries, reducing the risk of cardiovascular diseases such as atherosclerosis. Berberine has also been shown to have beneficial effects on blood pressure regulation. It may help relax and dilate blood vessels, improving blood flow and reducing hypertension. By supporting healthy blood pressure levels, Oregon grape root may help maintain optimal cardiovascular function and reduce the risk of cardiovascular complications.

10. **Oral Health:** The inclusion of Oregon grape root in oral care products stems from its recognized potential to enhance oral health. This botanical ingredient is believed to actively contribute to maintaining healthy gums, serving as a preventive measure against plaque formation. Berberine, a prominent alkaloid in Oregon grape root known for its antimicrobial and anti-inflammatory properties, has been studied for its potential in managing oral health issues by inhibiting the growth of bacteria associated with dental plaque and gingivitis. Additionally, other alkaloids present in Oregon grape root, such as berbamine and oxyacanthine, may contribute to its overall oral health effects.

While Oregon grape root is generally considered safe to consume, there are certain medical contradictions and drug interactions to be aware of. Oregon grape root may interact with certain medications, including anticoagulants and antiplatelet drugs, due to its potential antiplatelet and blood-thinning effects. It may interfere with the absorption of iron supplements, so it is recommended to separate the intake of Oregon grape root and iron supplements by a few hours. Allergy to Oregon grape root or plants belonging to the Berberidaceae family, such as barberry and goldenseal, is possible. Individuals with known allergies to these plants should avoid using Oregon grape root. Pregnant or lactating individuals should exercise caution and consult with their herbalist/practitioner before using Oregon grape root.

ORRIS ROOT

Orris root, scientifically known as Iris germanica, has a rich and fascinating history that spans centuries and is widely recognized for its aromatic properties. This herbaceous perennial, native to Europe, has been cultivated for its rhizomes, which contain the prized orris root. The use of orris root can be traced back to ancient civilizations, where it was highly valued for its diverse applications and potential health benefits. In ancient Egypt, orris root was revered for its sacred and mystical properties, being used in perfumes and cosmetics. It held a significant place in traditional medicine practices as well. Throughout history, orris root has remained a sought-after ingredient in perfumery, known for its delicate and captivating fragrance. The rhizomes are carefully harvested and processed to extract the aromatic compounds, which are used in creating perfumes, potpourri, and other fragrant products. Orris root has also found its place in culinary traditions, adding a unique floral and earthy flavor to dishes and beverages.

Now, let's explore ten extensive health and longevity benefits associated with orris root:

1. **Hair and Scalp Health:** Orris root aids scalp and hair health through its essential oils, including pinene, limonene, and myrcene, which have antimicrobial properties and help maintain a clean scalp environment. The antioxidants in orris root protect against oxidative stress, promoting hair follicle health. Additionally, the root contains essential minerals and vitamins like zinc, iron, and vitamins E and C, which nourish the hair follicles and support healthy hair growth. Overall, orris root strengthens the hair, improves texture, and enhances shine.
2. **Respiratory Health:** Orris root is known for its expectorant properties, which may help alleviate respiratory issues such as coughs, bronchitis, and congestion. Active compounds like saponins in orris root may help loosen mucus and phlegm, making it easier to expel and providing relief from respiratory congestion and discomfort.
3. **Anti-inflammatory Effects:** Orris root contains compounds that possess anti-inflammatory properties. These properties may help reduce inflammation in the body. The active compounds, including iridoids and flavonoids, help to modulate the body's inflammatory response, reducing inflammation and associated symptoms.

4. **Hormonal Balance:** This herb contains various plant compounds, including flavonoids and saponins, which have been found to act as natural hormone regulators. Flavonoids have estrogenic properties that may help balance hormonal levels by mimicking the effects of estrogen in the body. They can interact with hormone receptors and modulate hormonal activity, thus alleviating symptoms such as menstrual cramps and regulating menstrual cycles. Saponins, on the other hand, can support hormonal balance by promoting the production and regulation of hormones.
5. **Immune System Support:** Orris root contains antioxidants that may help strengthen the immune system, protecting the body against various infections and diseases. These antioxidants, including phenolic compounds and flavonoids, help to neutralize harmful free radicals and support the body's natural defense mechanisms, promoting a healthy immune system.
6. **Wound Healing:** Orris root possesses antiseptic properties that make it a valuable ingredient for addressing minor cuts, scrapes, and wounds. These properties may help prevent infections and promote faster healing. The antiseptic effects of orris root can be attributed to its various active compounds, including tannins, flavonoids, and phenolic acids.
7. **Oral Health:** Orris root possesses antimicrobial properties that may help maintain oral health by preventing the growth of harmful bacteria, reducing bad breath, and promoting healthy gums. The antimicrobial compounds in orris root, such as tannins and saponins, help to inhibit the growth of bacteria that can contribute to oral health issues, supporting a healthy oral microbiome.
8. **Antiseptic Effects:** Tannins present in orris root have astringent properties that help cleanse and tighten the skin, creating a barrier against harmful microorganisms. Flavonoids, such as rutin and quercetin, exhibit antimicrobial properties, inhibiting the growth of bacteria and preventing infection. Phenolic acids, including caffeic acid and ferulic acid, also contribute to the antiseptic activity of orris root by exerting antimicrobial effects. Together, these compounds work synergistically to provide an antiseptic effect, protecting the affected area from bacterial colonization and promoting optimal healing.

9. **Anxiety and Stress Relief:** Orris root is highly valued in aromatherapy for its delightful and soothing aroma, which is known to have profound effects on the mind and emotions. The aromatic compounds present in orris root, such as terpenes and sesquiterpenes, contribute to its therapeutic properties. These compounds interact with the olfactory system, stimulating the brain's limbic system and triggering emotional responses. The aromatic scent of orris root has a calming and relaxing effect on the nervous system, helping to reduce stress, anxiety, and tension.
10. **Graceful-aging Effects:** Orris root is highly regarded for its potential pro-aging effects on the skin. Its rich antioxidant content, including phenolic compounds and flavonoids, helps protect the skin from free radicals and oxidative stress caused by environmental factors such as pollution and UV radiation. These antioxidants neutralize harmful free radicals, preventing them from causing cellular damage and premature aging. By reducing oxidative stress, orris root helps maintain the skin's elasticity, firmness, and youthful appearance. Orris root contains natural moisturizing agents that help keep the skin hydrated, enhancing its overall texture and reducing the appearance of fine lines and wrinkles.

> While orris root is generally considered safe to consume, there are certain medical contradictions and precautions to consider. Orris root may interact with medications that are metabolized by the liver, such as certain statins, antiarrhythmics, and anticoagulants. Therefore, it is important to consult with a healthcare professional before using orris root if you are taking any medications that may be affected by liver metabolism. Individuals with known allergies or sensitivities to plants in the iris family (Iridaceae) should avoid the use of orris root. Pregnant and breastfeeding women should consult with their herbalist/practitioner prior to using orris root.

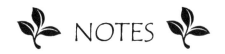

NOTES

OSHA ROOT

Osha root, scientifically known as Ligusticum porteri, is a perennial herb native to the Rocky Mountains of North America. It has a rich and storied history deeply rooted in the traditions of Native American tribes, who have long revered it for its exceptional medicinal properties. For centuries, these indigenous communities have utilized osha root as a versatile and potent herbal remedy. Osha root holds a sacred place in their traditional healing practices, where it is believed to possess spiritual as well as physical healing powers. The indigenous peoples of the region have used this remarkable herb to address a diverse range of health concerns, including respiratory ailments, digestive issues, and immune support. They recognized osha root as a powerful ally in promoting overall well-being and restoring balance in the body. The profound respect and deep understanding of osha root's therapeutic potential have been passed down through generations, cementing its significance in Native American healing traditions.

Now, let's explore ten extensive health and longevity benefits associated with osha root:

1. **Respiratory Health:** Osha root is renowned for its exceptional respiratory benefits. It contains active compounds such as coumarins, phenolic acids (including ferulic acid and caffeic acid), and polysaccharides. These compounds contribute to its expectorant properties, helping to alleviate coughs, bronchitis, and other respiratory conditions. Osha root promotes the expulsion of mucus, clears congested airways, and soothes respiratory tissues, providing relief and supporting respiratory health.
2. **Immune System Support:** Osha root contains antimicrobial compounds, specifically umbelliferone and saponins. Umbelliferone is a natural compound known for its antimicrobial activity against various pathogens, including bacteria, viruses, and fungi. It helps inhibit the growth and replication of these microorganisms, thereby supporting the body's defense against infections. Saponins, on the other hand, are bioactive compounds that possess immune-stimulating properties. They have the ability to activate immune cells, such as macrophages and natural killer cells, and enhance their response to pathogens. This helps to bolster the immune system's ability to identify and eliminate harmful microorganisms, ultimately promoting a strong and resilient immune system.

3. **Anti-inflammatory Effects:** Osha root possesses powerful anti-inflammatory properties attributed to its active compounds, such as ferulic acid, caffeic acid, and coumarins. These compounds help reduce inflammation in the body by inhibiting the production of inflammatory mediators. Osha root can be valuable for relieving pain, swelling, and inflammation associated with various conditions, including arthritis and muscle injuries, promoting overall well-being.
4. **Digestive Health:** Osha root has a long history of traditional use for supporting digestion and alleviating gastrointestinal discomfort. It contains active compounds like ferulic acid and caffeic acid, which possess digestive benefits. Osha root helps soothe stomachaches, cramps, and indigestion by promoting the secretion of digestive juices and supporting healthy digestion.
5. **Sinus Relief:** Osha root is highly regarded for its ability to provide relief from sinus congestion and sinusitis. This is primarily attributed to its active compounds, including saponins. These compounds exhibit decongestant properties that help alleviate nasal congestion and reduce swelling in the sinus cavities. By clearing the nasal passages, osha root promotes better airflow and eases the discomfort associated with sinus-related symptoms. Additionally, osha root's expectorant properties assist in loosening and expelling excess mucus, further contributing to sinus relief.
6. **Cardiovascular Health:** Osha root has been associated with promoting healthy blood circulation and cardiovascular function. It contains active compounds like ferulic acid, caffeic acid, and coumarins, which support circulatory health by improving blood flow and protecting blood vessels from oxidative damage.
7. **Minor Burn Support:** Osha root's cooling and soothing properties make it an excellent choice for topical application on minor burns. When applied to the affected area, osha root may help provide immediate relief from pain and discomfort caused by the burn. Its cooling effect helps to reduce inflammation and soothe the burned skin. Additionally, osha root's compounds, including saponins, possess antimicrobial properties that may help protect the burned area from potential infections. By supporting the healing process, osha root promotes the regeneration of healthy skin cells and minimizes the risk of scarring. Its natural properties also help to keep the burn moisturized and prevent excessive dryness, allowing the skin to heal more effectively.

8. **Acne Support:** Osha root's antimicrobial properties make it a potential candidate for the treatment of acne when applied topically. Acne is often caused by the proliferation of bacteria, such as Streptococcus and/or Propionibacterium acnes, which can lead to inflammation and the formation of pimples. Osha root's antimicrobial activity helps to combat these acne-causing bacteria, reducing their population on the skin and potentially preventing the development of new breakouts.
9. **Wound Healing:** Osha root possesses properties that make it beneficial for wound healing when applied topically. It contains active compounds, such as saponins and tannins, that contribute to its wound-healing properties. These compounds have antimicrobial effects, helping to prevent infection by inhibiting the growth of bacteria and other microorganisms on the wound site. Osha root has soothing and anti-inflammatory properties that may help reduce inflammation, swelling, and pain associated with wounds. It also supports the formation of new tissue, aiding in the regeneration and repair of damaged skin. This promotes the healing process and can result in faster wound closure.
10. **Muscle and Joint Pain Relief:** Osha root has been traditionally used topically for its analgesic properties, making it beneficial for relieving muscle and joint pain. When applied to the affected area, osha root can provide a soothing and numbing sensation, helping to alleviate discomfort and reduce pain. This effect is attributed to the presence of active compounds, such as saponins and alkaloids, which possess analgesic and anti-inflammatory properties. These compounds work by blocking pain signals and reducing inflammation in the muscles and joints.

While osha root is generally considered safe to consume, there are specific medical contradictions and precautions to consider. Osha root may interact with certain medications, including anticoagulant or antiplatelet drugs, as it contains coumarin compounds that can have blood-thinning effects. Individuals taking these medications should exercise caution and consult with a healthcare professional before using osha root. Individuals with bleeding disorders or scheduled surgeries should avoid osha root due to its potential to affect blood clotting. Osha root should also be avoided by individuals with hormone-sensitive conditions, as it contains natural plant compounds that could potentially affect hormonal balance. Women who are pregnant should avoid this root. Women who are breastfeeding should consult with their herbalist/practitioner prior to using osha root.

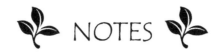# NOTES

PAPAYA SEED

Papaya, scientifically known as Carica papaya, boasts a fascinating history with origins in Central America and Mexico. Cultivated by ancient Mayan and Aztec civilizations, papaya gradually expanded its presence to various tropical regions. In historical contexts, papaya seeds were esteemed not only for their potential health benefits but also for their multifaceted applications in agriculture and cultural practices. Farmers ingeniously harnessed the power of crushed papaya seeds as an eco-friendly solution to repel pests and safeguard crops. Additionally, in certain cultures, these seeds carried symbolic weight, being associated with fertility and considered auspicious. They became integral in rituals and ceremonies, invoked to attract positive energies and blessings.

Now, let's explore ten extensive health and longevity benefits associated with papaya seed:

1. **Digestive Health:** Papaya seeds offer exceptional benefits for digestive health due to their rich content of the enzymes papain and chymopapain. These enzymes are potent proteolytic enzymes, meaning they have the ability to break down proteins. When consumed, papain and chymopapain assist the digestive system in efficiently breaking down complex proteins from the foods we eat. By doing so, they aid in the digestion and absorption of nutrients. These enzymes are particularly helpful in digesting meat and other protein-rich foods that can be challenging for some individuals to break down properly. Additionally, papain and chymopapain may support the digestive tract's overall health by reducing the likelihood of harmful bacteria and parasites taking hold in the intestines. Their antiparasitic properties may help combat intestinal worms and other harmful organisms, promoting a balanced gut environment. As a result, consuming papaya seeds or papain supplements has been associated with improved digestive function, reduced bloating, and relief from indigestion.
2. **Immune System Support:** Papaya seeds indeed contain vitamin C, a well-known immune system booster. They provide a range of other essential nutrients that collectively contribute to immune support. In addition to vitamin C, papaya seeds supply vital minerals such as magnesium, potassium, and calcium, all of which play integral roles in overall health and immune function. These minerals contribute to the body's ability to maintain a robust immune response and support various physiological processes essential for immune system effectiveness.

3. **Antimicrobial Effects:** Papaya seeds contain a bioactive alkaloid known as carpaine, which contains antimicrobial and antiparasitic properties. Carpaine exhibits a wide spectrum of activity against various pathogens, including bacteria, fungi, and parasites. Carpaine's antimicrobial effects are particularly valuable in promoting gastrointestinal health, as it may aid in controlling the growth of harmful bacteria and parasites in the digestive tract. Its antiparasitic properties suggest that carpaine could be beneficial in supporting the body's defense against parasitic infections.
4. **Detoxification:** Papaya seeds offer remarkable benefits for liver health due to the presence of various bioactive compounds. Among these, carpaine, a unique alkaloid found in papaya seeds, has been shown to possess hepatoprotective properties, aiding the liver in its natural detoxification processes. The seeds contain flavonoids, such as quercetin, and saponins, which act as potent antioxidants, supporting the liver's ability to neutralize harmful free radicals and reduce oxidative stress. These compounds help improve liver function and support detoxification.
5. **Anti-inflammatory Effects:** Papaya seeds offer significant anti-inflammatory effects thanks to the phenolic acids, flavonoids, and isothiocyanates found in papaya seeds. These compounds work synergistically to combat inflammation by inhibiting the activity of pro-inflammatory enzymes and molecules. As a result, papaya seeds may help alleviate symptoms associated with inflammatory conditions such as arthritis, joint pain, and muscle soreness.
6. **Collagen Support:** Papaya seeds contain essential nutrients like vitamin C and vitamin E, which are known to play a role in collagen synthesis. Vitamin C is a powerful antioxidant that supports the body's natural collagen production process by aiding in the conversion of proline, an amino acid, into collagen fibers. Vitamin E, another antioxidant, helps protect collagen fibers from damage caused by free radicals, preserving their structural integrity. Prolyl hydroxylases in papaya seeds play a crucial role in collagen synthesis. These enzymes require vitamin C as a cofactor to facilitate the hydroxylation of specific proline residues in procollagen chains. This modification allows the chains to fold into a stable triple helix structure, contributing to the strength and integrity of collagen. With the aid of papaya seeds' prolyl hydroxylases and their vitamin C content, collagen synthesis is supported, benefiting skin, bones, and connective tissues.

7. **Cardiovascular Health:** Papaya seeds contain antioxidants like phenolic acids and flavonoids, which have been associated with promoting heart health and reducing the risk of cardiovascular diseases.
8. **Antioxidant Powerhouse:** The antioxidant boost provided by papaya seeds stems from their rich content of beneficial phytonutrients, including flavonoids, phenolic acids, and isothiocyanates. These compounds play a crucial role in scavenging harmful free radicals in the body, neutralizing their damaging effects, and reducing oxidative stress. By doing so, papaya seeds help protect cells from damage, support cellular health, and promote overall well-being. Antioxidants are essential for maintaining a healthy immune system and reducing the risk of chronic diseases associated with oxidative damage, such as heart disease and cancer.
9. **Exfoliation Tool:** For exfoliation purposes, papaya seeds are typically used in their dried and ground form rather than raw. The drying process helps preserve the enzymes and compounds present in the seeds, making them effective for exfoliating the skin. To release the enzymes and compounds from inside the seeds, it is often recommended to crush or grind the dried papaya seeds before use. By breaking down the seeds, you ensure that the papain enzyme and other beneficial components are readily available for exfoliating the skin.
10. **Antiparasitic Effects:** These small, potent seeds contain bioactive compounds such as carpaine and benzyl isothiocyanate that have demonstrated promising abilities to combat various parasites, particularly intestinal worms. Carpaine, a natural alkaloid present in papaya seeds, has been studied for its anthelmintic properties, meaning it may help expel or destroy parasitic worms from the gastrointestinal tract. Additionally, benzyl isothiocyanate, another bioactive compound found in papaya seeds, has shown significant antiparasitic activity against certain types of parasites. The antiparasitic properties of papaya seeds make them a valuable natural remedy to support the body's defense against parasitic infections and promote gastrointestinal health

While papaya seeds are generally safe to consume, there are certain medical contradictions and warnings to consider. Papaya seeds may have blood-thinning properties due to their high content of papain, an enzyme that can interfere with blood clotting. Therefore, individuals taking anticoagulant or antiplatelet medications, such as warfarin or aspirin, should consult with a healthcare professional before consuming papaya seeds to avoid potential interactions and increased bleeding risks. Papaya seeds have been traditionally used as a natural vermifuge to expel intestinal worms. While this can be beneficial, individuals with known gastrointestinal disorders, such as irritable bowel syndrome or inflammatory bowel disease, should exercise caution, as the vermifuge properties may exacerbate symptoms. Papaya seeds contain compounds called alkaloids, which have been found to possess contraceptive effects in animal studies. Therefore, individuals trying to conceive or undergoing fertility treatments should avoid consuming papaya seeds. Individuals who have a known allergy to papaya or latex should avoid consuming papaya seeds, as they may experience allergic reactions. It is generally recommended that pregnant and lactating individuals avoid consuming papaya seeds in large therapeutic doses or for prolonged periods. Consult with your herbalist/practitioner prior to using papaya seeds during this period.

PAPRIKA

Paprika, scientifically known as Capsicum annuum, is a vibrant and flavorful spice with a history deeply rooted in Central and South America. Believed to have originated in the region that is now Mexico, paprika has a colorful journey that spans centuries and continents. Spanish explorers encountered paprika in the 16th century during their travels to the Americas, and they were intrigued by its unique taste and vibrant red color. They brought the spice back to Europe, where it quickly became popular and found its way into various cuisines. Today, paprika is an essential ingredient in many dishes around the world, adding not only a delightful taste but also a beautiful hue to food presentations. Interestingly, paprika comes in different varieties, each offering a distinct flavor profile, ranging from sweet and mild to hot and pungent. It is often made from dried and ground red bell peppers or chili peppers, and the intensity of its flavor is influenced by the type of pepper used and the processing methods. Now, let's explore ten extensive health and longevity benefits associated with paprika.

1. **Antioxidant Powerhouse:** Paprika contains various antioxidants, including carotenoids like beta-carotene, which convert to vitamin A in the body. These antioxidants help protect cells from oxidative damage, supporting healthy aging and reducing the risk of chronic diseases.
2. **Immune System Support:** Paprika is a good source of vitamin C, which is crucial for a strong immune system. Vitamin C enhances the production of white blood cells, which play a vital role in defending against infections and maintaining overall health.
3. **Cognitive Support:** Paprika is particularly abundant in vitamin B6, which plays a crucial role in brain function and the synthesis of neurotransmitters. It contains vitamin E, a potent antioxidant that helps protect brain cells from oxidative stress. Paprika also provides significant amounts of vitamin C, potassium, and magnesium, which are essential nutrients for brain health due to its involvement in neurotransmitter production and supporting cognitive abilities.
4. **Skin Health:** The antioxidants in paprika, along with its vitamin E content, promote healthy skin by protecting against free radicals and supporting collagen production. These properties may help maintain skin elasticity, reduce signs of aging, and support overall skin health.

5. **Cardiovascular Health:** The presence of capsaicin in hot paprika varieties may have beneficial effects on cardiovascular health. Capsaicin has been associated with improved blood circulation, reduced blood pressure, and a lower risk of heart disease.
6. **Anti-inflammatory Effects:** The antioxidants present in paprika, such as beta-carotene and vitamin C, have anti-inflammatory effects that help reduce inflammation in the body. Chronic inflammation is linked to various diseases and accelerated aging.
7. **Digestive Health:** Paprika stimulates the secretion of digestive enzymes, which enhances digestion and nutrient absorption. It can also help alleviate digestive discomfort and support a healthy gut.
8. **Stimulates Energy Expenditure:** Hot paprika varieties contain capsaicin, a compound that can stimulate energy expenditure in the body. This thermogenic effect may help increase calorie burning and promote a healthy energy balance.
9. **Detoxification:** Paprika contains specific compounds that can assist in the process of detoxification, such as carotenoids, including beta-carotene, which support liver function and aid in the body's natural detoxification processes. The antioxidants in paprika help enhance its detoxification abilities. Additionally, paprika contains other bioactive compounds like flavonoids, which have been shown to have hepatoprotective properties, meaning they may help protect the liver from damage caused by toxins.
10. **Antimicrobial Effects:** Paprika exhibits antimicrobial effects, including antibacterial and antifungal properties. These properties may help combat certain pathogens and promote a healthy immune system.

While paprika is generally considered safe to consume, individuals with known allergies to peppers or other members of the Solanaceae family should exercise caution as they may be sensitive to paprika. It is important to note that paprika does not typically have significant interactions with medications. Safety during pregnancy and lactation is generally acceptable when paprika is consumed in culinary servings.

PASSIONFLOWER

Passionflower, scientifically known as Passiflora incarnata, is an enchanting flowering plant that traces its origin to the Americas. This captivating plant has a long and rich history of traditional use, spanning centuries, where it has been treasured for its numerous health benefits and contributions to longevity. Native to the Americas, passionflower has been revered by indigenous cultures for its remarkable properties and has earned its place as an important herbal remedy. The plant's stunning and intricate blooms not only capture the attention of botanists and horticulturists but also symbolize its significance in cultural rituals and traditional medicine. Throughout history, various tribes and civilizations have utilized passionflower to support relaxation, promote restful sleep, soothe nervousness, and address a myriad of ailments. Its legacy as a revered herbal remedy continues to thrive as modern research sheds light on the plant's active compounds and their potential therapeutic effects.

Now, let's explore ten extensive health and longevity benefits associated with passionflower:

1. **Anxiety and Stress Relief:** Passionflower contains specific compounds like flavonoids such as chrysin, alkaloids such as harmol, and GABA (gamma-aminobutyric acid) that contribute to its calming properties. Flavonoids interact with receptors in the brain associated with anxiety, promoting relaxation and reducing stress. Alkaloids, particularly harmol, exhibit anxiolytic effects by modulating neurotransmitter activity, which helps ease nervous tension. GABA acts as an inhibitory neurotransmitter, promoting feelings of calmness and tranquility.
2. **Sleep Support:** Passionflower is rich in compounds like flavonoids (apigenin and chrysin), alkaloids (harmane), and gamma-aminobutyric acid (GABA). These compounds have calming and sedative effects on the central nervous system, which may help reduce anxiety and promote relaxation, making passionflower beneficial for improving sleep quality and managing sleep disturbances. The flavonoids, particularly apigenin, are known to bind to specific receptors in the brain, enhancing the effects of GABA, which is an inhibitory neurotransmitter that helps induce sleep and reduce insomnia symptoms. The alkaloids in passionflower may contribute to its anxiolytic and sedative properties, further supporting its role as a natural sleep aid.

3. **Mood Support:** Passionflower's mood-enhancing properties can be attributed to its flavonoids, specifically chrysin, which may increase the availability of mood-regulating neurotransmitters like serotonin. By modulating these neurotransmitters, passionflower helps alleviate symptoms of depression and promotes an overall sense of well-being.
4. **Cognitive Support:** Passionflower's positive impact on cognitive function is attributed to its specific flavonoids, including apigenin, luteolin, and quercetin. These bioactive compounds possess neuroprotective effects, supporting brain health by reducing oxidative stress and inflammation while enhancing focus, concentration, and memory. Apigenin and luteolin have been shown to improve synaptic plasticity and promote efficient neural communication, which is crucial for learning and memory processes. Quercetin acts as a potent antioxidant, neutralizing harmful free radicals and preserving brain cells from damage, which aids in preventing cognitive decline.
5. **Pain Relief:** Passionflower's analgesic properties stem from specific compounds, including harmane, harmol, and flavonoids like apigenin. Harmane and harmol are alkaloids found in passionflower, and they may work by interacting with pain receptors in the brain and central nervous system, thereby reducing pain perception. Flavonoids like apigenin possess anti-inflammatory effects, which can further contribute to pain relief by reducing inflammation and swelling that often accompanies painful conditions.
6. **Menopausal Relief:** The relief of menopausal symptoms by passionflower can be linked to its ability to interact with neurotransmitters, including serotonin and GABA. By modulating these neurotransmitters, passionflower may help alleviate hot flashes, night sweats, mood swings, and irritability commonly experienced during menopause.
7. **Skin Health:** Its flavonoids and phenolic acids exhibit antioxidant and anti-inflammatory properties, making passionflower suitable for topical application on the skin. When applied externally, passionflower may help soothe the skin, reduce redness, and promote a youthful appearance by combating oxidative stress and inflammation. These bioactive compounds work together to protect the skin from free radical damage, support collagen production, and maintain skin elasticity.

8. **Blood Pressure Management:** Passionflower's potential to regulate blood pressure is associated with its alkaloids, particularly harmane. Harmane acts as a vasodilator, helping to relax blood vessels and improve blood flow, thus contributing to maintaining healthy blood pressure levels.
9. **Digestive Health:** Passionflower's support for digestive wellness is linked to its flavonoids, such as chrysin and apigenin, which exhibit antispasmodic effects on the gastrointestinal tract. These compounds may help relieve indigestion, bloating, and gastrointestinal spasms, while also promoting a healthy digestive system.
10. **Anti-inflammatory Effects:** The flavonoids present in passionflower, such as apigenin, luteolin, and quercetin, have been extensively studied for their potent anti-inflammatory properties. These compounds help modulate the activity of inflammatory enzymes and signaling molecules in the body, leading to a reduction in inflammation. They also act as antioxidants, neutralizing free radicals that contribute to inflammatory processes and tissue damage. Isovitexin, another beneficial flavonoid found in passionflower, also contributes to its anti-inflammatory potential. Isovitexin acts on multiple inflammatory pathways, dampening the production of inflammatory molecules and cytokines.

While passionflower is generally considered safe to consume, there are certain medical contradictions and precautions to be aware of. Passionflower may potentiate the sedative effects of medications that have similar properties, such as sedatives, tranquilizers, or central nervous system depressants, leading to excessive drowsiness or dizziness. It is important to exercise caution if taking these medications concurrently. Individuals with a history of low blood pressure or hypotension should use passionflower with caution, as it may further lower blood pressure levels. People with liver disease or impaired liver function should consult with their herbalist/practitioner before using passionflower in large quantities. Individuals with a known allergy to passionflower or other plants in the Passifloraceae family should also avoid its use. Passionflower should be avoided during pregnancy and lactation.

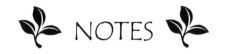

NOTES

PAU D'ARCO

Pau d'Arco, scientifically known as Tabebuia impetiginosa, is a remarkable herb with a history deeply intertwined with the cultures of the Amazon rainforest and various regions of South America. For centuries, indigenous communities revered this plant for its remarkable medicinal properties, using it to address a wide array of health concerns. The tree from which pau d'Arco is derived, with its striking pinkish-purple flowers, has been a symbol of strength and resilience in these ancient cultures. Indigenous tribes carefully harvested the inner bark of the pau d'Arco tree, recognizing its potential to promote health and well-being. They utilized this herb in traditional healing practices to address various ailments, including infections, inflammation, and digestive issues. Pau d'Arco's legacy of traditional use was eventually recognized by explorers and settlers, who marveled at its healing prowess and adopted it into their own pharmacopeias.

Now, let's explore ten extensive health and longevity benefits associated with pau d'Arco:

1. **Immune System Support:** Pau d'Arco's immune-enhancing properties are attributed to the presence of active compounds such as lapachol, quercetin, and beta-lapachone. These compounds help strengthen the immune system by boosting the activity of immune cells and promoting the production of antibodies, supporting the body's defense against pathogens.
2. **Digestive Health:** Pau d'Arco's beneficial effects on digestive health are attributed to compounds like lapachol and beta-lapachone. These compounds help promote a healthy gut environment by inhibiting the growth of harmful bacteria and fungi, supporting digestive wellness, and alleviating gastrointestinal issues such as bloating, indigestion, and diarrhea.
3. **Antifungal Effects:** Pau d'Arco's natural antifungal properties are mainly due to the compound lapachol. It has been shown to be effective against various fungal infections, including candida overgrowth and athlete's foot, making it a potential remedy for these conditions.
4. **Blood Cleansing:** Pau d'Arco's blood purifying and detoxifying properties are attributed to lapachol and other active compounds. These compounds help cleanse the blood, promote liver function, and aid in the removal of toxins from the body, contributing to overall detoxification.

5. **Anti-inflammatory Effects:** Pau d'Arco's potent anti-inflammatory effects can be attributed to specific compounds present in the herb, primarily lapachol, a naphthoquinone with notable anti-inflammatory properties. Additionally, pau d'Arco contains other phenolic compounds like quercetin and beta-lapachone, which also contribute to its anti-inflammatory action. These compounds work synergistically to inhibit pro-inflammatory enzymes, such as cyclooxygenase (COX) and lipoxygenase (LOX), which are responsible for the production of inflammatory molecules like prostaglandins and leukotrienes. By reducing the production of these inflammatory mediators, pau d'Arco helps alleviate inflammation in the body, potentially leading to improved joint health and reduced pain commonly associated with inflammatory conditions.
6. **Antioxidant Powerhouse:** Pau d'Arco's rich antioxidant content, including quercetin and lapachol, helps neutralize free radicals and reduce oxidative stress. By protecting cells from damage caused by free radicals, these antioxidants contribute to cellular health and may help prevent age-related damage.
7. **Respiratory Health:** Pau d'Arco's benefits for respiratory health are mainly due to lapachol and quercetin. These compounds possess anti-inflammatory and antimicrobial properties that may help alleviate symptoms of respiratory conditions such as bronchitis and coughs.
8. **Anti-cancer Effects:** Lapachol and beta-lapachone have demonstrated potential anti-cancer and anti-tumor properties. These compounds work by inhibiting the growth of certain cancer cells and tumors, showing potential for cancer prevention and treatment.
9. **Pain Relief:** Pau d'Arco's potential analgesic effects are attributed to several bioactive compounds, including lapachol, beta-lapachone, and additional constituents found in the herb. These compounds collectively contribute to its pain-relieving properties, offering potential relief from conditions such as arthritis, rheumatism, menstrual cramps, and nerve-related discomfort.
10. **Skin Health:** Pau d'Arco's topical benefits for skin health are linked to its anti-inflammatory and wound-healing properties, mainly due to lapachol. When applied topically, it may help soothe skin irritations, reduce inflammation, and support the healing process of wounds, promoting overall skin health.

While Pau d'Arco is generally considered safe to consume, there are certain medical contradictions and precautions to be aware of. Pau d'Arco may interact with certain medications, including anticoagulant or antiplatelet drugs, which can increase the risk of bleeding. Individuals with bleeding disorders or those scheduled for surgery should exercise caution and consult with a healthcare professional before using Pau d'Arco. This herb may have potential immunosuppressive effects, so individuals taking immunosuppressive medications should avoid its use or consult with a healthcare professional. Individuals with known hypersensitivity to Pau d'Arco or other plants in the Bignoniaceae family, such as Trumpet Trees (Tabebuia spp.), Jacaranda (Jacaranda mimosifolia), Catalpa (Catalpa spp.), Yellow Bells (Tecoma stans), Desert Willow (Chilopsis linearis), Queen's Wreath (Petrea volubilis), and Trumpet Vine (Campsis spp.), may experience skin rashes, itching, or respiratory reactions when exposed to the herb. Pau d'Arco should be avoided during pregnancy. Those who are lactating should consult with their herbalist/practitioner prior to using this herb.

NOTES

PEPPERMINT LEAF

Peppermint leaf, scientifically known as Mentha x piperita, has a rich and fascinating history that stretches back to ancient civilizations. Its origins can be traced to Europe and the Middle East, where it was believed to have been first cultivated. Peppermint is a hybrid of two mint species, watermint (Mentha aquatica) and spearmint (Mentha spicata), combining the best qualities of both plants. Throughout the ages, peppermint has been valued for its unique and refreshing aroma, which invigorates the senses and enlivens the mind. Its versatility and delightful flavor have made it a cherished ingredient in various culinary delights, from teas and beverages to desserts and savory dishes. Beyond its culinary uses, peppermint has been highly esteemed for its numerous health benefits. Ancient civilizations, such as the ancient Egyptians, Greeks, and Romans, valued peppermint for its medicinal properties, using it to address various ailments and promote well-being.

Now, let's explore ten extensive health and longevity benefits associated with peppermint leaf:

1. **Digestive Health:** Peppermint leaf's digestive benefits stem from its active compounds, particularly menthol and menthone. Menthol has antispasmodic properties that help relax the muscles of the gastrointestinal tract, alleviating symptoms of indigestion, bloating, and gas. It can also soothe stomach discomfort by reducing muscle contractions in the intestines, promoting healthy digestion.
2. **Nausea Relief:** Peppermint leaf's soothing effect on the stomach can be attributed to its menthol content. Menthol helps calm the stomach lining and reduces feelings of nausea. It is especially beneficial for alleviating morning sickness during pregnancy and motion sickness when inhaled or consumed as a tea.
3. **Respiratory Health:** Peppermint leaf's menthol acts as a natural decongestant, helping to clear the airways and ease sinus congestion. It also has mild expectorant properties, facilitating the expulsion of mucus and alleviating coughs.
4. **Headache and Migraine Relief:** Peppermint leaf's cooling properties are effective in reducing headache symptoms. The essential oil of peppermint contains menthol, which can dilate blood vessels and improve blood flow, providing relief from tension headaches and migraines when applied topically or inhaled.

5. **Muscle Relaxation:** Peppermint leaf essential oil's analgesic properties, mainly due to menthol, may help soothe muscle pain and reduce soreness. When applied topically, it can relax tense muscles and provide relief from discomfort.
6. **Cognitive Support:** Peppermint leaf's invigorating aroma, particularly its menthol component, can enhance mental clarity and focus. Inhaling the scent of peppermint can stimulate alertness and combat mental fatigue, promoting cognitive performance.
7. **Oral Health:** Peppermint leaf's essential oil is a powerhouse of oral health benefits due to its potent antimicrobial properties. The key active compounds responsible for these effects include menthol, menthone, and limonene. These compounds have been shown to exhibit significant antibacterial and antifungal activities, making peppermint leaf an effective natural aid for promoting oral hygiene and combating oral bacteria that can cause bad breath and various dental issues.
8. **Anxiety and Stress Relief:** Peppermint leaf's calming and relaxing effects are attributed to its menthol content. Inhaling peppermint's aroma or consuming it in tea form may help reduce stress and anxiety and promote a sense of calmness.
9. **Skin and Hair Health:** Peppermint leaf's skin and hair benefits can be attributed to its rich content of essential oils, primarily menthol and menthone, which provide its unique soothing and cooling properties. When applied topically, peppermint leaf can effectively alleviate itching and reduce inflammation in the skin, making it an excellent remedy for minor skin irritations like insect bites, rashes, and sunburns. Its cooling sensation can bring instant relief and comfort to irritated skin, leaving it feeling refreshed and revitalized. Peppermint leaf's topical application is also beneficial for maintaining a healthy scalp and promoting healthy hair. Its soothing properties may help soothe an itchy scalp and reduce scalp inflammation, making it an ideal solution for those experiencing discomfort due to dryness or dandruff.
10. **Antimicrobial Effects:** Peppermint leaf possesses antimicrobial properties, primarily attributed to its essential oil. These antimicrobial properties may help inhibit the growth of certain bacteria and fungi both internally and externally. When consumed as a tea or used in culinary applications, peppermint leaf's antimicrobial effects can potentially support digestive health by reducing harmful bacteria in the gut. On the skin, peppermint leaf's essential oil may help combat skin infections and irritation caused by certain microbes.

While peppermint leaf is generally considered safe to consume, there are certain medical contradictions and precautions to consider. Peppermint may interact with certain medications, such as antacids, proton pump inhibitors, and medications that are metabolized by the liver. It is advisable to consult with a healthcare professional if you have any of these specific medical conditions or are taking medications. People with a history of gallbladder disorders or gallstones should exercise caution, as peppermint may stimulate gallbladder contractions. Individuals with a hiatal hernia, a condition where part of the stomach pushes through the diaphragm, may experience worsened symptoms. This herb is generally considered safe to use during pregnancy and lactation.

NOTES

PERIWINKLE

Periwinkle, scientifically known as Vinca minor, is an enchanting evergreen herbaceous plant that traces its origins to Europe but has since established itself in various regions worldwide through naturalization. Admired for its stunning violet-blue flowers, periwinkle boasts a fascinating and extensive history in traditional herbal medicine. Throughout the ages, this remarkable herb has been cherished for its versatile array of health benefits and renowned age-reversal properties. Its traditional use spans centuries, where it has been employed as a remedy for various ailments and celebrated for its potential to enhance overall well-being. Today, periwinkle continues to captivate with its allure and remains a cherished botanical treasure, contributing to the world of herbal remedies and health support. Now, let's explore ten extensive health and longevity benefits associated with periwinkle:

1. **Diuretic Effects:** Periwinkle has the ability to enhance the elimination of excess fluids and toxins from the body. This diuretic action is thought to be beneficial for individuals dealing with conditions related to fluid retention or edema, as it can help reduce swelling and the accumulation of fluids in tissues. By increasing urine production and frequency, periwinkle may assist in maintaining fluid balance and supporting overall kidney function. Additionally, the diuretic properties of periwinkle may contribute to detoxification by aiding in the removal of waste products and harmful substances from the body.
2. **Anti-inflammatory Effects:** Vincamine has been found to possess anti-inflammatory effects. Vincamine may help inhibit the production of pro-inflammatory molecules, such as cytokines and prostaglandins, thereby reducing overall inflammation in the body. Periwinkle contains tannins, which also possess anti-inflammatory properties. Tannins may help soothe and protect tissues by reducing inflammation and promoting tissue repair.
3. **Neuroprotective Effects:** Vincamine plays a crucial role in safeguarding brain health. Vincamine has exhibited significant neuroprotective properties by shielding brain cells from oxidative damage and inflammation. It actively inhibits oxidative stress, which is detrimental to brain cells, while also promoting cellular energy production. These combined actions are pivotal in promoting optimal brain health and potentially slowing down the progression of degenerative brain diseases.

4. **Cardiovascular Health:** Periwinkle has been traditionally used to support a healthy cardiovascular system. One of the key active compounds responsible for these benefits is vincamine. Vincamine has been shown to have vasodilatory properties, meaning it helps widen blood vessels, leading to improved circulation.
5. **Graceful-aging Effects:** Periwinkle contains active compounds such as flavonoids, alkaloids, and phenolic acids, which work harmoniously as antioxidants to neutralize harmful free radicals that accumulate in the body due to various factors like exposure to pollution, unhealthy diet, and stress. By neutralizing these free radicals, periwinkle helps shield cells from oxidative damage, which is a significant contributor to aging and age-related conditions.
6. **Wound Healing:** Periwinkle leaves harbor an array of active compounds, including alkaloids, tannins, and flavonoids, that contribute to their remarkable wound-healing abilities. These compounds work synergistically to promote the regeneration of damaged skin tissue and aid in the clotting process, effectively helping wounds to close faster. Additionally, the anti-inflammatory properties of periwinkle help reduce swelling and redness around the wound, minimizing discomfort and providing a conducive environment for the healing process. Whether it's minor cuts, bruises, or skin irritations, the application of periwinkle-infused ointments or poultices can expedite the recovery of the affected area and ensure a smooth and efficient healing response.
7. **Antimicrobial Effects:** Periwinkle contains potent antimicrobial properties attributed to its bioactive compounds, including alkaloids, flavonoids, and tannins. These properties enable periwinkle to inhibit the growth of certain bacteria, fungi, and viruses.
8. **Vasodilatory Effects:** One of the key constituents responsible for these effects is a group of alkaloids known as vincamajines. These alkaloids have been shown to promote vasodilation, which means they help widen the blood vessels, allowing for improved blood flow throughout the body. This enhancement in blood circulation can be beneficial for various aspects of health, including supporting cardiovascular function, reducing blood pressure, and enhancing nutrient and oxygen delivery to different organs and tissues. Periwinkle contains flavonoids like quercetin and kaempferol, which also contribute to vasodilation and may further support improved blood flow.

9. **Digestive Health:** By promoting improved blood circulation, vincamine may enhance blood flow to the gastrointestinal tract, supporting the digestive process. Periwinkle contains alkaloids, such as ajmalicine and serpentine, which have been linked to smooth muscle relaxation. This relaxation effect may help alleviate gastrointestinal spasms and reduce bloating, providing relief from digestive discomfort. Periwinkle contains tannins, which have astringent properties that may help tone and tighten the tissues of the gastrointestinal tract, potentially aiding in digestion. These tannins may also have a protective effect on the digestive lining, contributing to a healthy gut.
10. **Auditory Support:** Periwinkle has garnered attention for its potential role in supporting auditory health, primarily due to its rich alkaloid content, particularly vincamine and vinpocetine. These compounds have been studied for their potential vasodilatory effects, which means they may help increase blood flow, including blood circulation to the inner ear. Improved blood flow to the cochlea and other auditory structures can support the maintenance of healthy hearing and may aid in addressing certain auditory conditions, such as tinnitus (ringing in the ears) or age-related hearing loss.

While periwinkle is generally considered safe to consume, there are some medical contradictions and drug interactions that individuals should be aware of. People with low blood pressure or hypotension should exercise caution, as periwinkle may further lower blood pressure. It may also interact with medications used to treat high blood pressure or antihypertensive drugs, potentially leading to adverse effects. Periwinkle may inhibit platelet aggregation, so individuals taking blood-thinning medications or anticoagulants should avoid excessive consumption to reduce the risk of bleeding. Periwinkle contains alkaloids, which may have sedative effects, so it is advised to avoid using it in combination with sedative medications to prevent excessive drowsiness. Allergy warnings include potential hypersensitivity to periwinkle or other plants in the Apocynaceae family, such as dogbane and oleander. Individuals with known allergies to these plants may experience skin rashes, itching, or respiratory reactions upon exposure. Pregnant or breastfeeding individuals should exercise caution and consult with their herbalist/practitioner before using periwinkle.

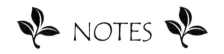

NOTES

PERSIMMON LEAF

Persimmon leaf, scientifically known as Diospyros kaki, is derived from the persimmon tree. This is an herb with a long history of traditional use and cultural significance. The persimmon tree is native to China, where it has been cultivated for thousands of years, and its leaves are known for their unique flavor and aroma, often used in teas and herbal preparations. There are different varieties of persimmon leaves, each with its own distinct characteristics and medicinal properties. In traditional Chinese medicine, persimmon leaves have been highly valued for their potential to support digestive health, promote respiratory wellness, and aid in managing blood sugar levels. In Korean culture, persimmon leaves have served as a natural dye for fabrics and a pesticide for preserving food. In Japan, they hold cultural significance, are used in tea ceremonies, and are believed to possess purifying properties.

Now, let's explore ten extensive health and longevity benefits associated with persimmon leaf:

1. **Antioxidant Powerhouse:** Persimmon leaf contains various antioxidants, including catechins, flavonoids, and carotenoids. These compounds help neutralize harmful free radicals, reducing oxidative stress and supporting healthy aging.
2. **Cardiovascular Health:** Persimmon leaf has been found to have potential cardio-protective effects. It contains flavonoids and tannins that may help maintain healthy blood pressure levels and support overall heart health.
3. **Skin Health:** The antioxidants and vitamin C in persimmon leaf contribute to skin health by protecting against free radicals and supporting collagen synthesis, promoting a youthful and radiant complexion.
4. **Liver Health:** Persimmon leaf contains antioxidants like catechins and flavonoids, which benefit liver health by shielding liver cells from oxidative damage and reducing inflammation. This supports the liver's crucial detoxification role by safeguarding its cells and improving toxin elimination, ultimately promoting optimal liver function and overall detoxification.
5. **Digestive Health:** Persimmon leaf has been traditionally used to support digestive health. It contains tannins that may help alleviate symptoms of diarrhea and soothe gastrointestinal irritation.

6. **Blood Sugar Regulation:** Certain compounds in persimmon leaf, such as flavonoids and tannins, may aid in blood sugar regulation by improving insulin sensitivity and reducing insulin resistance.
7. **Anti-inflammatory Effects:** Persimmon leaf contains compounds with anti-inflammatory properties, such as catechins and flavonoids. These properties may help reduce inflammation in the body, which is linked to various chronic diseases.
8. **Antimicrobial Effects:** Persimmon leaf has demonstrated antimicrobial activity against certain bacteria and fungi, suggesting its potential as a natural antimicrobial agent. The antimicrobial activity of persimmon leaf can be attributed to its bioactive compounds, such as tannins, flavonoids, and phenolic acids. These compounds have been found to possess antimicrobial properties and can inhibit the growth and proliferation of harmful microorganisms.
9. **Cognitive Support:** Persimmon leaf contains calming properties, which can contribute to improved mental clarity and focus. When consumed as a beverage extracted in water (herbal infusion, herbal decoction), persimmon leaf releases compounds that have a soothing effect on the nervous system, helping to reduce stress and anxiety. One specific compound found in persimmon leaf is gamma-aminobutyric acid (GABA). GABA is an inhibitory neurotransmitter that plays a crucial role in regulating brain activity and promoting relaxation.
10. **Immune System Support:** Persimmon leaf infusions and decoctions are thought to offer immune system support due to its rich content of bioactive compounds, including antioxidants, polyphenols, and tannins which can help bolster the body's defense mechanisms. These compounds may neutralize harmful free radicals, reduce oxidative stress, and thus contribute to a more robust immune response.

While persimmon leaf is generally considered safe to consume, there are some medical contradictions and drug interactions to be aware of. Individuals with a history of blood clotting disorders or those taking anticoagulant medications should exercise caution, as persimmon leaf may interact with these medications and potentially increase the risk of bleeding. Individuals with diabetes or those taking medications to lower blood sugar levels should monitor their blood glucose closely when using persimmon leaf, as it may enhance the effects of these medications. Allergy warnings include potential hypersensitivity to persimmon or other plants in the Ebenaceae family, which include ebony and ebony trees. Some individuals may experience skin rashes, itching, or respiratory reactions in response to exposure. Pregnant and lactating individuals should consult with their herbalist/practitioner before consuming persimmon leaf.

NOTES

PINE NEEDLES

Pine needles, obtained from a variety of pine tree species, hold a fascinating history of traditional use and are known for their myriad health benefits. Pine trees, being evergreen conifers, are abundant in different regions worldwide. The vast diversity of pine species yields an array of distinctive pine needle varieties, each boasting unique characteristics and potential therapeutic properties. From the aromatic Pinus sylvestris to the fresh Pinus radiata, the realm of pine needles offers a diverse range of sensory experiences. These needles are treasured for their pleasant scent and find common use in infusions, tinctures, and essential oils. However, due to the multitude of pine species and their respective histories, it becomes challenging to pinpoint specific details about the origin and history of each pine needle variety. Nonetheless, their long-standing presence in traditional practices and their valuable health attributes make pine needles a cherished and sought-after herbal resource.

Now, let's explore ten extensive health and longevity benefits associated with pine needles.

1. **Immune System Support:** Pine needles are rich in immune-supportive compounds, notably vitamin C, known for its role in bolstering the immune system and providing defense against pathogens. Additionally, they contain shikimic acid, a compound of interest due to its association with antiviral properties. Shikimic acid is a key component in the synthesis of Tamiflu, a medication used to treat influenza. The combination of vitamin C and shikimic acid contributes to the overall immune-boosting potential of pine needles.
2. **Respiratory Health:** Generally speaking, the inhalation of pine needle-infused steam can provide soothing benefits for the respiratory system. The steam helps to loosen mucus and congestion, making it easier to breathe and providing relief for individuals with respiratory conditions such as sinus congestion, bronchitis, or asthma. The aromatic compounds present in pine needles, including pinene and limonene, contribute to their beneficial effects on the respiratory system. These compounds possess expectorant properties, helping to clear the airways and promote easier breathing.
3. **Detoxification:** The antioxidants present in pine needles, along with their potential diuretic properties, can support the body's natural detoxification processes and help eliminate toxins.

4. **Antioxidant Powerhouse:** Pine needles are rich in polyphenols and flavonoids, crucial antioxidants that effectively neutralize harmful free radicals in the body. Free radicals, unstable molecules, can cause cellular damage and oxidative stress. The scavenging action of polyphenols and flavonoids in pine needles protects cells from oxidative damage, reducing the risk of chronic diseases and promoting healthy aging.
5. **Cognitive Support:** Some compounds found in pine needles, such as terpenes and monoterpenes, have been shown to have potential cognitive-enhancing effects, supporting memory, focus, and overall brain health.
6. **Skin Health:** Pine needle extracts possess antimicrobial and anti-inflammatory properties that can benefit the skin. They may help soothe irritation, reduce redness, and support a healthy complexion.
7. **Muscle Relief:** Pine needle essential oil contains terpenes which contribute to its muscle-relaxing properties. When applied topically through massage oils or added to bath soaks, the aromatic molecules of the essential oil are absorbed through the skin and inhaled, reaching the olfactory system. Once in contact with the skin, pine needle essential oil interacts with receptors and nerve endings, initiating a cascade of relaxation responses. Additionally, the chemical constituents in the oil have a mild analgesic effect, helping to alleviate soreness and discomfort in tired muscles.
8. **Digestive Health:** Pine needles contain certain compounds, such as tannins and flavonoids, which can aid in digestion and provide relief from gastrointestinal discomfort. These bioactive compounds help to stimulate the production of digestive enzymes, promoting efficient breakdown of food and enhancing nutrient absorption. Pine needle leaf extracts (herbal decoction) may possess anti-inflammatory properties, which may help soothe digestive inflammation and alleviate symptoms such as bloating and abdominal pain.
9. **Antimicrobial Effects:** Pine needle extracts, (herbal decoction) may exhibit antimicrobial effects against certain bacteria and fungi, making them potentially beneficial for maintaining a healthy microbial balance.

10. **Relaxation and Stress Relief:** The invigorating aroma of pine needles has long been associated with a sense of relaxation and stress reduction. The aroma is believed to have mood-enhancing properties, uplifting the spirit and creating a peaceful atmosphere. The unique blend of aromatic compounds found in pine needles, including various terpenes, contribute to their therapeutic aroma and potential stress-relieving effects.

> While pine needles are generally considered safe to use, there are a few medical contradictions and precautions to be aware of. Individuals taking medications that have interactions with blood clotting or blood pressure regulation, such as anticoagulants or antihypertensive medications, should exercise caution as pine needle may have potential interactions. It is advisable to consult with a healthcare professional before using pine needle products or infusions if you are taking any medications or have any underlying health conditions. Individuals with allergies to pine trees or pine pollen may experience allergic reactions to pine needle products and infusions. It is important to note that other plants belonging to the same family as pine, such as spruce and fir, may also have similar properties and potential allergenicity. Women who are pregnant or lactating should consult with their herbalist/practitioner prior to consuming pine needle infusions.

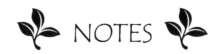

NOTES

PLANTAIN LEAF

Plantain leaf, scientifically known as Plantago major, is a hardy herbaceous plant with a fascinating history and global presence. Despite being considered a common weed in many regions, plantain leaf holds a significant place in the realm of traditional herbal medicine. Its origins can be traced back to Eurasia, but it has since spread across the world, adapting to diverse climates and environments. Throughout history, various cultures have recognized the potent healing properties of plantain leaf, incorporating it into their traditional remedies for a wide range of ailments. This versatile herb has been cherished for its numerous health and longevity benefits, contributing to overall well-being and vitality. From ancient times to modern days, plantain leaf remains a treasured botanical in the practice of herbal medicine, celebrated for its exceptional therapeutic qualities and its ability to promote a pro-aging lifestyle.

Now, let's explore ten extensive health and longevity benefits associated with plantain leaf:

1. **Respiratory Health:** Plantain leaf's soothing properties for the respiratory system can be attributed to its diverse array of compounds. Flavonoids, tannins, phenolic acids, iridoid glycosides, and mucilage found in plantain leaf possess anti-inflammatory properties, which help reduce inflammation in the airways and alleviate respiratory discomfort. These compounds can soothe coughs, reduce congestion, and promote clear breathing, making it a valuable ally, especially in environments with poor air quality or exposure to smoke.
2. **Skin Health:** Plantain leaf's skin-soothing properties are beneficial for topical applications. Compounds like allantoin and mucilage found in plantain leaf support the healing of minor wounds, cuts, insect bites, and skin irritations. These compounds aid in tissue regeneration and have anti-inflammatory effects, promoting faster healing and soothing irritated skin.
3. **Digestive Health:** Plantain leaf has been used to promote healthy digestion, thanks to its constituents like tannins and mucilage. Tannins contribute to astringent effects, which may help alleviate symptoms of indigestion and reduce bloating. Mucilage acts as a demulcent, forming a protective layer on the digestive tract's mucous membranes, soothing and alleviating discomfort caused by diarrhea.

4. **Detoxification:** Plantain leaves are often suggested as a natural remedy to help remove toxic heavy metals from the body. The primary way to remove heavy metals from the body is through the liver and kidneys' natural detoxification processes. Plantain leaves are thought to contain compounds with chelating properties, which means they may have the ability to bind to heavy metals and help facilitate their elimination from the body. Plantain leaves contain antioxidants, which can help reduce oxidative stress caused by heavy metal exposure. Oxidative stress can exacerbate the toxicity of heavy metals, so reducing their levels can be beneficial.
5. **Immune System Support:** Plantain leaf's immune-supportive properties are attributed to its bioactive compounds, particularly flavonoids and tannins. Flavonoids act as antioxidants, neutralizing free radicals and supporting immune function by promoting the production of immune cells. Meanwhile, tannins provide astringent effects, creating a protective barrier against infections in the respiratory and gastrointestinal tracts. Plantain leaf also promotes the production of cytokines, coordinating the immune response and regulating inflammation and immune cell activity.
6. **Urinary Tract Health:** Plantain leaf has been traditionally used to support urinary tract health due to its anti-inflammatory properties. Compounds like aucubin and allantoin found in Plantain leaf may help alleviate urinary tract infections, reduce inflammation, and support kidney function.
7. **Oral Health:** Plantain leaf's potential benefits for oral health stem from its constituents like tannins and mucilage, which have astringent and demulcent properties, respectively. These properties may help soothe gum inflammation, promote oral hygiene, and alleviate mouth ulcers.
8. **Antioxidant Powerhouse:** Plantain leaf contains antioxidants, such as flavonoids and phenolic acids, that help protect cells from oxidative damage caused by free radicals. These antioxidants contribute to graceful aging and overall well-being.
9. **Blood Sugar Regulation:** Plantain leaf has been traditionally used to support healthy blood sugar levels, partly due to its flavonoids, which may help regulate glucose metabolism and improve insulin sensitivity.

10. **Eye Health:** Plantain leaf's potential benefits for eye health are linked to its abundance of anti-inflammatory compounds. Among these compounds are flavonoids, tannins, and iridoid glycosides, which collectively contribute to the herb's eye-soothing properties. Inflammation is a common underlying factor in various eye conditions, and the anti-inflammatory effects of these compounds may help alleviate redness, irritation, and discomfort in the eyes. The mucilage present in plantain leaf may provide a protective and lubricating effect, helping to soothe dry eyes and maintain optimal eye moisture. Regular use of plantain leaf may promote overall eye wellness and comfort, making it a valuable natural remedy for those seeking to maintain their eye health.

> While plantain leaf is generally considered safe to consume, there are certain medical contradictions and considerations to be aware of. Plantain may interact with certain medications, including blood thinners or antiplatelet drugs, due to its potential mild anticoagulant effects. Individuals taking such medications should exercise caution and consult with a healthcare professional before using plantain leaf. Individuals with known allergies to plants in the Plantaginaceae family or other related plants, such as plantains or bananas, should avoid the use of plantain leaf to prevent allergic reactions. It is also important to note that plantain may have a mild diuretic effect, which can increase urine production, so individuals with kidney conditions or taking medications that affect kidney function should use plantain leaf with caution. Pregnant or breastfeeding women should consult with their herbalist/practitioner before using plantain leaf.

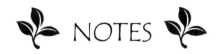

PSYLLIUM SEED

Psyllium seed, derived from the Plantago ovata plant, has a fascinating origin and a long history of use in traditional medicine. It is important to understand the difference between psyllium seed and psyllium husk, as they have distinct characteristics and health benefits. The seed refers to the small, reddish-brown seeds of the plant, while the husk refers to the fibrous outer covering of the seed. While both the seed and the husk offer health benefits, they differ in terms of their composition and uses.

Now, let's explore ten extensive health and longevity benefits associated with psyllium seed:

1. **Hemorrhoid Prevention:** Psyllium seeds' ability to promote soft and regular bowel movements can help prevent the development or exacerbation of hemorrhoids. Psyllium seeds contain soluble fiber, which absorbs water and forms a gel-like substance in the intestines. This gel helps soften stools, making them easier to pass without straining. When stools are soft and easy to pass, there is less pressure on the veins in the rectal area, reducing the risk of hemorrhoid development.
2. **Cholesterol Management:** Psyllium seed's cholesterol-lowering effects stem from its soluble fiber, which binds to cholesterol in the digestive system and prevents its absorption into the bloodstream. The soluble fiber, specifically beta-glucans and hemicellulose, acts as a sponge, trapping LDL (bad) cholesterol and escorting it out of the body through excretion. By reducing LDL cholesterol levels, psyllium seed supports cardiovascular health and helps reduce the risk of heart disease.
3. **Blood Sugar Control:** Psyllium seed's potential benefits in blood sugar regulation are linked to its soluble fiber content, which forms a gel-like substance when combined with water in the digestive system. This gel slows down the absorption of glucose from food, preventing rapid spikes in blood sugar levels. The slower glucose absorption also enhances insulin sensitivity, making psyllium seed a valuable aid for individuals with diabetes or those seeking to maintain stable blood sugar levels.
4. **Cardiovascular Health:** Psyllium seed's role in reducing cholesterol levels, particularly LDL cholesterol, directly impacts heart health. Lowering LDL cholesterol levels decreases the risk of atherosclerosis and heart disease, making psyllium seed a beneficial addition to a heart-healthy lifestyle.

5. **Weight Management:** The abundance of fiber in psyllium seed contributes to feelings of fullness and satiety. When consumed before meals, the fiber expands in the stomach, leading to a sense of satisfaction and reduced appetite. By promoting a feeling of fullness, psyllium seed aids in weight management by curbing overeating and supporting portion control.
6. **Colon Cleansing:** Psyllium seed's cleansing properties are closely related to its high fiber content. As the fiber absorbs water and forms a gel, it efficiently binds to waste materials, toxins, and other harmful substances in the colon. This gel-like bulk facilitates their elimination from the body, promoting detoxification and supporting colon health.
7. **Digestive Health:** The soluble fiber in psyllium seed functions as a prebiotic, providing nourishment to beneficial gut bacteria. By supporting the growth and activity of probiotic microorganisms, psyllium seed contributes to a thriving gut microbiome, enhancing overall gut health and optimizing digestive function.
8. **Anti-inflammatory Effects:** Psyllium seed contains compounds such as hemicellulose and mucilage, which have demonstrated anti-inflammatory properties. These compounds work to reduce inflammation in the body, alleviating symptoms associated with inflammatory conditions.
9. **Diabetes Management:** Psyllium seed's impact on diabetes management is partly due to its fiber content, which slows down the absorption of glucose, preventing rapid spikes in blood sugar levels. The improved insulin sensitivity resulting from the consistent use of psyllium seed may contribute to better glycemic control in individuals with diabetes.
10. **Nutrient Absorption:** The gel-forming properties of psyllium seed can delay the digestion and absorption of nutrients, allowing for better absorption of essential vitamins and minerals.

While psyllium seed is generally considered safe to consume, there are some medical contradictions and potential interactions to be aware of. People with certain gastrointestinal conditions, such as esophageal narrowing, bowel obstructions, or difficulty swallowing, should avoid using psyllium seeds as they may worsen these conditions. Psyllium seed can also interfere with the absorption and effectiveness of certain medications, including oral medications, as it forms a gel-like substance that can slow down the absorption of drugs. Therefore, it is important to take medications at least two hours before or after consuming psyllium seed to minimize this interaction. Psyllium seeds are part of the Plantaginaceae family, and individuals with known allergies to plants within this family may need to exercise caution when using psyllium seeds or products containing psyllium. It is also important to follow the recommended dosage and drink plenty of water when using psyllium seed, as inadequate fluid intake may lead to potential complications, such as bowel obstruction or choking. Those who are pregnant or lactating should consult with their herbalist/practitioner prior to using psyllium seeds.

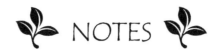

NOTES

RED CLOVER

Red clover, scientifically known as Trifolium pratense, is a flowering plant that boasts a fascinating history and origin. Believed to be native to Europe, Western Asia, and Northwest Africa, red clover has gradually spread its presence across the globe due to its adaptability and diverse applications. With its vibrant red flowers and characteristic clover-shaped leaves, red clover is easily recognizable and has become a beloved herb in various cultures. Throughout history, red clover has held a prominent place in traditional medicine systems, cherished for its potential health benefits and therapeutic properties. As time progressed, red clover's reputation and popularity have grown, making it a widely cultivated and utilized herb in contemporary herbal practices worldwide.

Now, let's explore ten extensive health and longevity benefits associated with red clover:

1. **Hormonal Balance:** Red clover contains isoflavones, such as genistein and daidzein, which are phytoestrogens that mimic the effects of estrogen in the body. These compounds may help alleviate menopausal symptoms like hot flashes and mood swings.
2. **Bone Health:** The isoflavones in red clover also support bone health by promoting bone density and reducing the risk of osteoporosis. This can be especially beneficial for postmenopausal women who are more prone to bone loss.
3. **Cardiovascular Health:** Red clover has been shown to support heart health by reducing LDL (bad) cholesterol levels and improving overall cardiovascular function. It may also help maintain healthy blood pressure levels.
4. **Skin Health:** The isoflavones and antioxidants present in red clover can contribute to healthier, more youthful-looking skin. They help protect against oxidative stress and may improve skin elasticity and hydration.
5. **Digestive Health:** Red clover has mild diuretic and detoxifying properties that can support healthy digestion and help cleanse the body of toxins. It may also aid in relieving digestive discomfort and promoting regular bowel movements.
6. **Respiratory Health:** Red clover has traditionally been used to support respiratory health, particularly in cases of coughs, bronchitis, and asthma. Its expectorant properties may help loosen phlegm and relieve congestion.

7. **Immune System Support:** The antioxidants found in red clover may help strengthen the immune system and protect the body against oxidative damage. Red clover also contains immunomodulatory properties, meaning it may help regulate immune responses. This can be beneficial in promoting a balanced immune system and preventing excessive immune reactions or imbalances. This can contribute to overall immune support and improved resistance to infections.
8. **Anti-inflammatory Effects:** Red clover contains specific constituents that contribute to its anti-inflammatory effects, making it beneficial for conditions such as arthritis and inflammatory skin conditions. The herb is rich in isoflavones, including genistein and daidzein, which reduce the production of inflammatory molecules. Additionally, red clover contains flavonoids like quercetin and kaempferol, which possess antioxidant and anti-inflammatory properties by neutralizing free radicals. Coumarins, such as scopoletin, and phenolic acids, such as chlorogenic acid and caffeic acid, further enhance its anti-inflammatory benefits by inhibiting pro-inflammatory enzymes. The combination of these compounds helps alleviate inflammation throughout the body, and the reduction of chronic inflammation also supports the normal functioning of the lymphatic system, which is crucial for immune function and detoxification processes.
9. **Lymphatic Support:** Red clover contains specific constituents that support lymphatic system function and detoxification processes. The herb is rich in flavonoids, such as quercetin and kaempferol, which have antioxidant properties that help neutralize free radicals and reduce oxidative stress. These antioxidants contribute to the body's natural detoxification processes by supporting the elimination of toxins, waste products, and cellular debris. Red clover contains phenolic compounds like chlorogenic acid and caffeic acid, which also possess antioxidant properties and aid in detoxification. By promoting the elimination of harmful substances, red clover indirectly supports the proper functioning of the lymphatic system, which is essential for removing metabolic waste and maintaining a healthy immune system.

10. **Wound Healing:** Red clover contains several constituents that contribute to its wound-healing properties when applied topically. One of the key components is isoflavones, including genistein and daidzein, which are powerful antioxidants. These isoflavones help neutralize free radicals that can damage cells and impede the healing process. By reducing oxidative stress, red clover facilitates the body's natural healing mechanisms, allowing wounds to close more efficiently and promoting tissue repair. Red clover contains flavonoids, such as quercetin and kaempferol, which also exhibit antioxidant and anti-inflammatory effects. These flavonoids aid in reducing inflammation at the wound site, which is crucial for supporting a healthy healing process. By minimizing inflammation, red clover helps to prevent excessive tissue damage and promotes a smoother healing process, thereby reducing the appearance of scars.

> While red clover is generally considered safe to consume, there are certain medical contradictions and precautions to be aware of. Individuals with hormone-sensitive conditions, such as breast, uterine, or ovarian cancer, should exercise caution as red clover contains compounds called isoflavones that may have estrogenic effects. It is advisable to consult with a healthcare professional before using red clover in such cases. Individuals taking medications that affect blood clotting or have a history of blood clotting disorders should use red clover with caution, as it may have anticoagulant properties. Red clover may interact with immunosuppressant drugs and medications metabolized by the liver, so it is important to consult with a healthcare professional if taking these medications. Pregnant or breastfeeding women should consult with their herbalist/practitioner prior to using red clover.

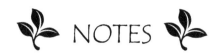

NOTES

RED DRAGON FRUIT (POWDER)

Red dragon fruit, scientifically known as Hylocereus costaricensis, but also recognized as pitaya or pitahaya, is a tropical fruit belonging to the cactus family. Believed to have originated in Central America and parts of South America, today, red dragon fruit is widely cultivated in various tropical regions around the world, including Southeast Asia, Australia, and the United States. Indigenous communities have long valued red dragon fruit for its liver protective properties. This versatile fruit can be transformed into red dragon fruit powder through a process that involves harvesting, cleaning, dehydration, and milling. The resulting powder retains the fruit's vibrant color, flavor, and nutritional components, offering a convenient and concentrated form for various culinary applications.

Now, let's explore ten extensive health and longevity benefits associated with red dragon fruit (powder):

1. **Antioxidant Powerhouse:** Red dragon fruit is rich in antioxidants, such as vitamin C, carotenoids, and flavonoids. These antioxidants help protect the body's cells from oxidative stress and damage caused by free radicals.
2. **Cardiovascular Health:** The fiber, potassium, and vitamin C content in red dragon fruit contribute to heart health. Potassium helps regulate blood pressure, while fiber and antioxidants help reduce cholesterol levels and improve overall cardiovascular function.
3. **Cognitive Support:** The high levels of antioxidants in red dragon fruit, especially vitamin C, support brain health and may help enhance cognitive function and memory.
4. **Immune System Support:** Red dragon fruit is a potent source of immune-enhancing nutrients that work synergistically to fortify the body's defense mechanisms. Vitamin C, a prominent component of red dragon fruit, plays a crucial role in bolstering immune function by stimulating the production of white blood cells, the body's primary defenders against infections. The abundance of antioxidants, such as betalains and flavonoids, further contributes to immune system enhancement. These antioxidants act as scavengers, neutralizing harmful free radicals that could otherwise weaken the immune response.
5. **Skin Health:** The antioxidants in red dragon fruit help combat oxidative stress and protect the skin from damage caused by environmental factors, promoting healthy aging and a vibrant complexion.

6. **Digestive Health:** Red dragon fruit contains phytochemicals such as betalains, which possess anti-inflammatory properties and may help soothe digestive inflammation. Additionally, the powder contains electrolytes like potassium, which helps maintain fluid balance and proper muscle function within the digestive system.
7. **Detoxification:** Red dragon fruit offers a range of beneficial compounds that support detoxification processes in the body. Its high antioxidant content, including vitamin C and various phytochemicals like betalains, aids in neutralizing harmful free radicals and reducing oxidative stress. These antioxidants contribute to cellular health and support the body's natural detoxification pathways.
8. **Liver Health:** Red dragon fruit contains various compounds and constituents that contribute to liver health. One of the key components is betacyanins, which are responsible for the fruit's vibrant red color. These natural pigments act as potent antioxidants and have been shown to have hepatoprotective properties, helping to shield the liver cells from oxidative stress and damage caused by free radicals. Additionally, red dragon fruit is rich in flavonoids, such as quercetin and catechin, which have anti-inflammatory and antioxidant effects, further supporting liver function by reducing inflammation and neutralizing harmful molecules.
9. **Eye Health:** The compounds and constituents found in red dragon fruit provide numerous benefits for eye health. Red dragon fruit is a rich source of antioxidants, such as vitamin C, beta-carotene, and lycopene. These antioxidants play a crucial role in protecting the eyes from oxidative stress and free radical damage, which can contribute to age-related eye conditions like cataracts and macular degeneration. Vitamin C, in particular, is known to support blood vessel health within the eyes and may help prevent the development of retinopathy. Red dragon fruit contains zeaxanthin and lutein, two essential carotenoids that are specifically beneficial for eye health. Zeaxanthin and lutein are found in high concentrations in the retina, where they act as natural filters that absorb harmful blue light and protect the delicate cells in the macula from damage. These carotenoids are also known to improve visual acuity and may reduce the risk of age-related vision loss.

10. **Anti-inflammatory Effects:** Red dragon fruit contains natural compounds, such as betacyanins and flavonoids, which possess potent anti-inflammatory properties. These compounds help inhibit the production of pro-inflammatory molecules in the body, thus reducing inflammation and its associated risks.

> While red dragon fruit and/or powder is generally considered safe to consume, it is important to be aware of certain medical contradictions and potential interactions with specific conditions and medications. Individuals with a known allergy to cacti or other plants in the Cactaceae family should exercise caution when consuming red dragon fruit, or its powder, as it may trigger an allergic reaction. Individuals with diabetes or those taking medications for blood sugar control should monitor their blood glucose levels closely, as red dragon fruit may have an impact on blood sugar levels. Individuals with kidney disorders or those taking medications that affect kidney function should exercise caution, as excessive consumption of red dragon fruit may pose a risk due to its potassium content. Red dragon fruit is generally considered safe for those who are pregnant and lactating.

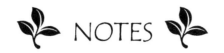

NOTES

RED RASPBERRY LEAF

Red raspberry leaf, scientifically known as Rubus idaeus, has a fascinating history and origin that traces back to ancient civilizations. Native to Europe and parts of Asia, red raspberry leaf has been a cherished herbal remedy for centuries. The use of red raspberry leaf in traditional medicine can be traced back to ancient Greek, Roman, and Egyptian cultures, where it was highly regarded for its medicinal properties. In medieval Europe, red raspberry leaf gained popularity as a medicinal herb, and its uses expanded to support various health conditions. It was commonly utilized to ease discomfort during pregnancy and childbirth, leading to its reputation as a "women's herb." In Native American cultures, the leaves of the red raspberry plant were used for their soothing properties, promoting overall well-being.

Now, let's explore ten extensive health and longevity benefits associated with red raspberry leaf:

1. **Adrenal Support:** Red raspberry leaf's beneficial effects on adrenal support can be attributed to its rich content of B vitamins, particularly vitamin B5, also known as pantothenic acid. The adrenal glands, located on top of the kidneys, play a vital role in the body's stress response and the synthesis of essential hormones, including cortisol and adrenaline. Vitamin B5 is a crucial component in the production of coenzyme A (CoA), a molecule involved in various metabolic processes. Specifically, in the context of adrenal support, vitamin B5 plays a significant role in the synthesis of adrenal hormones, aiding in the production of cortisol, the primary stress hormone. During times of stress, the body requires higher levels of cortisol to cope with the demands of the situation. Vitamin B5 helps in the conversion of cholesterol to pregnenolone, a precursor to cortisol, and thus contributes to maintaining balanced hormone levels during stress responses.

2. **Pregnancy Support:** Some herbalists suggest that red raspberry leaf may promote more efficient contractions during labor. Red raspberry leaf is commonly consumed during the third trimester of pregnancy, although some women start drinking red raspberry leaf tea in the second trimester. It is advisable to consult with your herbalist or midwife before incorporating red raspberry leaf tea into your pregnancy routine to determine the most appropriate timing for your specific situation.

3. **Adaptogenic Effects:** Red raspberry leaf is a remarkable herbal source of adaptogenic support, thanks to its abundant polyphenols, including ellagic acid and quercetin, as well as tannins. These bioactive compounds work synergistically to empower the body's ability to cope with stress, both physically and emotionally. By scavenging harmful free radicals and reducing oxidative stress, ellagic acid offers vital antioxidant support to cells under stress. Quercetin, on the other hand, possesses potent anti-inflammatory properties that help soothe inflammation resulting from stressors, further promoting overall well-being. The astringent properties of tannins play a role in toning and supporting body tissues, providing structural integrity even during challenging times. This combination of polyphenols and tannins within red raspberry leaf contributes to its adaptogenic potential, regulating stress hormones and promoting a balanced physiological response to stress.
4. **Uterine Toning:** When consumed, the tannins in red raspberry leaf interact with the body's tissues, particularly the uterine muscles. These compounds have a gentle yet effective tonic effect on the uterine walls, helping to tighten and strengthen the muscle fibers. The uterine toning properties of red raspberry leaf can be particularly valuable during pregnancy preparation. As a woman's body prepares for conception and pregnancy, the uterine muscles need to be in optimal condition to support a fertilized egg and facilitate healthy implantation. The toning effects of the tannins in red raspberry leaf may help create a supportive environment for the embryo's attachment and development, which is crucial during the early stages of pregnancy. During labor and childbirth, the uterine muscles undergo intense contractions to facilitate the delivery process. The toning properties of red raspberry leaf are thought to be helpful during this time as well.
5. **Fertility Enhancement:** Red raspberry leaf is believed to have a positive impact on fertility by improving the quality of cervical mucus, creating a more fertile environment for sperm transport, and increasing the likelihood of successful conception. This herbal ally is highly regarded for its nourishing properties, containing essential nutrients such as vitamin C, vitamin E, calcium, iron, and folate, all of which are important for reproductive health and fertility. The presence of phytoestrogens, particularly ellagitannins, in red raspberry leaf is thought to have a balancing effect on hormone levels, further supporting fertility.

6. **Skin Health:** Red raspberry leaf offers a potent combination of antioxidants that work together to benefit the skin. Vitamin C safeguards the skin's collagen, a crucial protein responsible for maintaining firmness and elasticity, thus supporting skin suppleness and resilience while reducing the appearance of fine lines and wrinkles. Alongside vitamin C, red raspberry leaf also contains vitamin E and various flavonoids that play a vital role in shielding the skin from the damaging effects of oxidative stress caused by environmental pollutants and UV radiation.
7. **Liver and Gallbladder Health:** Red raspberry leaf contains flavonoids, such as quercetin and kaempferol, which have been associated with potential liver-protective effects and support liver health. Red raspberry leaf may have a mild relaxing effect on the gallbladder and help support healthy bile flow.
8. **Cervical Mucus Quality:** One key group of compounds present in red raspberry leaf that contributes to this effect is the flavonoids. Flavonoids are a diverse class of phytochemicals known for their antioxidant and anti-inflammatory properties. Among the flavonoids found in red raspberry leaf are quercetin, kaempferol, and rutin. These flavonoids are believed to have a positive influence on cervical mucus quality by promoting optimal viscosity and texture. By supporting the consistency of cervical mucus, these flavonoids help facilitate the movement and motility of sperm within the female reproductive tract. When cervical mucus is of high quality, it provides a nourishing and protective medium for sperm, enhancing their viability and longevity. This creates a more conducive environment for the sperm's journey, increasing the likelihood of successful fertilization.
9. **Digestive Health:** Red raspberry leaf contains tannins, which are astringent compounds that may help support the gastrointestinal system as well as soothe and tone the digestive system. It may aid in relieving symptoms of indigestion, diarrhea, and gastrointestinal discomfort.
10. **Cardiovascular Health:** Red raspberry leaf may help maintain healthy blood pressure levels and improve circulation. It's also rich in flavonoids, such as quercetin and kaempferol, which have antioxidant properties that could support cardiovascular health.

While red raspberry leaf is generally considered safe to consume, there are certain medical contradictions and precautions to consider. Red raspberry leaf may interact with medications that have hormonal effects or affect blood clotting, such as anticoagulants or hormonal contraceptives. It is advisable to consult with a healthcare professional if you are taking any medications or have underlying medical conditions before incorporating red raspberry leaf into your routine. Individuals with a history of hormone-sensitive conditions, such as breast cancer, ovarian cancer, or uterine fibroids, should exercise caution and consult with a healthcare professional before using red raspberry leaf, as it may have estrogen-like effects. Additionally, individuals with a history of preterm labor should seek medical advice before using red raspberry leaf. It is important to note that while red raspberry leaf is often recommended for pregnant women to support the reproductive system, its safety during early pregnancy (first trimester) has not been sufficiently studied. Therefore, it is advisable to consult with your herbalist/practitioner before using red raspberry leaf during various stages of pregnancy.

REDROOT

Redroot, scientifically known as Ceanothus americanus, holds a significant place in the history of traditional herbal medicine. Indigenous to North America, this perennial plant has been an essential part of Native American healing practices for countless generations. Revered for its medicinal properties, redroot derives its name from the strikingly vibrant red hue of its roots, a characteristic that has intrigued herbalists and healers for centuries. The rich history of redroot's use by Native American tribes underscores its cultural significance and deep-rooted connection to the land. These tribes valued the plant for its diverse range of health benefits, which extended beyond physical well-being to include emotional and spiritual aspects of human existence. The wisdom passed down through generations recognized the potent healing potential held within this unassuming plant.

Now, let's explore ten extensive health and longevity benefits associated with redroot:

1. **Lymphatic Support:** Redroot's reputation as a lymphatic support herb is supported by its active constituents, including alkaloids such as ceanothine and ceanothidine. These alkaloids are thought to contribute to redroot's ability to promote lymphatic drainage and improve lymphatic circulation.
2. **Immune System Support:** Redroot's potential as an immune system booster can be attributed to its rich antioxidant profile, prominently featuring quercetin and other flavonoids. Quercetin, a powerful antioxidant, helps neutralize harmful free radicals and reduce oxidative stress, which can otherwise compromise immune function. By safeguarding immune cells from damage, redroot enhances the body's ability to respond to infections and support overall immune function.
3. **Respiratory Health:** Redroot, with its potential respiratory benefits, contains compounds such as flavonoids and tannins that may soothe respiratory discomfort and promote healthy lung function. Flavonoids, including quercetin and kaempferol, possess anti-inflammatory properties that may help reduce inflammation in the airways, providing relief from congestion and respiratory symptoms. Additionally, tannins contribute to redroot's astringent properties, which may help tighten and tone respiratory tissues, further supporting respiratory health and well-being.

4. **Digestive Health:** Redroot's traditional use as a digestive aid is supported by its active constituents, including alkaloids and flavonoids. These compounds may stimulate digestion and support a healthy gastrointestinal system by aiding in the breakdown of food and easing indigestion. Redroot's potential to alleviate digestive discomfort can be attributed to its tannin content, which exhibits a mild astringent effect on the digestive tract, promoting soothing relief.
5. **Anti-inflammatory Effects:** Redroot contains several compounds with potent anti-inflammatory effects. Ceanothic acid has been studied for its potential to reduce inflammation in the body. Ursolic acid has demonstrated its ability to modulate the inflammatory response and alleviate symptoms associated with inflammatory conditions. Oleanolic acid inhibits the activity of specific inflammatory molecules. Redroot is also rich in polyphenolic compounds, such as flavonoids and phenolic acids, which collectively contribute to its anti-inflammatory effects. These compounds work together to help combat inflammation and may offer relief from inflammatory conditions.
6. **Detoxification:** Redroot is considered a natural detoxifier due to its active compounds, including alkaloids and flavonoids, which support the liver's detoxification processes. The liver plays a crucial role in filtering and removing harmful substances from the body, and redroot's detoxification support aids in the elimination of toxins, promoting overall well-being.
7. **Cardiovascular Health:** Redroot's positive impact on cardiovascular health may be attributed to its flavonoid content, particularly quercetin and kaempferol, which possess antioxidant properties. These antioxidants help reduce oxidative stress and support healthy blood pressure levels and improved circulation, contributing to overall heart health and reducing the risk of cardiovascular issues.
8. **Antioxidant Powerhouse:** Redroot's rich antioxidant profile, including flavonoids like quercetin and kaempferol, and tannins, provides protection against oxidative stress and age-related damage caused by free radicals. By neutralizing harmful free radicals, redroot helps prevent cellular damage, supporting healthy aging and overall cellular health.

9. **Urinary Tract Health:** Redroot's potential diuretic properties are linked to its alkaloid content, which may support kidney and urinary tract health by promoting urine flow and flushing out toxins from the urinary system. The diuretic action of redroot aids in maintaining healthy urine production and promoting a healthy urinary system.
10. **Oral Health:** Redroot's traditional use in oral care can be attributed to its potential astringent properties, primarily due to the presence of tannins. These compounds may help alleviate symptoms of gum inflammation, promote gum health, and contribute to fresher breath by reducing bacteria in the mouth.

> While redroot is generally considered safe to consume, there are some medical contradictions and drug interactions to be aware of. Individuals with hypotension (low blood pressure) should exercise caution when using redroot, as it may further lower blood pressure. Redroot may also interact with antihypertensive medications and other drugs that lower blood pressure, potentially leading to adverse effects. Additionally, redroot may affect blood clotting, so individuals taking anticoagulant or antiplatelet medications should avoid using this herb without medical supervision. Allergic reactions to redroot are rare but possible, especially for individuals with known allergies to plants in the Rhamnaceae family, to which redroot belongs. Some other plants in the Rhamnaceae family include cascara sagrada (Rhamnus purshiana) and jujube (Ziziphus jujuba). Pregnant and lactating individuals should consult with their herbalist/practitioner before using redroot due to its potential effects on the uterus. Redroot is believed to have uterine-stimulating properties, which means it may stimulate contractions in the uterus. For pregnant individuals, this can be a concern as it might trigger premature contractions or increase the risk of miscarriage. The herb's ability to promote contractions may lead to reduced milk supply or interfere with the body's natural hormonal balance during the lactation period.

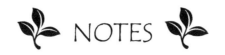

NOTES

REISHI MUSHROOM

Reishi mushroom, scientifically known as Ganoderma lucidum, is a powerful medicinal fungus with a rich history dating back thousands of years. Originating in Asia, particularly in China and Japan, reishi mushroom has been revered in traditional Chinese medicine for its numerous health benefits. Often referred to as the "mushroom of immortality" or the "elixir of life," reishi mushroom has been used to promote longevity and overall well-being. It has been treasured for its ability to enhance vitality, boost the immune system, and promote healthy aging.

Now, let's explore ten extensive health and longevity benefits associated with reishi mushroom:

1. **Immune System Support:** Reishi mushroom contains bioactive compounds such as polysaccharides, triterpenes, and beta-glucans, which enhance immune function and support the body's defense against pathogens.
2. **Antioxidant Powerhouse:** Reishi mushroom is rich in antioxidants, including ganoderic acids, which help neutralize harmful free radicals and protect cells from oxidative damage. Ganoderic acids in reishi mushroom have been studied extensively for their ability to scavenge free radicals and counteract oxidative stress. By donating electrons to free radicals, they stabilize these reactive molecules, preventing them from triggering a chain reaction of cellular damage. As a result, oxidative damage to tissues and organs is reduced, and the risk of various health conditions related to oxidative stress, such as cardiovascular diseases, neurodegenerative disorders, and certain cancers, may be mitigated.
3. **Anti-inflammatory Effects:** The active compound found in reishi mushroom, which exhibits potent anti-inflammatory effect, is ganoderic acid, which may help reduce chronic inflammation and associated diseases. Ganoderic acids are triterpenes specific to reishi mushroom and are believed to play a crucial role in its anti-inflammatory effects. These compounds are known for their ability to modulate various signaling pathways in the body, including those involved in inflammation. By interacting with key molecules and enzymes in the inflammatory process, ganoderic acids may help regulate the body's immune response and reduce excessive inflammation.

4. **Liver Health:** Triterpenes, including ganoderic acids have been shown to possess hepatoprotective properties. These triterpenes help support liver function by promoting the production of antioxidant enzymes, reducing inflammation, and enhancing detoxification processes. Additionally, polysaccharides present in reishi mushroom have been found to stimulate liver cell regeneration and improve liver health.
5. **Cardiovascular Health:** Triterpenes, including ganoderic acids, have been shown to possess hypotensive properties, helping to lower blood pressure levels. These compounds also have cholesterol-lowering effects by inhibiting cholesterol synthesis and promoting the removal of LDL (low-density lipoprotein) cholesterol. The polysaccharides found in reishi mushroom have been associated with improved circulation and the maintenance of healthy blood vessel function.
6. **Anti-cancer Effects:** Reishi mushroom has been extensively studied for its potential anti-cancer properties. Its bioactive compounds have shown promising effects in inhibiting tumor growth, boosting the immune response against cancer cells, and reducing the side effects of chemotherapy.
7. **Cognitive Support:** Reishi mushroom contains triterpenes, including ganoderic acids, which have been found to possess neuroprotective properties. These compounds help to reduce inflammation, oxidative stress, and the accumulation of beta-amyloid plaques, which are associated with cognitive decline and neurodegenerative disorders such as Alzheimer's disease. Reishi mushroom is also a source of polysaccharides, which have been shown to support brain health by enhancing neuronal communication, promoting the growth of nerve cells, and modulating neurotransmitter activity.
8. **Anti-radiation Effects:** Anecdotally, reishi mushrooms have garnered attention for their potential supportive role in mitigating the effects of radiation exposure. Some traditional and alternative medicine practitioners suggest that reishi's immune-modulating and antioxidative properties may help the body cope with radiation-induced stress and damage. It is believed that the bioactive compounds in reishi, including polysaccharides and triterpenoids, could potentially assist in reducing inflammation, scavenging free radicals, and bolstering the immune system, thereby aiding in the body's natural recovery process after radiation exposure.

9. **Skin Health:** Reishi mushroom offers a host of benefits for skin health and pro-aging due to its rich content of antioxidants and anti-inflammatory compounds. These bioactive components work in tandem to combat oxidative stress, a primary culprit in skin aging. By neutralizing harmful free radicals, reishi mushroom helps protect skin cells from damage, thus promoting a more youthful appearance. Additionally, this mushroom's anti-inflammatory properties help to reduce skin redness and irritation, contributing to a calmer and healthier complexion. Another significant advantage lies in reishi mushroom's ability to support collagen production, a crucial protein responsible for skin elasticity and firmness. By enhancing collagen synthesis, the mushroom aids in maintaining the skin's resilience and minimizing the appearance of fine lines and wrinkles.
10. **Respiratory Health:** The anti-inflammatory and immune-boosting properties of reishi mushroom may contribute to improved respiratory health, particularly in individuals with respiratory conditions such as asthma or bronchitis.

> While reishi mushroom is generally considered safe to consume, there are some medical contradictions and precautions to be aware of. Individuals with bleeding disorders or those taking anticoagulant medications should exercise caution, as reishi mushroom may have blood-thinning effects. Additionally, individuals with low blood pressure should monitor their blood pressure levels when consuming reishi mushroom, as it may further lower blood pressure. Allergy to mushrooms is also possible, so individuals with known mushroom allergies should avoid reishi mushroom. Reishi mushroom is generally considered safe in culinary quantities for those who are pregnant or breastfeeding. Consult with your herbalist/practitioner prior to using reishi mushroom in large therapeutic doses.

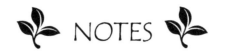

RHODIOLA ROOT

Rhodiola root, scientifically known as Rhodiola rosea, is an herb with a rich history dating back thousands of years. Originating in the mountainous regions of Europe and Asia, it has been used in traditional medicine for its adaptogenic properties and numerous health benefits. In ancient times, it was highly valued for its ability to enhance physical and mental endurance, combat fatigue, and promote longevity. Rhodiola root was particularly revered in Siberian and Scandinavian cultures, where it was consumed as a tea to improve resilience and overall well-being. Today, this remarkable herb continues to be recognized for its potent therapeutic properties and its role in supporting healthy aging.

Now, let's explore ten extensive health and longevity benefits associated with rhodiola root:

1. **Adrenal Support:** Rhodiola contains a compound called salidroside, known for its stress-reducing effects. Salidroside helps regulate the production of stress hormones, such as cortisol, by modulating the activity of the hypothalamic-pituitary-adrenal (HPA) axis. This regulation promotes a balanced stress response and helps mitigate the negative effects of chronic stress on the body.
2. **Cognitive Support:** The active compounds in rhodiola root, such as rosavin and salidroside, have been shown to enhance cognitive function, improve memory, and increase mental focus. They also have neuroprotective properties that may help prevent age-related cognitive decline.
3. **Cardiovascular Health:** Rhodiola has been associated with improved blood circulation, which is essential for ensuring that oxygen and nutrients reach all parts of the body efficiently. By enhancing blood flow, rhodiola root may contribute to better cardiovascular function and overall vitality. Inflammation plays a significant role in the development of cardiovascular diseases, and rhodiola's anti-inflammatory properties may help reduce inflammation in blood vessels and arterial walls, potentially mitigating the risk of heart-related issues. Rhodiola root has been suggested to support healthy blood pressure levels, which is critical for maintaining cardiovascular health and reducing the risk of hypertension-related complications.

4. **Adaptogenic Effects:** By acting as an adaptogen, rhodiola root helps the body adapt to various stressors, whether physical, emotional, or environmental, and fosters a more resilient response to challenging situations. It achieves this by regulating the release of stress hormones and neurotransmitters, promoting a sense of calm and stability in the face of adversity. As a result, individuals may experience improved mood, reduced feelings of anxiety, and an enhanced ability to manage emotional challenges.
5. **Energy Boost:** Rhodiola root contains specific compounds such as rosavins and salidroside, which contribute to its energizing properties. These compounds have been found to increase the production of ATP (adenosine triphosphate), the primary energy molecule in cells. By enhancing ATP synthesis and utilization, rhodiola root can effectively combat fatigue, improve physical endurance, and boost overall energy levels.
6. **Immune System Support:** Rhodiola root is rich in antioxidants, such as flavonoids and phenolic compounds, which play a crucial role in supporting a healthy immune system. These antioxidants help neutralize harmful free radicals and protect cells from oxidative damage, enhancing the body's defense against infections and diseases. Rhodiola root also contains bioactive compounds like rosavin and salidroside, which have been found to modulate immune responses and promote immune cell activity.
7. **Liver Health:** Rhodiola root has been found to exhibit protective effects on the liver, guarding it against damage induced by toxins and oxidative stress. By acting as an antioxidant, rhodiola root helps neutralize harmful free radicals that can otherwise cause cellular damage and compromise liver function. Additionally, rhodiola root supports the liver's detoxification processes, aiding in the elimination of waste products and potentially reducing the burden on this vital organ.
8. **Graceful-aging Effects:** As an adaptogen, rhodiola root helps the body cope with stress and maintain a state of balance, reducing the negative impact of chronic stress on cellular health. Chronic stress can lead to cellular damage and accelerated aging, and rhodiola's adaptogenic effects may help mitigate these effects. Rhodiola root is rich in antioxidants, such as salidroside and quercetin, which play a crucial role in neutralizing harmful free radicals and reducing oxidative stress. By protecting cells from oxidative damage, rhodiola root supports cellular health and promotes cellular repair mechanisms, potentially slowing down the aging process at a cellular level.

9. **Anti-inflammatory Effects:** The anti-inflammatory effects of rhodiola root can be attributed to its bioactive compounds, which include salidroside, rosavin, quercetin, and kaempferol. These compounds work synergistically to exert anti-inflammatory actions within the body, targeting inflammatory pathways and molecules. Salidroside has been studied for its ability to inhibit inflammation, while rosavin supports a balanced immune response. Quercetin acts as a powerful antioxidant, neutralizing free radicals and reducing oxidative stress. It also inhibits the activity of certain enzymes involved in inflammation, modulating the body's immune response and reducing the release of pro-inflammatory molecules. Similarly, kaempferol, another flavonoid, exhibits strong anti-inflammatory properties by acting as an antioxidant and suppressing the production of pro-inflammatory cytokines.
10. **Skin Health:** Rhodiola root contains specific compounds like kaempferol, quercetin, rosavin, and salidroside that contribute to its skin-protective properties. These antioxidants play a vital role in neutralizing free radicals, reducing oxidative stress, and preventing premature aging. Additionally, rhodiola root supports collagen synthesis, which helps maintain skin elasticity and firmness while improving skin tone and texture, promoting a youthful and radiant complexion.

While rhodiola is generally considered safe to consume, there are a few medical contradictions and drug interactions to be aware of. Rhodiola should not be used by individuals with bipolar disorder or certain anxiety disorders, as it may exacerbate symptoms. Additionally, those with bleeding disorders or taking anticoagulant medications should exercise caution, as rhodiola may increase the risk of bleeding. The herb may also interact with antidepressant medications, potentially altering their effects. Individuals taking stimulant medications should also be cautious, as rhodiola may enhance stimulant effects. Allergic reactions to rhodiola may occur, especially in individuals sensitive to plants in the Crassulaceae family, which includes Sedum, Sempervivum, and Kalanchoe. If you are pregnant or lactating, consult with your herbalist/practitioner prior to using this root.

NOTES

ROSE BUD AND PETALS

Rose buds and petals, derived from the beautiful and fragrant Rosa species, boast a fascinating history that spans thousands of years and transcends various cultures worldwide. Their origin can be traced back to regions such as the Middle East, Asia, and Europe, where they have been cherished for their aesthetic beauty, enchanting fragrance, and valuable medicinal properties. In ancient times, roses were not only admired for their ornamental use in gardens and celebrations but were also highly regarded for their therapeutic benefits. Across different civilizations, rose buds and petals were employed in traditional herbal medicine for their soothing and calming effects, making them a popular choice in remedies aimed at alleviating stress, anxiety, and emotional imbalances. Their captivating fragrance and symbolism of love and beauty earned them a place in rituals, ceremonies, and cultural traditions, making roses an integral part of art, literature, and folklore throughout history. Today, the reverence for rose buds and petals endures as they continue to be cherished and celebrated for their cultural significance and the myriad of ways they enrich our lives.

Now, let's explore ten extensive health and longevity benefits associated with rose buds and petals:

1. **Facial Toning:** The toning effect of rose buds and petals can be attributed to the presence of specific compounds, such as tannins, which act as natural astringents. Tannins, polyphenolic compounds found in roses, work by constricting and firming the skin's tissues and blood vessels, resulting in a temporary tightening effect. This helps reduce the appearance of enlarged pores and gives the skin a smoother and more refined texture. Additionally, rose buds and petals contain flavonoids like quercetin and kaempferol, which possess antioxidant and anti-inflammatory properties that contribute to the toning effect. By reducing oxidative stress and inflammation in the skin, these compounds support collagen production and promote a more elastic and toned complexion.
2. **Exfoliation Effects:** When finely ground, rose buds and petals serve as a gentle yet effective exfoliant due to their natural texture, providing mild abrasion that aids in removing dead skin cells, dirt, and impurities from the skin's surface. This physical exfoliation promotes a smoother texture and enhances cell turnover, improving the skin's appearance.

3. **Skin Health:** Rose buds and petals offer a plethora of skincare benefits, primarily due to their active compounds. These delicate buds and petals are rich in natural oils, including essential fatty acids, which moisturize and nourish the skin, leaving it soft and supple. Rose buds and petals contain vitamin C, a powerful antioxidant that supports collagen production, promoting a youthful complexion and reducing the appearance of wrinkles and fine lines. The presence of tannins in roses provides astringent properties, which help tighten and tone the skin, leading to a smoother and firmer appearance. The natural anti-inflammatory effects of compounds like quercetin, kaempferol, and various flavonoids, can further soothe skin irritation and reduce redness and inflammation associated with conditions like acne and eczema.
4. **Anti-inflammatory Effects:** Rose buds and petals contain bioactive compounds such as quercetin and kaempferol. These compounds act as natural anti-inflammatory agents by inhibiting the release of pro-inflammatory molecules and reducing the activation of inflammatory pathways. As a result, rose buds and petals may help soothe skin irritation and alleviate redness and inflammation associated with various skin conditions, making them a gentle and effective remedy for those with sensitive or inflamed skin.
5. **Antimicrobial Effects:** One of the key compounds responsible for these effects is the presence of essential oils in rose petals, such as citronellol and geraniol. These essential oils have demonstrated potent antimicrobial activity against various strains of bacteria and fungi. They work by disrupting the cell membranes of harmful microorganisms, leading to their inhibition and potential elimination. The polyphenolic compounds in rose petals, including flavonoids and tannins, also contribute to the antibacterial and antimicrobial properties.
6. **Digestive Health:** Rose buds and petals have been traditionally used for their mild laxative effect, which can be attributed to the presence of quercetin. These compounds help stimulate bowel movements and aid digestion, relieving discomfort such as bloating and cramping. Additionally, the natural soothing properties of roses may help calm digestive inflammation, making them a gentle and beneficial option for promoting digestive health.

7. **Immune System Support:** Rose buds and petals contain vitamin C, an essential nutrient known for its immune-boosting properties. Vitamin C supports the body's natural defense mechanisms by enhancing the production and function of immune cells, helping to protect against infections and illnesses. The antioxidants present in roses, including quercetin, kaempferol, and polyphenols, help neutralize harmful free radicals, reducing oxidative stress and supporting overall health and immunity.
8. **Respiratory Health:** In traditional medicine, rose buds and petals have been used to alleviate respiratory symptoms due to their natural aromatic and anti-inflammatory properties. The inhalation of rose-infused steam may help soothe the respiratory tract, providing relief from coughs, congestion, and sore throat. The anti-inflammatory effects of compounds like quercetin and kaempferol further contribute to a clear breathing experience, making rose buds and petals a valuable aid for respiratory health.
9. **Cardiovascular Health:** The antioxidants present in rose buds and petals, such as flavonoids and phenolic compounds, play a crucial role in supporting cardiovascular health. These compounds help reduce oxidative stress and inflammation in blood vessels, promoting healthy circulation and reducing the risk of cardiovascular diseases. The natural ability of rose buds and petals to support healthy blood vessels contributes to overall heart health and may help maintain proper blood pressure levels.
10. **Aromatherapy Benefits:** Rose buds and petals are highly valued in aromatherapy for their aromatic qualities. Inhaling the delightful scent of roses may help reduce stress and anxiety and promote a sense of well-being. The aromatic compounds found in rose buds and petals, including phenethyl alcohol, geraniol, and citronellol, contribute to their mood-enhancing effects. Aromatherapy with roses can uplift the spirits, improve mood, and create a soothing and harmonious ambiance, making them a treasured choice in aromatherapy practices.

While rose buds and petals are generally considered safe to consume, there are some medical contradictions and potential drug interactions to be aware of. Individuals with bleeding disorders or taking anticoagulant medications should consult a healthcare professional before consuming rose buds and petals, as they may have mild blood-thinning properties that could interact with anticoagulant drugs. Individuals with a history of allergies to roses or other plants in the Rosaceae family should exercise caution when using rose buds and petals internally, as allergic reactions may occur. As for pregnancy and lactation, while rose buds and petals are generally considered safe when used in culinary amounts, pregnant and breastfeeding individuals should consult with their herbalist/practitioner before using them medicinally or in larger quantities.

ROSEHIPS

Rosehips, the fruit of the wild rose plant, boast a captivating history that stretches far back in time and spans across diverse cultures. These petite, round, and brightly colored fruits have held significant medicinal importance for centuries. Originating from regions encompassing Europe, North America, and Asia, rosehips have long been revered for their abundance of nutrients and diverse therapeutic benefits. Ancient civilizations and indigenous communities recognized the remarkable potential of these small fruits and integrated them into traditional healing practices. From ancient herbal remedies to folk medicine, rosehips have played a vital role in supporting health and well-being. Their versatility and adaptability made them a valuable resource, as they could be harvested from various wild rose species growing abundantly in different climates. The historical significance and continued use of rosehips as a potent source of nutrients and healing compounds have contributed to their enduring popularity in modern herbal medicine.
Now, let's explore ten extensive health and longevity benefits associated with rosehips:

1. **Eye Health:** Rosehips contain lutein and zeaxanthin; these carotenoids act as natural filters for blue light. Prolonged exposure to blue light from digital screens, sunlight, and artificial lighting can lead to retinal damage and visual discomfort. The presence of lutein and zeaxanthin in rosehips helps filter out harmful blue light and protects the retina from potential damage.
2. **Skin Health:** Rosehips are one of the richest, most bioavailable plant sources of vitamin C. This vitamin is a powerful antioxidant that helps protect against oxidative stress, supports collagen synthesis for skin elasticity, and aids in overall skin health. Rosehips contain provitamin A carotenoids, including beta-carotene, which can be converted into vitamin A in the body. Vitamin A is essential for maintaining healthy skin and promoting cell regeneration. Rosehips contain vitamin E, another antioxidant that helps protect cells from oxidative damage. Vitamin E is involved in maintaining healthy skin and may contribute to reducing the appearance of wrinkles and fine lines. Rosehips contain various polyphenols, including ellagic acid and gallic acid, which have antioxidant and healthy aging effects. These compounds may support collagen synthesis and contribute to skin rejuvenation.

3. **Joint Health:** In addition to their antioxidant properties, the flavonoids and polyphenols in rosehips have been found to possess anti-inflammatory effects. They may help modulate the immune response and inhibit the production of pro-inflammatory substances, such as cytokines and enzymes involved in joint inflammation. By reducing inflammation, rosehips may help alleviate symptoms associated with inflammatory joint conditions and support joint comfort.
4. **Immune System Support:** Rosehips are high in bioavailable vitamin C, and are a source of carotenoids such as beta-carotene, lycopene, and lutein. Carotenoids are known for their immune-boosting properties and their role in supporting the body's defense against infections and diseases. They help modulate immune responses and promote the production of immune cells that combat pathogens. Rosehips also contain various polyphenolic compounds, including ellagic acid and gallic acid. Polyphenols possess antioxidant and anti-inflammatory properties that support immune health. They help neutralize harmful free radicals, reduce inflammation, and support the body's immune response against pathogens.
5. **Digestive Health:** Rosehips offer valuable support for digestive health due to their content of prebiotic compounds, notably galactolipids. These prebiotics act as nourishment for beneficial gut bacteria, fostering a balanced and diverse gut microbiome. By cultivating a healthy gut environment, rosehips facilitate the growth and activity of beneficial probiotics, such as Lactobacillus and Bifidobacterium species, which are crucial for maintaining digestive health. A well-balanced gut microbiome plays a pivotal role in breaking down food particles, synthesizing essential nutrients, and supporting proper nutrient absorption.
6. **Anti-inflammatory Effects:** Rosehips contain polyphenols, including gallic acid and ellagic acid. Gallic acid works by inhibiting the activity of certain enzymes and signaling pathways that promote inflammation in the body. By reducing the production of pro-inflammatory molecules, gallic acid helps alleviate inflammation and its associated symptoms. Ellagic acid has been recognized for its antioxidant and anti-inflammatory effects. It helps neutralize free radicals, which are reactive molecules that can trigger inflammation. By reducing oxidative stress and inhibiting inflammation, ellagic acid contributes to the overall anti-inflammatory properties of rosehips.

7. **Anti-cancer Effects:** The antioxidants found in rosehips, particularly vitamin C and various flavonoids, play a pivotal role in potential cancer prevention. These powerful compounds neutralize harmful free radicals in the body, which can cause oxidative stress and cellular damage, ultimately leading to the development of cancer. By reducing oxidative stress, rosehips may help safeguard DNA integrity and inhibit mutations that can trigger cancerous growth. Additionally, the presence of polyphenols in rosehips contributes to their anti-cancer properties, as they have been shown to inhibit the growth of cancer cells and impede the formation of new blood vessels that supply nutrients to tumors.
8. **Cardiovascular Health:** Rosehips have been associated with numerous benefits for heart health, making them a valuable addition to a heart-healthy diet. One of the key factors contributing to their heart-supportive properties is their high antioxidant content, particularly flavonoids like quercetin and kaempferol. These powerful antioxidants help combat oxidative stress and reduce the risk of damage to blood vessels and heart tissues caused by harmful free radicals. By neutralizing free radicals, rosehips may help prevent the development of atherosclerosis, a condition characterized by the buildup of plaque in the arteries, which can lead to heart disease. The presence of vitamin C in rosehips can contribute to heart health by promoting the synthesis of collagen, a protein essential for maintaining the integrity of blood vessels. Strengthened blood vessels are less susceptible to damage and more capable of supporting proper blood flow, reducing the risk of hypertension and other cardiovascular issues.
9. **Graceful-aging Effects:** Rosehips contain natural oils and fatty acids, such as linoleic acid and oleic acid, which help to nourish and hydrate the skin. These compounds help to maintain the skin's moisture barrier, preventing water loss and promoting a supple and plump complexion. Proper hydration is crucial for preventing the formation of fine lines and maintaining a youthful glow. Vitamin C is a vital nutrient for collagen synthesis, which is essential for maintaining the skin's elasticity and firmness. Collagen is a protein that provides structure and support to the skin. By supplying a highly bioavailable form of vitamin C, rosehips support collagen production, helping to reduce the appearance of wrinkles and improve skin elasticity.

10. **Antioxidant Powerhouse:** Rosehips are a rich source of antioxidants, including flavonoids, along with a highly bioavailable form of vitamin C. This form of vitamin C helps to neutralize harmful free radicals and protect against oxidative stress. The bioavailability of vitamin C in rosehips is influenced by the presence of other compounds, such as flavonoids. Flavonoids can enhance the absorption and utilization of vitamin C in the body, allowing it to exert its antioxidant activity more effectively. This means that when vitamin C is consumed from rosehips, the presence of flavonoids and other antioxidants enhances its overall effect in the body.

> While rosehips are generally considered safe to consume, there are some medical contradictions and considerations to be aware of. Individuals with iron overload disorders, such as hemochromatosis, may want to avoid rosehips due to their high vitamin C content, which can enhance iron absorption. Those with known allergies to roses should avoid rosehips as they may trigger allergic reactions. Rosehip seeds, also known as "hairs" or "itching powder," can cause irritation and discomfort if ingested in larger quantities. These hairs contain small amounts of chemicals called irritants, such as oxalate crystals and trichomes. Ingesting large quantities of rosehip seeds may lead to gastrointestinal upset, including irritation of the digestive tract, stomach pain, and potentially allergic reactions. Rosehip herbal infusions are generally considered safe for those who are pregnant and lactating.

ROSEMARY

Rosemary, a fragrant and versatile herb, boasts a fascinating history that traces back to the ancient Mediterranean region. Revered for both its culinary and medicinal properties, rosemary has been a treasured part of human civilization for centuries. Its name is derived from the Latin words "ros," meaning dew, and "marinus," meaning sea, highlighting its natural inclination for thriving in coastal areas and its connection to the sea's misty breeze. Rosemary's distinct aroma and unique flavor have made it a beloved herb in numerous cuisines, where it has been used to add depth and character to an array of dishes. Beyond its culinary significance, rosemary has held a prominent place in traditional medicine, where its various therapeutic benefits were recognized and utilized. Throughout history, rosemary has symbolized different meanings, ranging from remembrance and fidelity in ancient cultures to protection and purification during ceremonial rituals. Its long and storied history is a testament to the enduring popularity and significance of rosemary as a cherished herb that continues to captivate both the culinary and herbal worlds to this day. Now, let's explore ten extensive health and longevity benefits associated with rosemary:

1. **Respiratory Health:** The respiratory support provided by rosemary can be attributed to its bioactive constituents, including camphor, which has expectorant properties to relieve congestion, 1,8-cineole (eucalyptol), known for its bronchodilator and mucolytic effects, and rosmarinic acid, an antioxidant and anti-inflammatory compound that may help reduce inflammation in the respiratory system. Rosemary also contains various flavonoids with antioxidant properties that protect the respiratory system from oxidative damage.
2. **Cardiovascular Health:** Rosemary's potential to support healthy blood circulation lies in its bioactive compounds and their effects on the cardiovascular system. The presence of compounds like rosmarinic acid and carnosic acid in rosemary contributes to its positive impact on blood flow. Rosmarinic acid, as an antioxidant and anti-inflammatory agent, helps reduce oxidative stress and inflammation, which can improve blood vessel function and promote smoother blood flow. Carnosic acid, on the other hand, has been studied for its vasodilatory properties, meaning it may help dilate blood vessels, allowing for better nutrient and oxygen delivery throughout the body.

3. **Digestive Health:** Rosemary's digestive health benefits stem from its bioactive compounds, including camphor, carnosic acid, and rosmarinic acid. These compounds, along with bitter diterpenes like carnosol and rosmanol, contribute to improved digestion, relief from indigestion, and soothing gastrointestinal discomfort. The bitter compounds in rosemary stimulate the production of digestive enzymes and bile, supporting the breakdown and absorption of nutrients. They also encourage the secretion of gastric juices, aiding in the digestive process.
4. **Antimicrobial Effects:** Rosmarinic acid has demonstrated strong antimicrobial effects against various bacteria and viruses. Another significant compound is 1,8-cineole (eucalyptol), known for its antiviral and antibacterial properties, which is particularly effective against respiratory viruses and bacteria. Additionally, rosemary contains camphor, which exhibits antiviral activity. These active constituents work synergistically to combat harmful pathogens and support the body's immune system. When used topically, rosemary-infused products may help protect the skin from bacterial infections, aid in wound healing, and soothe skin irritations. Internally, consuming rosemary or its extracts may contribute to boosting the immune response and aiding the body in fighting off infections.
5. **Cognitive Support:** Rosemary contains various bioactive compounds that contribute to its potential cognitive benefits. One of the key compounds is rosmarinic acid, which exhibits antioxidant and anti-inflammatory properties. These properties are thought to protect the brain from oxidative stress and inflammation, which are associated with cognitive decline and neurodegenerative diseases. Rosemary also contains essential oils, including 1,8-cineole (also known as eucalyptol). 1,8-cineole has been shown to have positive effects on cognitive function. It is believed to increase cerebral blood flow and enhance neurotransmitter activity, specifically acetylcholine, which is important for learning and memory processes.
6. **Immune System Support:** Rosemary contains potent antioxidants like rosmarinic acid and caffeic acid, which play a crucial role in supporting the immune system by neutralizing harmful free radicals that can damage cells and weaken immune responses. Rosemary's immune-enhancing effects are attributed to its ability to modulate immune responses. Rosemary extracts may stimulate the production and activity of immune cells, including lymphocytes and natural killer cells, bolstering the body's natural defense against pathogens.

7. **Anti-inflammatory Effects:** Rosmarinic acid, a polyphenolic compound abundant in rosemary, is known for its potent antioxidant and anti-inflammatory effects. By neutralizing harmful free radicals and modulating inflammatory pathways, rosmarinic acid may help mitigate the effects of oxidative stress and reduce inflammation associated with chronic conditions, such as arthritis and cardiovascular diseases. Similarly, carnosic acid, another key constituent in rosemary, may target specific inflammatory molecules and signaling pathways. Carnosic acid may contribute to the overall anti-inflammatory effects of rosemary, making it a valuable herb for supporting a balanced inflammatory response and potentially easing symptoms related to inflammation-induced conditions.
8. **Hair and Scalp Health:** Rosemary oil is often used in hair care products due to its ability to stimulate hair growth, improve scalp health, and help combat dandruff.
9. **Joint and Muscle Pain Relief:** Rosemary oil's topical application for joint and muscle health is attributed to its potent analgesic and anti-inflammatory properties. Individuals dealing with conditions like arthritis can benefit from this natural remedy. When massaged onto sore muscles, rosemary oil helps alleviate tension, reduce muscle pain, and improve blood circulation, promoting faster recovery after physical activity. Furthermore, its anti-inflammatory effects can provide relief from joint pain and swelling, enhancing mobility and comfort for those with inflammatory joint issues.
10. **Headache Relief:** Rosemary has shown potential in supporting headache management due to its diverse bioactive compounds and therapeutic properties. One key compound in rosemary is 1,8-cineole, also known as eucalyptol, which has been studied for its analgesic and anti-inflammatory effects. When inhaled or applied topically, 1,8-cineole may help alleviate headache discomfort by relaxing tension in the head and neck muscles and reducing inflammation in the blood vessels surrounding the brain. Additionally, rosemary contains rosmarinic acid, a polyphenolic compound with antioxidant and anti-inflammatory properties that may help ease headache symptoms by reducing oxidative stress and calming inflammation in the nervous system.

While rosemary is generally considered safe to consume, there are certain medical contradictions and precautions associated with this herb. Individuals with bleeding disorders or those taking anticoagulant medications, such as warfarin, should consult their healthcare provider before using rosemary in large volumes. Similarly, individuals with a history of seizures or epilepsy should exercise caution, as rosemary contains camphor, which can potentially trigger seizures in susceptible individuals. People with high blood pressure should also be cautious when using rosemary in large volumes, as it may have a mild hypertensive effect. Additionally, individuals with allergies to plants in the Lamiaceae family, such as mint, basil, or oregano, may be at an increased risk of allergic reactions to rosemary. Pregnant and lactating women can safely consume very small amounts of rosemary as a culinary herb. Consult with your herbalist/practitioner before using high volumes of rosemary consistently during pregnancy.

SAGE

Sage, a herb with a rich and storied history, can be traced back to the Mediterranean region, where it has been cultivated and valued for millennia. Its prominence in ancient cultures is evident in its diverse uses, ranging from medicinal applications to culinary delights. The name "sage" itself carries a profound meaning, originating from the Latin word "salvare," which translates to "to save" or "heal." This etymology highlights the esteemed status of sage as a healing plant in traditional healing practices. Throughout history, sage has been highly revered for its aromatic properties, emitting a distinct fragrance that has captivated the senses and held cultural significance in various rituals and ceremonies. Additionally, its culinary uses have delighted palates across different cuisines, adding depth of flavor and a touch of herbal sophistication to dishes.

Now, let's explore ten extensive health and longevity benefits associated with sage:

1. **Hormonal Balance:** Sage has a long history of traditional use in relieving menopause-related symptoms such as hot flashes and night sweats, offering valuable hormonal support. Sage contains phytoestrogens, including flavonoids like apigenin and luteolin, which have estrogenic activity and may help balance hormone levels during menopause. These phytoestrogens bind to estrogen receptors, mimicking the effects of estrogen in the body and potentially reducing hot flashes and other menopausal discomforts. Rosmarinic acid helps regulate the hypothalamic-pituitary-adrenal (HPA) axis, which plays a role in the body's stress response and hormone regulation. By supporting the HPA axis, rosmarinic acid in sage may help alleviate symptoms associated with menopause. Sage is also a rich source of vitamins and minerals, including vitamin K, vitamin A, calcium, and magnesium, which contribute to overall hormonal and bone health.
2. **Mood Support:** Sage contains thujone, a terpene that has been associated with mood-enhancing properties. Thujone is believed to act as a GABA receptor antagonist, which could result in increased alertness and improved mood. By interacting with GABA receptors in the brain, thujone may modulate neurotransmitter activity, potentially leading to a positive impact on mood regulation.

3. **Cognitive Support:** Sage contains rosmarinic acid, a polyphenolic compound known for its antioxidant and anti-inflammatory properties. It helps protect the brain from oxidative stress and inflammation, which are implicated in age-related cognitive decline and neurodegenerative diseases. Another key compound found in sage is carnosic acid, which has been shown to have neuroprotective effects. It may enhance memory and cognitive function by promoting the production of nerve growth factors, which are essential for the growth and maintenance of brain cells. Sage contains compounds that inhibit the activity of acetylcholinesterase, an enzyme that breaks down acetylcholine, a neurotransmitter involved in memory and learning. By inhibiting acetylcholinesterase, sage may increase the availability of acetylcholine in the brain, potentially improving cognitive function.
4. **Digestive Health:** Sage offers notable digestive support through its various bioactive constituents. One of the key compounds responsible for its digestive benefits is rosmarinic acid, which helps soothe the digestive tract by reducing inflammation and irritation, thereby alleviating gastrointestinal discomfort. Sage also contains essential oils like cineole and camphor, which possess carminative properties, promoting the expulsion of gas from the digestive system and reducing bloating. Sage has also been shown to stimulate the production of digestive enzymes, aiding in the breakdown of food and enhancing nutrient absorption. Its antimicrobial properties may also help combat harmful bacteria that could disrupt gut health.
5. **Oral Health:** Sage's oral health benefits are attributed to its natural antimicrobial properties and anti-inflammatory effects. The presence of compounds like thujone, camphor, and cineole in sage contributes to its ability to combat harmful bacteria that can lead to plaque formation and cavities. By inhibiting bacterial growth in the oral cavity, sage helps maintain a healthier balance of oral flora and reduces the risk of dental infections. Sage's anti-inflammatory properties help soothe gum tissues, reducing redness and swelling associated with gingivitis and other oral inflammations.
6. **Skin Health:** The natural astringent and antiseptic properties of sage make it beneficial for skin health, helping to cleanse pores, soothe irritation, and promote a clear complexion.

7. **Respiratory Health:** Sage is renowned for its expectorant properties, making it valuable in alleviating respiratory symptoms like coughs, flu strains, and sore throats. Thujone acts as an expectorant, helping to loosen and expel mucus from the respiratory tract. Sage's volatile oils, including cineole, camphor, and borneol, soothe respiratory passages, reduce inflammation, and promote easier breathing. Additionally, sage is rich in flavonoids like apigenin and luteolin, which possess anti-inflammatory properties and support the immune system's response to respiratory infections. The presence of vitamin C in sage further aids in boosting immune function and reducing the severity of respiratory symptoms.
8. **Immune System Support:** Sage's immune-boosting properties are attributed to various terpenes, such as thujone, camphor, and cineole. Thujone is believed to interact with GABA receptors, potentially influencing mood and alertness. Camphor contributes to immune health by exhibiting antimicrobial effects that hinder the growth of detrimental microorganisms. Cineole, also known as eucalyptol, plays a crucial role in immune support with its strong antibacterial and antiviral properties, aiding in the inhibition of specific pathogens. By curbing the presence of these harmful microorganisms, sage's terpenes collectively reinforce the immune system's resilience, helping protect against infections and promoting overall immune well-being.
9. **Anti-inflammatory Effects:** Rosmarinic acid contains potent anti-inflammatory effects. Rosmarinic acid helps inhibit the production of inflammatory compounds in the body, such as prostaglandins and leukotrienes. Sage also contains flavonoids, such as apigenin and luteolin, which exhibit anti-inflammatory activity by modulating immune responses and reducing oxidative stress. Sage is also rich in antioxidants like carnosic acid and caffeic acid, which help neutralize free radicals and protect against cellular damage caused by inflammation. These active compounds work synergistically to support the body's natural inflammatory response and may provide relief for conditions such as arthritis, allergies, and inflammatory bowel disease.

10. **Hair Health:** Rosmarinic acid may help to soothe the scalp and reduce scalp inflammation that may impede hair growth. Sage also contains essential oils such as cineole and camphor, which possess antimicrobial properties that may help combat dandruff-causing fungi and bacteria. Sage is also a natural source of vitamins and minerals, including vitamin A, vitamin C, calcium, and magnesium, which nourish the hair follicles, promote a healthy scalp environment, and support optimal hair growth. When applied as a hair rinse or used in hair care products, sage can provide a gentle and natural solution for maintaining a healthy scalp, stimulating hair growth, and addressing dandruff concerns, contributing to overall hair health.

While sage is generally considered safe to consume, there are certain medical contradictions and precautions to be aware of. Individuals taking medications that have sedative effects, such as benzodiazepines or barbiturates, should be cautious with sage, as it may have mild sedative properties that could enhance the effects of these medications. For individuals with epilepsy or a history of seizures, sage contains thujone, a compound that may exacerbate seizure activity if consumed in large quantities. Sage may interact with antiepileptic medications and should not be used concurrently without consulting a healthcare professional. Allergy to plants in the Lamiaceae family, which includes mint, basil, and rosemary, may also be a concern for some individuals, as it can lead to allergic reactions such as skin rash, itching, or respiratory symptoms. Pregnant and lactating women should also exercise caution with sage and only use it in culinary amounts, as it may stimulate uterine contractions in high doses.

SASSAFRAS ROOT

Sassafras root, obtained from the sassafras tree (Sassafras albidum), boasts a captivating history that dates back centuries, enriched by its extensive utilization in various cultures and traditions. Indigenous communities in North America were among the first to recognize the medicinal properties of sassafras root, using it to treat a wide array of ailments, including skin conditions, fevers, and digestive issues. With the arrival of European settlers, its reputation as a valuable herbal remedy spread rapidly, and it became an essential ingredient in traditional herbal medicine practices of the time. During the 16th and 17th centuries, sassafras root gained popularity in Europe and was considered a medicinal treasure. The aromatic properties of sassafras root also captured the interest of early explorers and colonists, leading to its inclusion in beverages such as "root beer" and herbal teas. As time passed, sassafras root continued to be cherished for its unique flavor and medicinal potential, cementing its place as a historically significant botanical with a long-lasting legacy.

Now, let's explore ten extensive health and longevity benefits associated with sassafras root:

1. **Digestive Health:** Sassafras root has a notable history in traditional medicine for supporting digestive health. It has been relied upon to alleviate indigestion, bloating, and stomach cramps due to its active constituents, such as safrole, eugenol, and quercetin. Safrole, one of the key compounds in sassafras root, has demonstrated antimicrobial properties, which may help combat harmful bacteria in the digestive tract, promoting a balanced gut environment. Eugenol, another active component, exhibits anti-inflammatory effects that can soothe inflammation in the gastrointestinal system, contributing to relief from discomfort. Quercetin may reduce oxidative stress in the digestive system, aiding in overall digestive health.
2. **Liver Health:** Safrole and eugenol help to support liver health and aid in detoxification processes. Safrole has been studied for its hepatoprotective properties, which can be beneficial when used in low doses for short spurts of time. Safrole helps to protect the liver from damage caused by toxins and oxidative stress. Eugenol has shown the potential to enhance liver function by promoting the production of liver enzymes that aid in detoxification. Together, these constituents assist the liver in efficiently eliminating toxins from the body, promoting overall well-being and optimal liver health.

3. **Immune System Support:** Sassafras root is a rich source of antioxidants, including phenolic compounds like safrole, eugenol, and quercetin. These powerful antioxidants play a crucial role in combating free radicals and reducing oxidative stress, which can weaken the immune system. Safrole, a key component of sassafras root, has demonstrated antimicrobial and antiviral properties, potentially enhancing the body's ability to fight off harmful pathogens. Additionally, eugenol exhibits immune-modulating effects and has been shown to enhance the activity of immune cells.
4. **Anti-inflammatory Effects:** Sassafras root exhibits notable anti-inflammatory effects, rendering it beneficial for individuals managing conditions like arthritis or inflammatory bowel disease. This can be attributed to the active compounds safrole and eugenol. Safrole has been studied for its ability to inhibit inflammatory pathways and reduce the production of pro-inflammatory molecules, helping to alleviate inflammation and its associated symptoms. Eugenol acts as an anti-inflammatory agent by suppressing inflammatory enzymes and signaling pathways in the body. By targeting these inflammatory processes, sassafras root can provide relief from inflammatory conditions and support overall inflammatory balance.
5. **Respiratory Health:** Sassafras root has a traditional use in easing respiratory conditions such as coughs and bronchitis. Its expectorant properties, mainly attributed to safrole, help loosen mucus and facilitate easier breathing. Safrole acts as a mild irritant to the respiratory tract, stimulating mucus production and secretion. By lubricating and soothing the airways, it aids in expelling mucus and phlegm from the lungs.
6. **Skin Health:** One of the key compounds found in sassafras root extract is safrole, which has demonstrated anti-inflammatory activity. Safrole helps reduce the production of inflammatory molecules, effectively alleviating redness, itching, and rashes caused by skin irritation. Eugenol also possesses anti-inflammatory properties that contribute to its skin-soothing effects. Eugenol helps to inhibit inflammatory enzymes and signaling pathways, further supporting the reduction of skin irritation and discomfort. When applied topically, sassafras root extract works synergistically with these active constituents to provide a calming and gentle solution for various skin irritations, leaving the skin feeling relieved and refreshed.

7. **Cardiovascular Health:** Safrole and eugenol may contribute to the cardiovascular benefits of sassafras. Safrole has been studied for its potential to dilate blood vessels, which could help improve blood circulation and lower blood pressure. Eugenol exhibits vasodilatory effects, promoting the relaxation and widening of blood vessels, further enhancing blood flow. Improved blood circulation and reduced blood pressure can be advantageous for heart health, as they reduce the workload on the heart and lower the risk of cardiovascular ailments.
8. **Antimicrobial Effects:** The antimicrobial activity of sassafras root extends to both internal and topical use. The active compounds found in sassafras root, such as safrole and eugenol, contribute to its potent antimicrobial effects. Safrole has been studied for its antimicrobial properties against various bacteria and fungi, making it effective in fighting off harmful pathogens both inside and outside the body. When ingested, sassafras root may help combat harmful microorganisms in the digestive system, supporting gut health and overall well-being. When applied topically, sassafras root extract may help inhibit the growth of bacteria and fungi on the skin's surface, aiding in the prevention and management of skin infections. The antimicrobial properties of sassafras root play a significant role in promoting microbial balance, helping the body maintain a healthy and robust defense against potential infections, regardless of whether it is used internally or externally.
9. **Antioxidant Powerhouse:** Sassafras root is a rich source of antioxidants that play a vital role in safeguarding the body against oxidative stress, a process linked to cellular damage and aging. Safrole, eugenol, and quercetin are key active constituents responsible for the root's antioxidant-rich properties. These compounds neutralize harmful free radicals, unstable molecules that can cause oxidative damage to cells and DNA. By scavenging free radicals, the antioxidants in sassafras root help maintain cellular integrity and protect the body from various environmental stressors. Their collective action contributes to overall longevity and may support healthy aging.

10. **Diaphoretic Effects:** Sassafras has a long history of use as a diaphoretic, which means it has the ability to induce sweating. This diaphoretic property of sassafras has been valued for its role in promoting natural detoxification and supporting the body's ability to eliminate toxins through the skin. When taken as a warm infusion or tea, sassafras can increase body temperature and promote sweating, which helps to open the pores and release accumulated waste products and toxins. The diaphoretic action of sassafras is believed to facilitate the elimination of metabolic waste, promote lymphatic drainage, and support the overall cleansing of the body. As a result, sassafras has been traditionally used to aid in the treatment of various conditions, including fevers, colds, and infections, where inducing sweating may help the body fight off pathogens and restore balance.

While sassafras root is generally considered safe to consume when it's used in small quantities (and not for prolonged periods), there are several medical contradictions and important warnings to consider. Sassafras root may interact with certain medications. It is known to induce the activity of cytochrome P450 enzymes, which can affect the metabolism and effectiveness of various drugs. Therefore, individuals taking medications metabolized by these enzymes, such as anticoagulants, anticonvulsants, certain antidepressants (e.g., selective serotonin reuptake inhibitors or SSRIs), and immunosuppressants, should exercise caution and consult with a healthcare professional before using sassafras root. Individuals with liver disease or impairment should avoid sassafras altogether, as sassafras contains safrole, a compound that can be hepatotoxic (harmful to the liver) if used in high doses or for prolonged periods. It's important to note that when the root itself is extracted in water (herbal infusion or herbal decoction), it has lower concentrations of safrole than the essential oil, which is derived from sassafras root (and its bark). That said, sassafras essential oil should never be ingested. Pregnant and breastfeeding women should avoid sassafras, as safrole has shown estrogenic and genotoxic effects in animal studies, which raises concerns about potential risks to the developing fetus or infant.

SAW PALMETTO BERRIES

Saw palmetto berries, scientifically known as Serenoa repens, is a small palm tree native to the southeastern regions of the United States. This remarkable herb has a rich history of traditional use by Native American tribes, particularly the Seminole Indians, who valued its medicinal properties. The berries of the saw palmetto tree have been used for centuries to promote health and well-being. In the early 20th century, saw palmetto gained popularity as a natural remedy for various conditions, particularly in relation to prostate health. Today, it continues to be widely recognized and extensively studied for its potential therapeutic benefits. Now, let's explore ten extensive health and longevity benefits associated with saw palmetto berries:

1. **Prostate Health:** Saw palmetto berries are widely recognized for its ability to support prostate health. It contains specific bioactive compounds like fatty acids such as lauric acid and oleic acid, flavonoids, and phytosterols, including beta-sitosterol. These compounds help maintain prostate health, support urinary function, and alleviate symptoms associated with benign prostatic hyperplasia (BPH).
2. **Hormonal Balance:** The phytochemicals in saw palmetto berries, including sterols and fatty acids, contribute to its ability to promote hormonal balance in men. It helps regulate the conversion of testosterone to dihydrotestosterone (DHT), thereby supporting hormonal equilibrium.
3. **Prostate Cancer Support:** Saw palmetto's ability to potentially inhibit the growth of prostate cancer cells by blocking the enzyme 5-alpha-reductase, responsible for converting testosterone into the more potent dihydrotestosterone (DHT), has sparked interest as a potential supportive strategy for individuals dealing with prostate cancer. By reducing DHT levels, it may slow the growth of cancer cells and help maintain a healthier hormonal balance within the prostate gland.
4. **Anti-inflammatory Effects:** Phytosterols, particularly beta-sitosterol, plays a significant role in saw palmetto's anti-inflammatory effects. Beta-sitosterol is a plant compound that bears structural similarities to cholesterol, leading it to compete with cholesterol absorption in the digestive tract. This competition not only contributes to reducing cholesterol levels but also helps modulate the immune response and dampen inflammatory reactions.

5. **Antioxidant Powerhouse:** Flavonoids, such as quercetin and kaempferol, are potent scavengers of free radicals, neutralizing their harmful effects and preventing cellular damage. Carotenoids, including beta-carotene and lutein, act as powerful antioxidants, shielding cells from oxidative damage caused by environmental factors like UV radiation and pollution. The antioxidant activity of saw palmetto berry is essential for maintaining the structural integrity of cell membranes and protecting vital cellular components, such as DNA and proteins, from damage. This cellular protection contributes to the preservation of optimal cell function and helps to slow down the aging process.
6. **Urinary Tract Health:** Compounds such as fatty acids and beta-sitosterol may promote urinary tract health and alleviate symptoms associated with urinary tract infections (UTIs). Beta-sitosterol has anti-inflammatory properties, which may help reduce inflammation in the urinary tract and ease discomfort caused by UTIs. Saw palmetto berries are believed to have a positive impact on urinary flow by supporting prostate health in men. As the prostate gland surrounds the urethra, any enlargement or inflammation of the prostate can lead to difficulties with urinary flow. Saw palmetto berry's ability to inhibit the conversion of testosterone to dihydrotestosterone (DHT) may help maintain healthy prostate size and function, thereby promoting improved urinary flow. For women, saw palmetto berry's anti-inflammatory and soothing properties may also contribute to overall urinary tract health and comfort.
7. **Cognitive Support:** Saw palmetto berry's flavonoids and carotenoids act as natural defenders against harmful free radicals and inflammation in the brain. Flavonoids are known for their potent antioxidant and anti-inflammatory effects, helping to neutralize free radicals and reduce inflammation in brain tissues. While saw palmetto's cognitive benefits are not as extensively studied as its effects on prostate health, its potential role in promoting a balanced redox environment in the brain is noteworthy. Redox balance refers to the equilibrium between oxidation and reduction reactions, where antioxidants play a crucial role in safeguarding neurons from oxidative damage caused by free radicals. By supporting redox balance, saw palmetto may contribute to maintaining healthy cellular function and protecting the brain from harmful oxidative stress.

8. **Liver Health:** The antioxidants, including flavonoids and carotenoids present in saw palmetto berries, neutralize harmful free radicals and prevent them from causing harm to liver tissues. Saw palmetto Berries contain essential fatty acids such as oleic acid and lauric acid, which also contribute to liver health. These fatty acids have been found to possess hepatoprotective properties, shielding the liver from various toxins and environmental pollutants. This fruit's active constituents facilitate the liver's detoxification processes, assisting in the breakdown and elimination of harmful substances from the body.
9. **Hair Health:** Saw palmetto extract is often used in hair care products due to its potential to support hair health. It is believed to help inhibit the enzyme responsible for converting testosterone to dihydrotestosterone (DHT), which is associated with hair loss. By blocking DHT, saw palmetto may promote hair growth and maintain healthy hair.
10. **Scalp Health:** Saw palmetto's potential benefits for scalp health are attributed to its ability to balance sebum production and support a healthier scalp environment. Sebum is an oily substance produced by the sebaceous glands in the scalp, and its excess production can lead to oily scalp conditions, clogged hair follicles, and the development of dandruff. The active compounds found in saw palmetto, such as fatty acids (like lauric acid and oleic acid) and phytosterols, contribute to this herb's scalp health-supportive properties. These compounds may help regulate sebum production, preventing both excessive oiliness and dryness, leading to a more balanced and nourished scalp.

While saw palmetto berries are generally considered safe to consume, there are certain medical contradictions and precautions to be aware of. Individuals taking medications that have hormonal effects, such as hormone replacement therapy or oral contraceptives, should exercise caution with saw palmetto, as it may interfere with hormonal balance. For individuals with a history of hormone-sensitive conditions, such as breast cancer or prostate cancer, saw palmetto's hormonal effects may not be appropriate. Saw palmetto may interact with anticoagulant or antiplatelet medications, potentially increasing the risk of bleeding. Individuals with bleeding disorders or scheduled for surgery should avoid saw palmetto. Allergy to saw palmetto or plants in the same family (Arecaceae) is possible, and individuals with known allergies should avoid its use. Regarding pregnancy and lactation, saw palmetto should be avoided, as it may have hormonal effects that could potentially impact fetal development or lactation.

SCHISANDRA BERRIES

Schisandra berries, scientifically known as Schisandra chinensis and referred to as the "five-flavor fruit," have a captivating history deeply rooted in traditional Chinese medicine. These petite and colorful berries are sourced from the Schisandra chinensis plant, which finds its origins in the regions of Northern China, Russia, and other parts of Asia. For centuries, Schisandra berries have been cherished for their multifaceted contributions to holistic health, earning them a reputation as an age-reversal tonic. Throughout history, these berries have been treasured and incorporated into various medicinal practices due to their intriguing taste profile encompassing all five fundamental flavors—sweet, sour, salty, bitter, and pungent. Their journey from ancient herbal remedies to a revered superfood highlights the enduring fascination with Schisandra's potential wellness benefits across diverse cultures and eras.

Now, let's explore ten extensive health and longevity benefits associated with Schisandra berries:

1. **Liver Health:** One of the key bioactive compounds in Schisandra berries has been shown to possess antioxidant and anti-inflammatory properties. These properties help protect liver cells from oxidative stress and reduce inflammation, thereby supporting the liver's overall well-being. Additionally, the berries contain lignans, such as schisandrin B and gomisin A, which exhibit hepatoprotective effects by enhancing liver cell regeneration, inhibiting liver fibrosis, and promoting detoxification enzyme activity. Schisandra berries are also rich in vitamin C, which acts as a potent antioxidant, further shielding the liver from free radicals and oxidative damage.
2. **Respiratory Health:** Schisandrin A, schisandrin B, and gomisin A, play a crucial role in supporting respiratory health through their demonstrated anti-inflammatory effects. These compounds help mitigate inflammation in the respiratory tract, which can be particularly beneficial for individuals dealing with coughs, bronchitis, or other respiratory conditions. By reducing inflammation, Schisandra berries contribute to the relief of respiratory discomfort, making it easier to breathe and promoting overall lung function. Furthermore, their anti-inflammatory properties extend to soothing irritated airways, facilitating mucus clearance, and potentially alleviating symptoms associated with respiratory ailments.

3. **Sustained Energy Levels:** Schisandrin A, schisandrin B, and gomisin A contribute to the energizing effects of these berries. These compounds have been scientifically studied for their adaptogenic properties, which help the body adapt to stress and improve overall energy regulation. By modulating the stress response and enhancing cellular energy production, Schisandra berries promote sustained energy throughout the day without the typical jitters or crashes experienced with caffeine or other stimulants.
4. **Adaptogenic Effects:** The adaptogenic benefits of Schisandra berries extend beyond their potent antioxidant properties. Schisandrin and gomisin, prominent constituents of these berries, not only shield cells from the harmful effects of oxidative stress induced by stressors but also intricately interact with various receptors and enzymes within the body. This interaction plays a pivotal role in modulating the body's response to stress, facilitating a profound sense of equilibrium and calm. Schisandrin and gomisin contribute to the body's adaptability in the face of both physical and emotional stressors, helping individuals better cope with life's challenges. These adaptogenic properties make Schisandra berries a valuable ally in promoting overall well-being, enhancing resilience, and maintaining a balanced state of mind even in demanding situations.
5. **Neuroprotective Effects:** Schisandrin has been shown to possess neuroprotective properties by reducing oxidative stress and inflammation in the brain. Schisandrin A and B have been found to enhance learning and memory by modulating neurotransmitters and improving synaptic plasticity. Additionally, the presence of antioxidants such as vitamins C and E in Schisandra berries helps combat free radicals and protect brain cells from damage.
6. **Enhanced Physical Performance:** The adaptogenic properties of Schisandra berries may help increase endurance, reduce fatigue, and improve physical performance, making them popular among athletes.
7. **Skin Health:** Schisandrin A, gomisin A, and schisandrin B possess potent antioxidant properties. These lignans help neutralize harmful free radicals, reducing oxidative damage to the skin and preventing premature aging. Schisandra berries contain vitamin C, a powerful antioxidant that plays a crucial role in collagen synthesis, helping to maintain skin elasticity and reduce the appearance of wrinkles. The berries also provide vitamins E and A, which further contribute to their antioxidant and skin-nourishing effects.

8. **UV Protection:** Schisandrin A and gomisin A may have potential protective effects against UV-induced skin damage. Antioxidants are essential in neutralizing harmful free radicals generated by UV radiation. By incorporating Schisandra berry extract into skincare products or using it topically, its antioxidant properties may help shield the skin from UV rays and potentially reduce the risk of UV-induced skin damage. The antioxidants in Schisandra berries work by scavenging and neutralizing free radicals, thereby mitigating oxidative stress and supporting overall skin health.
9. **Digestive Health:** Lignans, such as schisandrin and gomisin, are among the key elements found in Schisandra berries that contribute to their digestive benefits. These lignans have been studied for their ability to stimulate the production of digestive enzymes, including amylase, lipase, and protease. Amylase is responsible for breaking down carbohydrates into simpler sugars, lipase aids in the digestion of fats into fatty acids and glycerol, and protease assists in the breakdown of proteins into amino acids. By stimulating the production of these digestive enzymes, Schisandra berries facilitate the efficient breakdown of macronutrients, supporting optimal nutrient absorption and utilization. The active compounds in Schisandra berries help soothe gastrointestinal discomfort, reducing issues like bloating, gas, and indigestion. They can also aid in promoting a healthy gut environment by supporting beneficial gut bacteria, which further contributes to improved digestion and overall gut health.
10. **Immune System Support:** The unique combination of compounds found in Schisandra berries, including antioxidants and immune-modulating substances, may help strengthen the immune system and support overall wellness.

While Schisandra berries are generally considered safe to consume, there are certain medical contradictions and precautions to be aware of. Individuals taking medications that are metabolized by the liver's cytochrome P450 enzymes, such as certain antiviral, antifungal, and antidepressant medications, should exercise caution, as Schisandra berries may potentially interact with these drugs and affect their metabolism. Schisandra berries may interact with medications that affect blood sugar levels, so individuals with diabetes or on diabetic medications should consult their healthcare provider before using this herb. Individuals with bleeding disorders or taking anticoagulant medications should avoid Schisandra berries, as they may have mild anticoagulant properties that could increase the risk of bleeding. Allergy to Schisandra berries or other plants in the Schisandraceae family is possible, and individuals with known allergies to these plants should avoid their use. Women who are pregnant or breastfeeding should consult with their herbalist/practitioner before using Schisandra berries.

SEA BUCKTHORN (POWDER)

Sea buckthorn, scientifically known as Hippophae rhamnoides, is a small deciduous shrub with a rich history dating back thousands of years. Originating from the mountainous regions of Asia and Europe, sea buckthorn has been utilized for its medicinal properties in traditional medicine practices. This versatile herb has a long-standing presence in various cultures and has been recognized for its potent health benefits. Sea buckthorn powder is derived from the berries of the plant, which are known for their vibrant orange color and high nutrient content. The berries are carefully harvested and processed to create a fine powder that retains the beneficial compounds found in sea buckthorn.

Now, let's explore ten extensive health and longevity benefits associated with sea buckthorn:

1. **Skin Health:** Sea buckthorn is a powerhouse of antioxidants, including vitamins C and E, carotenoids, such as beta-carotene and lycopene, and flavonoids, such as quercetin and kaempferol. These active compounds work together to protect the skin from oxidative stress caused by free radicals, preventing premature aging and maintaining a youthful appearance. The high vitamin C content in sea buckthorn aids in collagen synthesis, promoting skin elasticity and smoothness, contributing to healthy and radiant skin.
2. **Immune System Support:** The impressive vitamin C content in sea buckthorn plays a crucial role in supporting the immune system. Vitamin C boosts the production and activity of white blood cells, strengthening the body's defense against infections and diseases. Sea buckthorn contains immune-modulating compounds like beta-sitosterol and quercetin, which help regulate immune responses, ensuring a balanced and efficient immune system.
3. **Cardiovascular Health:** Sea buckthorn is a rich source of heart-healthy nutrients, such as omega-3 fatty acids (alpha-linolenic acid), plus vitamin E, and other flavonoids, including isorhamnetin and kaempferol. These components collectively contribute to cardiovascular health by reducing inflammation in blood vessels, improving blood flow, and supporting healthy blood pressure levels. The omega-3 fatty acids in sea buckthorn have also been associated with a reduced risk of heart disease and promoting overall heart health.

4. **Digestive Health:** Sea buckthorn's bioactive compounds, including quercetin and isorhamnetin, and tannins (ellagitannins and proanthocyanidins) play a vital role in supporting digestive health. These compounds contribute to a balanced gut microbiome, fostering the growth of beneficial gut bacteria while alleviating gastrointestinal inflammation. As a result, sea buckthorn supports a healthy digestive system, optimizes nutrient absorption, and promotes overall gastrointestinal well-being.
5. **Anti-inflammatory Effects:** Quercetin and isorhamnetin, both flavonoids, have been extensively studied for their anti-inflammatory properties, as they help regulate inflammatory pathways and reduce the production of pro-inflammatory molecules. Additionally, ellagitannins and proanthocyanidins, known as polyphenols, contribute to the anti-inflammatory effects of sea buckthorn by neutralizing free radicals and modulating immune responses. The presence of beta-carotene, a carotenoid and precursor to vitamin A, adds to sea buckthorn's anti-inflammatory prowess, as it helps protect cells from oxidative stress and inflammation.
6. **Liver Health:** Sea buckthorn supports liver health by harnessing the power of antioxidants, such as vitamin E and flavonoids, alongside essential fatty acids like omega-3 and omega-6. These components actively participate in liver detoxification processes while shielding liver cells from harmful free radicals. The combination of antioxidants and essential fatty acids boosts liver function and overall liver health, facilitating the body's natural detoxification mechanisms.
7. **Neuroprotective Effects:** The high antioxidant content in sea buckthorn, particularly vitamins C and E, supports brain health and cognitive function. These antioxidants protect brain cells from oxidative stress, reducing the risk of neurodegenerative diseases. As a result, sea buckthorn's neuroprotective effects contribute to improved brain function and overall cognitive health.
8. **Wound Healing:** Sea buckthorn oil is renowned for its remarkable wound-healing properties. The oil's rich nutrient profile, including vitamins C and E, promotes tissue regeneration and collagen synthesis, accelerating the healing process of various skin wounds, burns, and other skin injuries. Sea buckthorn oil's anti-inflammatory effects help reduce inflammation and soothe damaged skin, further facilitating the wound-healing process.

9. **Eye Health:** Sea buckthorn contains essential carotenoids, such as lutein and zeaxanthin, which are beneficial for eye health. These compounds help protect the eyes from oxidative damage and age-related macular degeneration, promoting optimal vision and eye health.
10. **Eczema and Psoriasis Relief:** Sea buckthorn oil, derived from the berries of the sea buckthorn plant, is renowned for its therapeutic effects on various skin conditions, particularly eczema and psoriasis. Its ability to alleviate these conditions can be attributed to its rich composition of bioactive compounds. The oil is abundant in antioxidants like vitamin E, beta-carotene, and flavonoids, which exert powerful anti-inflammatory effects on the skin. By neutralizing harmful free radicals and modulating inflammatory pathways, these antioxidants help reduce the redness, itching, and inflammation commonly experienced in eczema and psoriasis.

> While sea buckthorn is generally considered safe to consume, it's important to be aware of certain medical contradictions and precautions. Individuals with specific conditions such as bleeding disorders or low blood pressure should exercise caution when using sea buckthorn, as it may interfere with blood clotting and blood pressure medications. Sea buckthorn may affect blood sugar levels, so individuals with diabetes or those taking diabetes medications should monitor their blood sugar closely. It's important to note that sea buckthorn may cause allergic reactions in individuals sensitive to plants in the Elaeagnaceae family, including Russian olive, oleaster, buffalo berry, and silverberry. Sea buckthorn is generally considered safe for consumption in culinary amounts by pregnant and lactating individuals.

NOTES

SEA LETTUCE

Sea lettuce, also known as Ulva lactuca, is a type of edible green seaweed with a rich history and origin. This herb is commonly found in coastal areas and has been used as a food source and traditional medicine in various cultures throughout history. Sea lettuce has long been valued for its nutritional profile and health benefits. It is packed with essential nutrients, including vitamins A, C, and K, as well as minerals such as iodine, iron, and calcium. This nutrient-rich seaweed also contains specific antioxidants, such as beta-carotene and chlorophyll, which contribute to its health-promoting properties.

Now, let's explore ten extensive health and longevity benefits associated with sea lettuce.

1. **Detoxification:** Sea lettuce contains chlorophyll, a green pigment that aids in detoxification processes by supporting liver function and assisting in the elimination of toxins from the body. Chlorophyll has been studied for its potential to bind to and remove heavy metals and other harmful substances from the body, promoting overall detoxification and cleansing.
2. **Graceful-aging Effects:** Sea lettuce is a rich source of antioxidants, including beta-carotene, vitamin C, and chlorophyll, which play a vital role in combating oxidative stress. Beta-carotene acts as a powerful antioxidant, protecting cells from damage caused by free radicals and promoting healthy aging. Vitamin C, known for its strong antioxidant properties, helps neutralize free radicals, supports collagen production, and maintains the overall health and vitality of the skin. Chlorophyll, the pigment responsible for the green color of sea lettuce, also possesses antioxidant properties that contribute to its ability to combat oxidative stress and promote healthy aging. Sea lettuce also contributes to maintaining the integrity and elasticity of the skin, promoting a healthy complexion and youthful appearance.
3. **Thyroid Health:** Sea lettuce is an excellent source of iodine, a vital mineral that is essential for proper thyroid function. Iodine plays a crucial role in the synthesis of thyroid hormones, which are responsible for regulating various bodily functions, including temperature regulation and regulating the metabolic processes of nearly all cells. Adequate iodine intake is necessary for maintaining a healthy thyroid gland and ensuring optimal hormone production.

4. **Immune System Support:** Sea lettuce is rich in vitamin C, which plays a crucial role in supporting immune function and defending against infections. Vitamin C is known to enhance the production and activity of immune cells, such as white blood cells, and help the body mount a robust immune response against pathogens.
5. **Cognitive Support:** Sea lettuce contains vitamin C and beta-carotene, which protect brain cells from oxidative stress and support overall cognitive function. Additionally, it provides minerals like magnesium and iron, which are essential for neurotransmitter synthesis and oxygen transport to the brain. These nutrients work synergistically to support brain health, cognition, and overall mental well-being.
6. **Protein Synthesis:** Protein synthesis is a fundamental process in the body that plays a critical role in maintaining overall health and well-being, and sea lettuce's abundance of amino acids contributes to this essential function. Amino acids, the building blocks of proteins, are involved in the synthesis of various proteins that serve as the structural foundation for tissues, organs, muscles, enzymes, and hormones. One of the key health benefits of sea lettuce is its support for protein synthesis, which is vital for the growth, repair, and maintenance of body tissues. Proteins are essential for building and repairing muscle mass, supporting muscle function, and ensuring the proper functioning of organs and bodily systems.
7. **Anti-inflammatory Effects:** Peptides found in sea lettuce possess potent anti-inflammatory properties that help regulate the body's immune response and counteract excessive inflammation. These peptides act as signaling molecules, modulating the inflammatory processes and promoting balance within the immune system. Additionally, the polyphenols in sea lettuce, including flavonoids and tannins, play a pivotal role in reducing inflammation by neutralizing free radicals and inhibiting pro-inflammatory enzymes. By targeting inflammatory pathways, sea lettuce's bioactive compounds help to reduce swelling, redness, and discomfort associated with inflammation.
8. **Cardiovascular Health:** Sea lettuce's nutrient content, particularly potassium and magnesium, supports heart health by regulating blood pressure and maintaining proper cardiovascular function. Potassium helps relax blood vessels and improve blood flow, while magnesium is essential for maintaining a healthy heart rhythm and preventing arrhythmias.

9. **Bone Health:** The calcium and vitamin K found in sea lettuce are essential for maintaining strong and healthy bones, reducing the risk of osteoporosis. Calcium is a crucial mineral for bone formation and density, while vitamin K plays a role in regulating calcium metabolism and promoting bone health.
10. **Antimicrobial Effects:** Sea lettuce contains specific bioactive compounds, such as peptides and polyphenols, that exhibit antimicrobial properties. These compounds have shown the ability to inhibit the growth of various bacteria and fungi, making sea lettuce a potential natural remedy for addressing microbial infections and promoting a healthy microbial balance in the body.

> While sea lettuce is generally considered safe to consume, it's important to be aware of potential medical contradictions and interactions. It's important to note that sea lettuce may interact with medications that affect the thyroid, such as thyroid hormone replacement therapy or medications for hyperthyroidism or hypothyroidism. Additionally, sea lettuce may have a blood-thinning effect, so individuals taking anticoagulant medications or with bleeding disorders should consult their healthcare provider before incorporating sea lettuce into their diet. Individuals with allergies to seafood or iodine should avoid consuming sea lettuce. It is also crucial to source the seaweed from the Atlantic Ocean to avoid higher levels of contamination from pollutants in the Pacific Ocean. Those who are pregnant or lactating should consult with their herbalist/practitioner prior to consuming sea lettuce in large quantities for prolonged periods during this time.

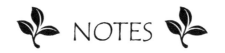

NOTES

SHANKHPUSHPI

Shankhpushpi, also known as Convolvulus pluricaulis, is a revered herb in traditional Ayurvedic medicine that has been used for centuries in India. This herb is derived from a small, creeping plant with beautiful blue or white flowers and is primarily found in the Himalayan region. Shankhpushpi has gained significant recognition for its potential health benefits and is often referred to as a brain tonic due to its impact on cognitive functions and mental well-being.

Now, let's explore ten extensive health and longevity benefits associated with Shankhpushpi:

1. **Cognitive Support:** Shankhpushpi contains flavonoids such as kaempferol and quercetin, known for their antioxidant and anti-inflammatory properties, which may play a role in improving cognitive function. These flavonoids have been studied for their potential to enhance blood flow to the brain, further contributing to improved cognitive function. By protecting neurons from oxidative damage and reducing neuroinflammation, Shankhpushpi supports brain health and fosters optimal cognitive performance.
2. **Neuroprotective Support:** Neuroprotective support is one of the significant benefits associated with Shankhpushpi, thanks to the presence of the primary active compound, scopoletin. As a natural coumarin derivative, scopoletin has garnered attention in scientific research due to its potential neuroprotective and antioxidant properties, believed to safeguard brain health and function. Oxidative stress, caused by an imbalance between free radicals and antioxidants in the body, can lead to damage and degeneration of brain cells over time. However, scopoletin antioxidant properties help neutralize harmful free radicals, reducing the risk of oxidative damage to brain cells.
3. **Anti-inflammatory Effects:** Shankhpushpi exhibits anti-inflammatory properties due to its constituents, including shankhpushpin, flavonoids such as kaempferol and quercetin, and alkaloids like convolvulusine A. These compounds play a role in inhibiting inflammatory processes, which can be beneficial for conditions like arthritis and joint pain. Flavonoids help regulate inflammatory pathways and mediators, while alkaloids suppress pro-inflammatory cytokines, collectively contributing to the herb's anti-inflammatory effects.

4. **Adaptogenic Effects:** One of the primary active compounds responsible for these benefits is shankhpushpin, a flavone glycoside found in the herb. Shankhpushpin acts as an adaptogen, helping the body adapt to physical and emotional stressors by modulating the body's stress response systems. By promoting a sense of calmness and relaxation, it can alleviate feelings of anxiety and tension. Shankhpushpi also contains other flavonoids, such as kaempferol and quercetin, which contribute to its adaptogenic and anxiolytic effects. These flavonoids interact with neurotransmitter systems in the brain, particularly the GABAergic system, enhancing GABAergic neurotransmission and promoting a calming effect on the nervous system. Additionally, Shankhpushpi contains alkaloids like convolvulusine A, which have been investigated for their anxiolytic effects.
5. **Immune System Support:** Shankhpushpi is abundant in bioactive compounds that contribute to its immune-modulating properties. Among these, alkaloids play a key role, believed to stimulate the production of essential immune cells, including macrophages and lymphocytes, crucial for the body's defense mechanism. Additionally, the herb contains glycosides, such as scopolin and scopoletin, which have demonstrated antimicrobial and antiviral activities, potentially aiding in combatting infectious agents.
6. **Nervous System Support:** Shankhpushpi is highly regarded as a nervine tonic, containing various bioactive compounds that nourish and fortify the nervous system. One of the key constituents, shankhpushpin, acts as a nerve-strengthening agent, providing support to the nervous system and enhancing its resilience to stress and daily challenges. By bolstering nerve health, Shankhpushpi may assist in maintaining optimal nerve functions, including the proper transmission of nerve impulses and communication between nerve cells. The herb also contains flavonoids like kaempferol and quercetin, known for their potential neuroprotective properties, helping shield nerve cells from oxidative damage caused by free radicals, essential for preserving nerve health and function. Another significant component of Shankhpushpi is scopoletin, a natural coumarin derivative that exhibits neuroprotective and antioxidant characteristics, further contributing to supporting the nervous system by defending nerve cells from oxidative stress and promoting overall nerve well-being.

7. **Cardiovascular Health:** Shankhpushpi is believed to have cardio-protective properties, benefiting heart health through its flavonoids like kaempferol and quercetin, known for their antioxidant and anti-inflammatory effects that reduce oxidative stress and inflammation in blood vessels. Alkaloids, including convolvulusine A, found in Shankhpushpi may help regulate blood pressure and enhance blood vessel function, supporting healthy circulation. The herb also provides essential minerals such as potassium and magnesium, crucial for maintaining heart health, with potassium aiding blood pressure regulation and magnesium promoting smooth muscle relaxation in blood vessels.
8. **Reduces Under-Eye Puffiness:** Shankhpushpi contains bioactive compounds, including flavonoids like kaempferol and quercetin, which contribute to its anti-inflammatory properties. When applied topically, these flavonoids may help reduce under-eye puffiness and dark circles by soothing and calming the delicate skin around the eyes. Flavonoids inhibit inflammatory processes in the skin, beneficial in minimizing puffiness caused by fluid retention and inflammation. Additionally, Shankhpushpi possesses antioxidant properties attributed to compounds like scopoletin and shankhpushpin, aiding in protecting the skin from oxidative stress and free radical damage. This antioxidant activity can further support the reduction of under-eye puffiness by maintaining skin health and elasticity. Applying Shankhpushpi as an overnight treatment can increase hydration, soothe the skin, and improve circulation, contributing to a refreshed appearance in the morning.
9. **Liver Health:** Shankhpushpi offers significant benefits for liver health and detoxification due to its diverse range of bioactive constituents. Among these compounds, shankhpushpin stands out as a primary active component, displaying hepatoprotective properties that shield the liver from toxins and oxidative stress by acting as an antioxidant and neutralizing harmful free radicals. In addition to shankhpushpin, the herb contains flavonoids like quercetin and kaempferol, known for their anti-inflammatory and antioxidant effects that further support liver health by reducing inflammation and combating oxidative damage. Shankhpushpi's alkaloids, particularly convolvulusine A, have also been studied for their hepatoprotective properties, contributing to the liver's overall function and integrity.

10. **Sleep Support:** This herb contains specific nutrients and compounds that support its potential benefits for insomnia, sleep quality, and sleep pattern regulation. One such compound is flavonoids, including kaempferol and quercetin, which possess sedative properties and help induce relaxation. Another key component is saponins, such as shankhpushpin, which have a calming effect on the nervous system, reducing anxiety and promoting tranquility conducive to sleep. Additionally, Shankhpushpi contains alkaloids like convolvulusine A, which exhibit neuroprotective and anxiolytic effects, working synergistically to support healthy sleep by calming the mind, reducing stress, and improving overall sleep quality.

While Shankhpushpi is generally considered safe to consume, there are some medical contradictions and precautions that should be considered. Shankhpushpi may have sedative effects, so individuals taking medications that have sedative properties, such as benzodiazepines, barbiturates, or certain antidepressants, should use Shankhpushpi with caution to avoid excessive sedation. Shankhpushpi may interact with blood-thinning medications, such as warfarin, and increase the risk of bleeding. It is advisable to consult with a healthcare professional if you are taking any medications that could potentially interact with Shankhpushpi. Individuals with certain medical conditions, such as diabetes, hypotension (low blood pressure), and bradycardia (slow heart rate), should exercise caution when using Shankhpushpi as it may interact with their existing medications and exacerbate these conditions. Pregnant or breastfeeding women should also exercise caution and consult with their herbalist/ practitioner before using Shankhpushpi.

SHATAVARI

Shatavari, scientifically known as Asparagus racemosus, is an ancient herb deeply rooted in Ayurvedic medicine. It is a climbing plant native to India and is highly regarded for its various health benefits and its association with longevity. Shatavari has been traditionally used for its rejuvenating and nourishing properties, particularly in women's health. Its name, "shatavari," translates to "she who possesses a hundred husbands," indicating its reputation for promoting vitality and fertility in women. However, the herb is also beneficial for men and offers a wide range of overall health benefits.

Now, let's explore ten extensive health and longevity benefits associated with shatavari:

1. **Hormonal Balance:** Shatavari's adaptogenic properties are attributed to its bioactive compounds, such as saponins like shatavarin and shatavaroside. These compounds help regulate hormone levels in the body, making it particularly beneficial for women. By balancing hormones, shatavari may alleviate symptoms associated with hormonal imbalances, such as menstrual irregularities, hot flashes, and mood swings.
2. **Reproductive Health:** Shatavari's role in enhancing reproductive health can be attributed to its rich nutrient profile, which includes saponins, phytoestrogens, and amino acids. Saponins, such as shatavarin and shatavaroside, are bioactive compounds known for their adaptogenic properties. These compounds help regulate hormone levels in the body, making shatavari particularly beneficial for women with hormonal imbalances. By supporting hormone regulation, shatavari may alleviate symptoms associated with menstrual irregularities, hot flashes, and mood swings. Shatavari contains phytoestrogens like diosgenin and isoflavones, which are plant-based compounds that mimic the actions of estrogen in the body. These phytoestrogens can nourish the reproductive organs and promote healthy fertility. By binding to estrogen receptors, they help maintain the balance of reproductive hormones and may aid in alleviating discomfort during menstruation. Shatavari is also a source of essential amino acids. Amino acids are the building blocks of proteins and play a crucial role in various physiological processes, including hormone synthesis. The availability of amino acids in shatavari can support the synthesis of hormones necessary for reproductive health.

3. **Immune System Support:** The immunomodulatory effects of shatavari can be attributed to its alkaloids, glycosides, and polysaccharides. These bioactive compounds enhance the body's immune response, making it more resilient against infections and diseases. By strengthening the immune system, shatavari reduces the risk of illnesses and improves overall well-being.
4. **Digestive Health:** Shatavari's calming effect on the digestive system is supported by its active compounds, including saponins and mucilage. These compounds help soothe gastrointestinal distress, such as bloating, acidity, and indigestion. Shatavari also supports the production of digestive enzymes, promoting better nutrient absorption and gut health.
5. **Respiratory Health:** Shatavari's expectorant properties can be attributed to its saponins and alkaloids, which help relieve respiratory congestion and cough. It may alleviate symptoms associated with respiratory conditions like asthma, bronchitis, and allergies, promoting clearer and healthier breathing.
6. **Adaptogenic Effects:** Shatavari, an adaptogenic herb, holds remarkable properties that help restore emotional equilibrium and foster mental well-being. Its active compounds, such as saponins and flavonoids, play a significant role in its mood-balancing effects. As an adaptogen, shatavari aids the body in adapting to stress, shielding it from the detrimental effects of heightened cortisol levels. By regulating neurotransmitters in the brain, shatavari promotes a calming influence, effectively reducing anxiety, irritability, and mood swings.
7. **Graceful-aging Effects:** Shatavari's rejuvenating properties are supported by its active compounds, including steroidal saponins and flavonoids. These compounds help maintain skin elasticity, promote a healthy complexion, and may reduce the appearance of fine lines and wrinkles, contributing to a youthful and radiant appearance.
8. **Nail Health:** This herb's ability to promote stronger and healthier nails is attributed to its rich content of nutrients, including vitamins A, C, and E, as well as minerals like zinc and iron. Vitamin A is crucial for maintaining the health of nail tissues and preventing dryness and brittleness. Vitamin C aids in collagen synthesis, which is essential for maintaining the structural integrity and strength of the nails. Vitamin E is a powerful antioxidant that helps protect the nails from oxidative damage, keeping them healthy and vibrant. The presence of minerals like zinc and iron in shatavari further contributes to nail growth and overall nail health.

9. **Cardiovascular Health:** Shatavari's cardioprotective effects are attributed to its flavonoids and saponins, particularly shatavarin. These compounds may help regulate blood pressure levels, reduce cholesterol levels, and improve overall cardiovascular function, supporting heart health.
10. **Hair and Scalp Health:** Shatavari's abundance of phytoestrogens, including diosgenin and isoflavones, further promotes hair health by nourishing hair follicles and supporting their growth. Additionally, shatavari contains antioxidants like ascorbic acid (vitamin C) and flavonoids, which help protect hair and the scalp from oxidative stress and damage caused by free radicals. The adaptogenic properties of shatavari also contribute to its hair and scalp support by reducing stress and anxiety, both of which can negatively impact hair health. By addressing stress, shatavari helps create a conducive environment for healthy hair growth and minimizes the risk of hair loss. This herb's anti-inflammatory effects, attributed to its saponins and flavonoids, may also play a role in alleviating scalp conditions like itching and irritation, promoting overall hair and scalp well-being.

While this herb is generally considered safe to consume, there are certain medical contradictions and precautions to be aware of. Individuals with estrogen-sensitive conditions such as breast, uterine, or ovarian cancer should avoid or use caution when using shatavari, as it possesses estrogenic properties that could potentially stimulate the growth of hormone-dependent tumors. Individuals with a history of hormone-related conditions or those who are on hormone replacement therapy should consult their healthcare provider before using shatavari. It is important to exercise caution when combining shatavari with medications that have estrogen-like effects, such as tamoxifen, as it may interfere with their efficacy. Individuals with allergies to plants in the Asparagaceae family, which includes asparagus, may also be allergic to shatavari. Pregnant and lactating women should consult with their herbalist/practitioner before using shatavari to ensure its safe and appropriate use during these times.

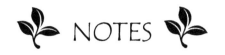

SHEEP SORREL

Sheep sorrel, scientifically known as Rumex Acetosella, is a perennial herb that belongs to the Polygonaceae family. It is native to Europe, Asia, and North America and has been used for centuries in traditional herbal medicine. The plant is characterized by its vibrant green leaves and small reddish flowers that bloom during the summer months. Sheep sorrel has been traditionally valued for its medicinal properties, and its use dates back to ancient times. It was widely recognized by Native American tribes, who used it for various purposes, including its potential as a diuretic, detoxifier, and digestive aid. The herb's tart and lemony flavor also made it a popular addition to salads and culinary dishes. Today, sheep sorrel continues to be appreciated for its potential health benefits and versatility. Now, let's explore ten extensive health and longevity benefits associated with sheep sorrel:

1. **Immune System Support:** Sheep sorrel contains potent antioxidants like quercetin and kaempferol, which help strengthen the immune system by neutralizing harmful free radicals and supporting the body's defense against infections and diseases. These antioxidants work to protect immune cells and enhance immune function, promoting overall health and well-being.
2. **Anti-inflammatory Effects:** Sheep sorrel's anti-inflammatory effects are attributed to the presence of flavonoids and phenolic compounds like rutin and chlorogenic acid. These bioactive compounds help reduce inflammation in the body by inhibiting pro-inflammatory enzymes and signaling pathways. By mitigating chronic inflammation, sheep sorrel may play a role in preventing or managing various inflammatory conditions and promoting optimal health.
3. **Antimicrobial Effects:** Sheep sorrel has shown promising antimicrobial activity against certain bacteria and fungi, highlighting its potential as a natural antimicrobial agent. This herb contains specific bioactive compounds that contribute to its antimicrobial properties. For instance, sheep sorrel is a rich source of various phenolic compounds, such as gallic acid, catechin, and quercetin. These phenolic compounds have been studied for their ability to inhibit the growth and spread of harmful microorganisms. Gallic acid, in particular, has demonstrated strong antibacterial activity against certain strains of bacteria.

4. **Digestive Health:** Sheep sorrel has a traditional role in promoting digestive health, assisting with digestion and providing relief from gastrointestinal discomfort. It may stimulate the release of digestive enzymes, improving the breakdown of food and enhancing nutrient absorption. Furthermore, its anti-inflammatory properties help soothe digestive inflammation and support a healthy gut environment.
5. **Detoxification:** Sheep sorrel's diuretic properties can aid in detoxification by supporting kidney function and promoting the elimination of waste products and toxins from the body. This diuretic action helps flush out accumulated toxins, contributing to the body's natural detoxification processes.
6. **Skin Health:** The antioxidant compounds found in sheep sorrel, such as quercetin and kaempferol, play a crucial role in promoting healthy skin. These antioxidants protect skin cells from oxidative damage caused by free radicals, helping to maintain skin elasticity and reduce the signs of aging, contributing to a vibrant and youthful complexion.
7. **Liver Health:** Sheep sorrel's hepatoprotective effects can be attributed to its rich composition of bioactive compounds, which include anthraquinones like emodin and rhein, as well as flavonoids such as quercetin and kaempferol, along with tannins. These compounds work in harmony to promote liver health by shielding liver cells from oxidative stress, curbing inflammation, and facilitating optimal liver function.
8. **Cardiovascular Health:** Sheep sorrel contains flavonoids, such as quercetin and kaempferol, which have been associated with cardiovascular benefits, including vasodilation and improved blood flow. The presence of tannins in sheep sorrel may also play a role in promoting cardiovascular health by reducing inflammation and supporting blood vessel function.
9. **Anti-cancer Effects:** Sheep sorrel contains anthraquinones like emodin and chrysophanol, which have shown potential anti-cancer properties in preliminary studies. However, further research is needed to fully understand their impact on cancer cells and potential applications in cancer treatment.
10. **Respiratory Health:** The presence of flavonoids like quercetin and kaempferol in sheep sorrel contributes to its respiratory health benefits. These compounds possess anti-inflammatory and antispasmodic effects, helping to reduce inflammation in the respiratory system and alleviate coughing and congestion, potentially benefiting individuals with respiratory conditions like asthma and bronchitis.

While sheep sorrel is generally considered safe to consume, there are certain medical contradictions and precautions to be aware of. Sheep sorrel may interact with certain medications, such as anticoagulants or blood-thinning drugs, due to its potential to affect blood clotting. Therefore, individuals taking such medications should consult a healthcare professional before using sheep sorrel. Allergy to sheep sorrel or plants in the Polygonaceae family is possible, and individuals with known allergies to these plants should avoid its use. Cross-reactivity with other plants in the same family, such as rhubarb and buckwheat, may occur, leading to allergic reactions. Women who are pregnant or lactating can generally consume fresh sheep sorrel in culinary amounts safely. Consult with your herbalist/practitioner prior to using this herb in large therapeutic doses during these times.

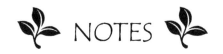

SHEPHERD'S PURSE

Shepherd's purse, scientifically known as Capsella Bursa-Pastoris, is an herb with a fascinating history and origin that stretches back to ancient times in Europe and Asia. This versatile plant has been deeply ingrained in traditional medicine and herbal remedies for centuries, and its usage can be found in various cultures throughout history. The name "shepherd's purse" is derived from the distinct shape of its seed pods, which indeed resemble small purses or pouches, giving the plant its unique and memorable identity. The origins of shepherd's purse are deeply interwoven with folklore and cultural beliefs. In some cultures, the herb was associated with protection and good luck, and it was believed to ward off evil spirits and bring blessings to those who carried it. In others, it was seen as a symbol of fertility and used in rituals related to childbirth and women's health. In ancient civilizations, shepherd's purse was revered for its medicinal properties and various practical uses. The herb's historical significance can be seen in records of traditional herbalism, where it was often mentioned as a valuable remedy for a range of health issues. Its widespread cultivation and use in different regions were a testament to its adaptability and effectiveness as a medicinal herb.

Now, let's explore ten extensive health and longevity benefits associated with shepherd's purse:

1. **Menstrual Support:** Shepherd's purse, with its long history of traditional use, has been sought after for its potential to regulate menstrual cycles, reduce heavy menstrual bleeding, and alleviate menstrual cramps. Its effectiveness in addressing these concerns can be attributed to the presence of compounds like flavonoids and tannins. Flavonoids, including quercetin, possess anti-inflammatory properties that may help reduce inflammation, easing menstrual discomfort. Tannins, on the other hand, have astringent properties that may help tighten and tone the uterine tissues, potentially reducing excessive bleeding during menstruation.
2. **Urinary Tract Health:** Shepherd's purse's diuretic properties make it beneficial for urinary health. The herb's ability to increase urine flow can be attributed to various bioactive compounds, including flavonoids, tannins, and alkaloids. These constituents may help alleviate urinary tract infections by promoting the elimination of harmful bacteria from the urinary system and supporting overall urinary system health.

3. **Wound Healing:** Shepherd's purse showcases remarkable hemostatic properties, making it a valuable aid in stopping bleeding and promoting wound healing. This ability can be attributed to its constituents like flavonoids, tannins, and alkaloids. Flavonoids, such as quercetin and kaempferol, possess antioxidant properties that may help protect and repair damaged tissues. Tannins have astringent effects that can promote blood clotting and facilitate wound closure. Alkaloids present in shepherd's purse, such as choline, contribute to the herb's wound healing properties by supporting tissue repair and regeneration.
4. **Digestive Health:** Shepherd's purse offers digestive support through its diverse array of compounds. The flavonoid quercetin, with its anti-inflammatory properties, may help reduce gastrointestinal inflammation, alleviating symptoms of indigestion and stomach cramps. Tannins contribute to the herb's astringent effects, potentially helping to alleviate diarrhea by toning the intestinal tissues. The alkaloid choline may stimulate appetite, aiding in digestion by supporting the production of acetylcholine, a neurotransmitter involved in regulating appetite and digestion.
5. **Blood Pressure Regulation:** Shepherd's purse has demonstrated hypotensive effects, suggesting potential benefits in regulating blood pressure levels. The specific compounds responsible for these effects are still under investigation, but the herb's therapeutic properties may offer support for maintaining healthy blood pressure.
6. **Respiratory Health:** With its expectorant properties, shepherd's purse can be valuable in relieving respiratory discomforts such as coughs, bronchitis, and congestion. These benefits may be attributed to certain compounds that support respiratory health by promoting the clearance of mucus and soothing the respiratory system.
7. **Liver Health:** Shepherd's purse has earned a well-deserved reputation for supporting liver health and promoting detoxification processes. The herb's abundance of flavonoids like quercetin, kaempferol, and rutin, as well as glucosinolates such as glucobrassicin, contribute to its hepatoprotective effects. These compounds exhibit antioxidant properties, helping protect liver cells from oxidative stress and supporting the organ's detoxification pathways. Phenolic acids found in shepherd's purse, like caffeic acid and p-coumaric acid, further contribute to liver protection by reducing inflammation and safeguarding liver cells from damage.

8. **Anti-inflammatory Effects:** Shepherd's purse contains compounds with anti-inflammatory properties, which may help reduce inflammation and provide relief from various inflammatory conditions in the body.
9. **Postpartum Support:** Shepherd's purse is believed to offer postpartum support due to its constituents, including flavonoids, tannins, alkaloids, and saponins. Flavonoids and tannins possess antioxidant and anti-inflammatory properties, which can aid in reducing postpartum inflammation and promoting tissue healing. Alkaloids and saponins may support hormonal balance and help alleviate postpartum discomfort. Shepherd's purse is often used in traditional medicine to assist in uterine contractions, reduce excessive bleeding, and support overall postpartum recovery.
10. **Antimicrobial Effects:** The antimicrobial effects of shepherd's purse are attributed to several key constituents found in the herb. Flavonoids, such as quercetin and kaempferol, are among the primary bioactive compounds responsible for these properties. These flavonoids have demonstrated broad-spectrum antimicrobial activity and can effectively combat various pathogens, including bacteria and fungi. Shepherd's purse contains tannins, which possess both astringent and antimicrobial properties. These tannins play a significant role in preventing microbial growth and providing additional support for the herb's antimicrobial effects. Together, the flavonoids and tannins present in shepherd's purse contribute to its potent antimicrobial properties, making it a potentially valuable natural remedy for combatting infections and promoting overall health.

While the herb shepherd's purse is generally considered safe to consume, there are several medical contradictions and precautions to be aware of. Individuals with bleeding disorders or those taking anticoagulant medications should avoid shepherd's purse due to its potential anticoagulant properties, as it may increase the risk of bleeding or interfere with the efficacy of blood-thinning medications. Individuals with a history of hypotension or low blood pressure should exercise caution when using shepherd's purse, as the herb may further lower blood pressure levels. Individuals with known allergies or sensitivities to the Brassicaceae family, which includes cruciferous vegetables like cabbage and mustard, should exercise caution when using shepherd's purse. It is also important to note that shepherd's purse may have uterotonic effects, which means it can stimulate uterine contractions. Consequently, pregnant women should avoid using this herb, as it may potentially cause miscarriage or premature labor.

SKULLCAP (AMERICAN)

Skullcap, scientifically known as Scutellaria lateriflora, holds a fascinating and rich history deeply rooted in North America, particularly the Eastern United States. This perennial herb's name is derived from the distinctive shape of its flowers, resembling small helmets or skullcaps, which adds to its unique allure. However, the significance of skullcap goes far beyond its charming appearance. Native American tribes have treasured skullcap for centuries, recognizing its therapeutic properties and incorporating it into their traditional medicinal practices. The herb was highly regarded for its potential to promote relaxation and calmness and support emotional well-being. Skullcap's traditional use by Native Americans serves as a testament to its long-standing reputation as a valuable botanical ally in times of stress and tension. Throughout history, skullcap has been admired as an age-reversal tonic, contributing to its allure as a potential agent for promoting healthy aging and longevity. Its intriguing past as a herb deeply entwined with cultural traditions and healing practices has contributed to its enduring fascination and continued use in modern times. Now, let's explore ten extensive health and longevity benefits associated with skullcap (American):

1. **Anxiety and Stress Relief:** Skullcap has been traditionally used as a mild sedative and anxiolytic (anti-anxiety agent). This herb is known for its calming and relaxing effects, helping to alleviate symptoms of stress, anxiety, and nervous tension. Flavonoids like apigenin and chrysin, alongside baicalin and scutellarin, contribute to its anxiolytic and calming effects.
2. **Sleep Support:** Skullcap is renowned for its gentle sedative effect, making it a valuable herb for promoting restful sleep and combating insomnia. Several nutrients and compounds present in American skullcap contribute to its sleep-enhancing properties. One of the key compounds is baicalin, a flavonoid with calming effects that promotes relaxation and soothes the nervous system. Baicalin interacts with neurotransmitters in the brain, such as gamma-aminobutyric acid (GABA), which helps regulate mood and reduce anxiety, contributing to a sense of calmness conducive to sleep. Additionally, skullcap contains other flavonoids like scutellarin, which exhibits anxiolytic properties, further reducing anxiety and enhancing its sleep-promoting effects. Flavones such as baicalein and wogonin further support its sedative properties, making skullcap an excellent choice for improving sleep quality and encouraging a restful night's sleep.

3. **Mood Support:** Baicalin interacts with neurotransmitters in the brain, such as gamma-aminobutyric acid (GABA), which helps regulate mood and reduce anxiety. Additionally, skullcap contains other flavonoids like scutellarin and wogonin, which possess neuroprotective properties and help modulate neurotransmitter activity. These compounds contribute to skullcap's ability to promote relaxation, ease nervous tension, and support emotional balance.
4. **Cognitive Support:** Skullcap contains compounds like scutellarin, catalpol, apigenin, baicalein, and wogonin, which have been studied for their potential neuroprotective effects. Neuroprotective compounds help protect brain cells from damage and promote their overall cognitive health and function.
5. **Anti-inflammatory Effects:** Skullcap's remarkable anti-inflammatory effects can be attributed to a diverse array of compounds found within the herb. Among these are flavonoids, such as baicalin, baicalein, wogonin, apigenin, and chrysin. These powerful flavonoids have demonstrated potent anti-inflammatory properties that may help mitigate neuroinflammation, contributing to improved cognitive function and overall brain health. By inhibiting the production of pro-inflammatory cytokines and reducing oxidative stress, these flavonoids act as natural defenders against harmful inflammation in the brain. Inflammation in the brain has been linked to various neurodegenerative diseases and cognitive decline, making the anti-inflammatory prowess of skullcap a promising avenue for supporting brain health and preserving cognitive abilities.
6. **Anti-itch Effects:** The potential anti-inflammatory and soothing properties of American skullcap may contribute to its ability to alleviate itchiness when applied topically. The herb contains several bioactive compounds, including flavonoids like baicalin, baicalein, and wogonin, which have demonstrated anti-inflammatory effects in some studies. These flavonoids may help reduce skin inflammation and irritation, which are often associated with itchiness. American skullcap's use in traditional medicine and anecdotal evidence suggest that it has been applied topically as a poultice or ointment to soothe irritated skin and provide relief from itching. Its historical use in topical formulations may have contributed to its reputation for this particular benefit.

7. **Antioxidant Powerhouse:** With its rich content of antioxidants, skullcap can protect cells from oxidative damage caused by free radicals, contributing to graceful aging and overall health. Compounds like baicalin and catalpol, alongside flavonoids, play essential roles in providing antioxidant support.
8. **Respiratory Health:** Skullcap's ability to soothe respiratory conditions, such as allergies, coughs, and bronchitis, can be attributed to its rich array of bioactive compounds. The herb contains flavonoids like baicalin, baicalein, wogonin, apigenin, and chrysin, which are known for their potent anti-inflammatory properties. By reducing inflammation in the respiratory tract, these flavonoids help alleviate irritation and discomfort, promoting healthier airways. Skullcap's expectorant properties, supported by the presence of baicalin and other compounds, aid in loosening and expelling mucus and phlegm, easing breathing difficulties and congestion. Additionally, the herb's calming effects, induced by compounds such as scutellarin and baicalein, contribute to respiratory support by reducing stress and tension, which can be beneficial during respiratory challenges.
9. **Muscle Relaxation:** Baicalein, wogonin, and scutellarin, possess muscle relaxant and antispasmodic activities. These flavonoids have been shown to interact with neurotransmitter systems in the body, such as GABA (gamma-aminobutyric acid), which plays a key role in regulating muscle activity. By enhancing GABAergic neurotransmission, skullcap helps to reduce muscle excitability and hyperactivity, leading to relaxation and relief from tension and spasms. The presence of flavonoids like baicalin and wogonin in skullcap contributes to its anti-inflammatory properties. Inflammation can cause muscle stiffness and pain, and the ability of skullcap to reduce inflammation can aid in easing muscle discomfort. In traditional medicine, skullcap has been used as a muscle relaxant to alleviate various conditions, including muscle cramps, headaches, and menstrual cramps. Its muscle-relaxing effects make it a valuable herbal remedy for individuals experiencing muscle tension and discomfort.

10. **Acne Support:** Topically, American skullcap has shown potential in reducing acne due to its anti-inflammatory and antioxidant properties which have been found to possess anti-inflammatory effects, making it effective in calming and soothing irritated skin. Additionally, its antioxidant activity helps neutralize free radicals, which can contribute to skin inflammation and acne formation. Some studies have indicated that the application of topical creams containing skullcap extracts may help reduce the severity of acne lesions and improve overall skin condition.

While American skullcap is generally considered safe to consume, there are some medical contradictions and potential drug interactions to be aware of. Individuals with liver disorders or impaired liver function should exercise caution when using American skullcap, as the herb may affect certain liver enzymes involved in drug metabolism. It is advised to avoid American skullcap if you are taking medications metabolized by these enzymes, as it may alter their effectiveness. Additionally, American skullcap may lower blood pressure, so individuals with hypotension or those taking antihypertensive medications should use this herb with caution. Allergy to plants in the Lamiaceae family, which includes mint, sage, and basil, may also extend to American skullcap, so individuals with known allergies to these plants should avoid its use. Women who are pregnant or breastfeeding should consult with their herbalist/practitioner prior to using this herb.

SLIPPERY ELM BARK

Slippery elm bark, scientifically known as Ulmus rubra, is an ancient and esteemed medicinal herb deeply rooted in the history of North America. Native American tribes and early settlers revered this remarkable herb for its versatile and healing properties, using it for a myriad of health purposes. The slippery elm tree, also known as red elm or Indian elm, is indigenous to the eastern parts of North America, primarily found in regions with rich, moist soils. The history of slippery elm as a medicinal herb can be traced back to the Native American tribes, who passed down their knowledge of its therapeutic benefits through generations. One of the primary uses of slippery elm bark was for its mucilaginous properties. When combined with water, the inner bark forms a mucilage-like substance that becomes gelatinous and viscous. This mucilage was prized for its soothing and demulcent properties, making it a go-to remedy for soothing sore throats, coughs, and other respiratory irritations. The early settlers in North America quickly recognized the efficacy of slippery elm bark and adopted its use from the Native Americans. During the American Revolution, slippery elm became known as the "liberty tree" because its mucilaginous infusion was used to treat wounded soldiers and provide relief from pain and inflammation.

Now, let's explore ten extensive health and longevity benefits associated with slippery elm bark:

1. **Digestive Health:** Slippery elm bark is renowned for its mucilaginous properties, forming a protective layer along the digestive tract, promoting healthy digestion, and soothing gastrointestinal discomfort. This remarkable herb contains several active compounds, including mucilage, which becomes gel-like and slippery when mixed with water. This mucilage coats the lining of the digestive tract, providing a protective barrier that helps alleviate irritation and inflammation. Additionally, slippery elm bark contains tannins with astringent properties that can further soothe the digestive lining and reduce inflammation. The presence of beta-sitosterol and caffeic acid in slippery elm bark further supports gastrointestinal health. Beta-sitosterol is known to have anti-inflammatory properties that can reduce gastrointestinal inflammation, while caffeic acid exhibits antioxidant effects, helping to combat oxidative stress in the digestive system.

2. **Soothes Sore Throat:** Slippery elm bark can provide relief for sore throats and coughs by coating the throat and reducing irritation. The key active compound responsible for this effect is mucilage, which, when mixed with water, becomes a soothing gel that coats the throat and provides relief from discomfort. Slippery elm bark contains antioxidants such as polyphenols, which help reduce oxidative stress and inflammation in the throat, further contributing to its soothing properties. Slippery elm bark contains antioxidants such as polyphenols, including ferulic acid and gallic acid, which help reduce oxidative stress and inflammation in the throat, further contributing to its soothing properties. These antioxidants may help protect the throat's delicate tissues from damage and reduce irritation.
3. **Respiratory Health:** It may help alleviate respiratory conditions such as bronchitis, asthma, and coughs due to its soothing effects on the respiratory system. The mucilaginous nature of slippery elm bark plays a crucial role in providing relief for respiratory conditions. The gel-like mucilage helps soothe and protect the respiratory lining, reducing irritation and inflammation. Additionally, slippery elm bark contains antioxidants like polyphenols, which contribute to overall respiratory health by combating oxidative stress and promoting lung health. Slippery elm bark contains antioxidants like polyphenols, including quercetin and rutin, which contribute to overall respiratory health by combating oxidative stress and promoting lung health. Quercetin, in particular, has been studied for its potential benefits in respiratory conditions due to its anti-inflammatory and antioxidant properties.
4. **Diarrhea Support:** Slippery elm is a traditional herbal remedy known for its potential to provide support for individuals experiencing diarrhea. The bark of the slippery elm tree contains a significant amount of mucilage, a gel-like substance that can coat the gastrointestinal tract, soothing irritation, and forming a protective barrier. This mucilage can also absorb excess water in the intestines, resulting in bulkier stool and slower transit time, which can help alleviate diarrhea symptoms.
5. **Nutrient Absorption:** Slippery elm bark is renowned for its ability to support nutrient absorption in the intestines by creating an environment conducive for beneficial gut bacteria to thrive. The mucilage acts as a protective coating, soothing and lubricating the digestive tract. It forms a gentle barrier that helps prevent irritation and inflammation, allowing the intestines to effectively absorb essential nutrients.

6. **Weight Management:** Slippery elm bark can assist in weight management by promoting feelings of fullness, reducing overeating, and supporting healthy digestion. The mucilaginous properties of slippery elm bark contribute to feelings of fullness and satiety, which may help reduce excessive food intake.
7. **Skin Health:** Slippery elm bark has a long history of topical use for its soothing and emollient properties, making it a valuable natural remedy for various skin conditions, including burns, rashes, and wounds. Slippery elm bark is rich in mucilage, a gel-like substance that becomes slippery and viscous when mixed with water. This mucilage forms a protective layer on the skin, helping to soothe irritation and provide a barrier against further damage. Slippery elm bark contains antioxidants such as polyphenols, which help combat oxidative stress and promote skin health. Additionally, the bark contains tannins that have astringent properties, contributing to the tightening of tissues and reducing inflammation.
8. **Oral Health:** Slippery elm bark may help maintain oral health by reducing inflammation in the mouth, soothing gum irritations, and relieving symptoms of mouth ulcers. The mucilaginous properties of slippery elm bark provide a soothing and protective effect on the mouth and gums, reducing irritation and inflammation. The herb's antioxidants, including polyphenols, further support oral health by combating oxidative stress in the mouth.
9. **Urinary Tract Health:** It may help alleviate urinary tract infections and support urinary system health due to its anti-inflammatory and diuretic properties. Slippery elm bark contains anti-inflammatory compounds like tannins and flavonoids, which may help reduce inflammation in the urinary tract and alleviate symptoms of urinary tract infections. This herb's diuretic properties may promote increased urine production, helping to flush out toxins and potentially reducing the risk of urinary tract infections.
10. **Stress Relief:** Beta-sitosterols have been studied for its potential anxiolytic effects, reducing anxiety. Additionally, the presence of caffeic acid in this herb may further contribute to stress relief by acting as an antioxidant, helping to combat oxidative stress associated with stress and anxiety.

While slippery elm bark is generally considered safe to consume, there are certain medical contradictions and precautions that should be considered. Slippery elm bark can potentially interfere with the absorption and effectiveness of medications due to its mucilage content, which can form a protective coating in the digestive tract. Therefore, it is important to separate the intake of slippery elm bark from medications by at least two hours. Individuals taking medications such as warfarin or other anticoagulants, as well as those with bleeding disorders, should be cautious, as slippery elm bark may have mild anticoagulant properties and could increase the risk of bleeding. Individuals with a history of gastrointestinal obstruction or narrowing should exercise caution when using slippery elm bark, as it may worsen these conditions. Women who are pregnant or lactating should consult with their herbalist/practitioner prior to using this herb.

SOLOMON'S SEAL

Solomon's seal, scientifically known as Polygonatum, has ancient origins and a rich history in traditional medicine. While folklore has associated it with King Solomon, there is no direct historical evidence linking the herb to the biblical figure. This versatile plant is native to regions across the globe, including North America and Asia, and it has played a significant role in the healing practices of various cultures, including Ancient Greece, China, and Native American traditions. Its enduring popularity among herbalists, holistic practitioners, and health enthusiasts today can be attributed to its historical use and well-documented versatile healing properties. Solomon's seal continues to be highly valued for its potential health benefits and its positive impact on overall well-being.

Now, let's explore ten extensive health and longevity benefits associated with Solomon's seal:

1. **Adrenal Support:** Solomon's seal is rich in saponins, which are natural plant compounds known for their adaptogenic properties. Adaptogens are substances that help the body adapt to various stressors, whether physical, emotional, or environmental. Saponins interact with the adrenal glands, which are responsible for producing hormones like cortisol and adrenaline in response to stress. By supporting the adrenal glands' function, saponins may enhance the body's ability to respond to stress in a balanced and controlled manner. By providing support to the adrenal glands, Solomon's seal can help individuals better adapt to stress, promoting a more balanced and resilient response.
2. **Cellular Regeneration and Repair:** Solomon's seal contains phytonutrients, most notably allantoin, which have been associated with improved organ health due to their capacity to facilitate cellular repair and regeneration. Allantoin is particularly renowned for its remarkable ability to promote the regeneration and repair of cells. In instances where organs are subjected to stress or damage, the cells within them may become compromised. Allantoin plays a pivotal role in stimulating the growth of new cells, thereby expediting the healing process in damaged tissues. This cellular regeneration is of paramount importance in sustaining the optimal functioning of organs, especially when they are confronted with the natural wear and tear that occurs over time.

3. **Brain Health:** Solomon's seal contains quercetin, kaempferol, and rutin, belonging to the flavonoid family, along with caffeic acid and ferulic acid, which are prominent phenolic acids, and vitamin C, all of which contribute to preserving brain health. These antioxidants play a vital role in shielding brain cells from oxidative stress, a process that occurs due to an imbalance between free radicals and the body's natural defense mechanisms. Solomon's seal may help to maintain the structural integrity of brain cells, protect against cellular damage, and potentially slow down the aging process of the brain.
4. **Wound Healing:** The allantoin in Solomon's seal stimulates tissue regeneration. When an preparation of this herb is applied to minor cuts, burns, or scrapes, the allantoin accelerates the formation of new skin cells and collagen production, promoting faster wound healing and minimizing scars.
5. **Bone and Joint Health:** Solomon's seal offers notable benefits for bone and joint health, owing to its valuable content of essential minerals, including calcium, phosphorus, and manganese, which collectively support the maintenance of strong bones and promote joint flexibility. Calcium is crucial for bone density and strength, while phosphorus contributes to bone formation and mineralization. Manganese plays a vital role in the synthesis of connective tissues, supporting cartilage and tendon health, along with acting as a cofactor for enzymes involved in bone metabolism.
6. **Immune System Support:** Solomon's seal contains polysaccharides and saponins which may help enhance the immune system's defenses against pathogens. Polysaccharides are complex carbohydrates known for their immunomodulatory properties, meaning they can regulate the immune system's response to infections and help enhance its overall efficiency. Saponins, on the other hand, are natural compounds with antimicrobial properties, making them effective against certain bacteria and viruses.
7. **Bile Production Support:** Saponins found in Solomon's seal have been shown to stimulate the liver's production and secretion of bile. Bile is essential for the digestion and absorption of dietary fats and fat-soluble toxins. By increasing bile production, Solomon's seal facilitates the elimination of toxins and waste products from the liver, promoting a more efficient detoxification process.

8. **Antimicrobial Effects:** The active phytochemicals in Solomon's seal, such as saponins, flavonoids, and alkaloids, have the ability to disrupt the integrity of microbial cell membranes. This disrupts their normal functioning and leads to the breakdown of essential cellular processes, ultimately causing the destruction of the microorganisms.
9. **Bruise Relief:** Solomon's seal contains a variety of anti-inflammatory compounds, including flavonoids such as quercetin and kaempferol. When a preparation of this herb is applied to the bruised area, these compounds work to inhibit the body's inflammatory response to the injury. By reducing inflammation in the affected area, Solomon's seal may help improve blood circulation around the bruise. Improved circulation helps disperse the pooled blood from the bruise more effectively, reducing the discoloration and accelerating the healing process.
10. **Graceful-aging Effects:** Solomon's seal is rich in antioxidants, including flavonoids, phenolic acids, and vitamin C. These antioxidants play a crucial role in neutralizing free radicals, which are unstable molecules that can cause cellular damage and lead to aging. By reducing oxidative stress and protecting cells from damage, the antioxidants in Solomon's seal help to maintain cellular health and slow down the aging process.

While Solomon's seal is generally considered safe to consume, there are some medical contradictions and drug interactions that should be taken into account. Individuals with bleeding disorders or those taking anticoagulant medications should exercise caution as Solomon's seal may possess mild antiplatelet properties, potentially increasing the risk of bleeding. Additionally, individuals with diabetes or taking medications to lower blood sugar levels should monitor their blood glucose closely, as the herb may have hypoglycemic effects. Those with kidney disease or taking medications that impact kidney function should consult a healthcare professional before using Solomon's seal due to its potential diuretic properties. Individuals with known allergies to plants in the Asparagaceae family, which Solomon's seal belongs to, should avoid its use to prevent adverse reactions. Those who are pregnant or lactating should consult with their herbalist/practitioner prior to using this herb.

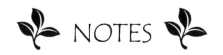

NOTES

SPEARMINT LEAF

Spearmint leaf, scientifically known as Mentha spicata, has a fascinating and ancient history dating back to ancient civilizations. Its origins can be traced to the Mediterranean region, where it was revered for its medicinal properties and culinary delights. The use of spearmint can be found in ancient texts, including the writings of Greek philosopher and naturalist Theophrastus, who described its aromatic and cooling qualities. Throughout history, spearmint has been cherished by various cultures for its refreshing aroma and cooling taste. The ancient Romans used spearmint to add flavor to their cuisine, while in ancient Egypt, it was a beloved herb used in culinary dishes and medicinal preparations. Traditional applications of spearmint in herbal medicine were wide-ranging, from aiding digestion and alleviating gastrointestinal discomfort to soothing headaches and respiratory ailments. Ancient cultures also utilized spearmint for its soothing properties, using it to create poultices and balms to relieve skin irritations and muscle pain.

Now, let's explore ten extensive health and longevity benefits associated with spearmint leaf:

1. **Digestive Health:** Spearmint leaf has been traditionally used to alleviate digestive discomfort, including bloating, gas, and indigestion. It may help soothe the stomach and support healthy digestion. The main constituents responsible for these benefits are the natural compounds found in spearmint, including menthol, carvone, and limonene. Menthol acts as a carminative, helping to relax the muscles of the digestive tract and reduce spasms, thereby relieving gas and bloating. Carvone and limonene also contribute to spearmint's digestive support by promoting the flow of bile, which aids in the digestion of fats and helps prevent indigestion.
2. **Antimicrobial Effects:** Spearmint leaf contains compounds such as carvone, limonene, and rosmarinic acid. These compounds possess antimicrobial properties against various bacteria and fungi, helping to combat infections and promote overall health.
3. **Detoxification:** Spearmint leaf is known for its diuretic properties, which may aid in flushing out toxins from the body and supporting kidney function. The diuretic effect is primarily attributed to compounds like menthol and flavonoids, which promote increased urine production and help the body eliminate waste products effectively.

4. **Oral Health:** The natural antimicrobial properties of spearmint leaf may help combat bacteria in the mouth, freshen breath, and promote oral hygiene. The primary compound responsible for these effects is carvone, which has been shown to possess antibacterial properties against certain oral pathogens.
5. **Respiratory Health:** Menthol helps to relax and open up the airways, allowing for easier breathing and relieving congestion. Additionally, spearmint leaf is rich in antioxidants, including flavonoids and phenolic compounds, which help reduce inflammation and oxidative stress in the respiratory system. These antioxidants support the body's natural defense mechanisms, helping to alleviate symptoms associated with respiratory conditions.
6. **Hormonal Balance:** Spearmint leaf has been associated with supporting hormonal balance, particularly in individuals with polycystic ovary syndrome (PCOS). It may help regulate androgen levels and improve symptoms such as excess hair growth and hormonal acne. The active compounds believed to be responsible for these effects are rosmarinic acid and flavonoids like luteolin. These compounds have been shown to modulate hormone levels and exert anti-androgenic effects.
7. **Stress Relief:** The aroma of spearmint has a calming effect on the mind and body, helping to reduce stress and anxiety and promote relaxation. The primary compound responsible for these relaxing properties in spearmint is menthol. Menthol interacts with receptors in the brain responsible for promoting a sense of calmness and well-being, leading to its stress-relieving effects.
8. **Cognitive Support:** Spearmint leaf contains rosmarinic acid, a phenolic compound with antioxidant and anti-inflammatory properties. It has been shown to cross the blood-brain barrier and exert neuroprotective effects by reducing oxidative stress and inflammation in the brain. Additionally, spearmint leaf contains other bioactive compounds, such as flavonoids, menthol, and limonene, which may also contribute to its cognitive benefits.
9. **Anti-inflammatory Effects:** Spearmint leaf contains compounds with anti-inflammatory properties that may help reduce inflammation in the body, potentially benefiting conditions such as arthritis and inflammatory bowel disease. The primary compounds responsible for these effects are rosmarinic acid and flavonoids, which work together to suppress inflammatory pathways and reduce the production of pro-inflammatory molecules.

10. **Skin Health:** Spearmint leaf has been used topically to soothe skin irritations, such as insect bites and rashes. Its cooling properties may help reduce redness and inflammation. The presence of antioxidants like rosmarinic acid and flavonoids in spearmint leaf also contributes to its skin-soothing effects by combating oxidative stress and supporting skin health.

While spearmint leaf is generally considered safe to consume, there are some medical contradictions and precautions to consider. Spearmint may interact with certain medications, such as antacids, proton pump inhibitors, and medications metabolized by the liver, potentially altering their effectiveness or increasing the risk of side effects. Spearmint may have estrogen-like effects and should be used with caution in individuals with hormone-sensitive conditions, such as breast cancer, uterine fibroids, or endometriosis. Individuals with known allergies to plants in the Lamiaceae family, including mint, basil, thyme, and oregano, should avoid spearmint to prevent allergic reactions. Pregnant or breastfeeding individuals should consult with their herbalist/practitioner before using spearmint in large therapeutic doses. Culinary amounts, however, are generally considered safe to use during these times.

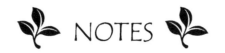

ST. JOHN'S WORT

St. John's wort, scientifically known as Hypericum perforatum, has a fascinating history in traditional medicine that spans centuries. Its use can be traced to ancient civilizations, including the Greeks and Romans, who held the plant in high regard for its potential therapeutic benefits. The name "St. John's wort" is said to have been derived from the belief that the plant's bright yellow flowers reached their peak bloom around the feast day of St. John the Baptist, which falls on June 24th. Throughout history, St. John's wort has been associated with various symbolic and superstitious beliefs. It was often regarded as a protective herb against evil spirits and was hung above doorways and windows to ward off malevolent forces. Additionally, the plant's bright yellow flowers were thought to represent the sun and its life-giving properties, further reinforcing its association with positive energy and healing. St. John's wort gained recognition for its potential mood-enhancing properties. It was believed to bring comfort to the spirit and was often used to alleviate feelings of sadness and promote emotional well-being. The plant was also associated with the notion of bringing light into darkness, both symbolically and in its applications for improving mood and emotional balance.

Now, let's explore ten extensive health and longevity benefits associated with St. John's wort:

1. **Sleep Support:** St. John's wort is believed to have sleep-inducing properties due to its influence on various neurotransmitters in the brain, particularly serotonin. Serotonin is a neurotransmitter that plays a key role in regulating mood, emotions, and sleep-wake cycles. St. John's wort contains hypericin, a compound that is thought to inhibit the reuptake of serotonin, essentially increasing its availability in the brain. This increase in serotonin levels may promote a sense of relaxation and calmness, making it easier for individuals to fall asleep. St. John's wort also contains hyperforin, another active compound that may contribute to its sleep-promoting effects. Hyperforin is believed to have sedative properties, which can further aid in inducing sleep and enhancing the overall quality of sleep. By calming the nervous system and promoting a sense of tranquility, St. John's wort may help individuals achieve a more restful and rejuvenating night's sleep.

2. **Mood Support:** Hypericin has been studied for its potential antidepressant properties and is believed to inhibit the reuptake of serotonin, dopamine, and norepinephrine in the brain. By modulating these neurotransmitters, hypericin may help regulate mood and alleviate symptoms of mild to moderate depression.
3. **Digestive Health:** Some of the active compounds found in St. John's wort, such as hyperforin and hypericin, have been studied for their potential effects on certain digestive enzymes. These compounds may help regulate the activity of enzymes involved in the breakdown of food, leading to improved digestion and nutrient absorption. The bitter compounds in this herb can stimulate the production of digestive juices, including stomach acid and enzymes, which are essential for proper digestion and nutrient assimilation.
4. **Antioxidant Powerhouse:** St. John's wort contains various flavonoids, including hyperoside, quercetin, and rutin. Flavonoids are known for their antioxidant and anti-inflammatory properties. These compounds help protect cells from oxidative stress and inflammation, which can have a positive impact on overall health and well-being.
5. **Nervous System Support:** St. John's wort contains constituents like flavonoids, including hyperoside, quercetin, and rutin, known for their antioxidant and anti-inflammatory effects. These compounds may help reduce inflammation and oxidative stress that may affect the nervous system. By mitigating inflammation and oxidative damage, St. John's wort may alleviate symptoms related to nerve pain and discomfort.
6. **Cognitive Support:** Hypericin also contains neuroprotective compounds. These neuroprotective compounds help protect brain cells from damage and promote their overall cognitive health and function. Hypericin may also influence neurotransmitter levels in the brain, specifically serotonin, dopamine, and norepinephrine. These neurotransmitters play essential roles in mood regulation, focus, and concentration. By inhibiting the reuptake of these neurotransmitters, hypericin helps maintain higher levels of these chemicals in the brain, which can lead to improved mood, enhanced focus, and better mental clarity. St. John's wort contains flavonoids like hyperoside, quercetin, and rutin, which possess antioxidant properties. Antioxidants help protect brain cells from oxidative stress, reducing the risk of age-related cognitive decline and supporting overall cognitive function.

7. **Antiviral Effects:** Hypericin has been shown to interfere with the replication process of HSV within infected cells. It works by inhibiting certain viral enzymes required for viral DNA replication, thereby limiting the virus's ability to multiply and spread. Hyperforin, another important compound in St. John's wort, plays a role in disrupting the formation of the viral envelope of HSV. The viral envelope is crucial for the virus's ability to enter and infect host cells. By interfering with this process, hyperforin helps prevent the virus from entering new cells and propagating further.
8. **Stress Relief:** In addition to hypericin and its influence on various neurotransmitters that support stress reduction, St. John's wort also contains flavonoids that possess antioxidant and anti-inflammatory properties. Oxidative stress and inflammation are often associated with increased stress levels and can negatively impact overall well-being. By combating oxidative stress and inflammation, the herb may contribute to a calmer physiological response to stress.
9. **Menopausal Support:** St. John's wort has the ability to interact with neurotransmitters and hormones in the body. During menopause, there is a significant fluctuation in hormone levels, particularly estrogen and progesterone, which can lead to uncomfortable symptoms like hot flashes and mood swings. St. John's wort contains active compounds like hypericin and hyperforin, which have been studied for their impact on serotonin and other neurotransmitters. Serotonin is a neurotransmitter that plays a crucial role in regulating mood, emotions, and body temperature. Hypericin is believed to inhibit the reuptake of serotonin, increasing its availability in the brain. This may help stabilize mood and reduce mood swings during menopause. This herb may also have an impact on other hormone-related pathways. St. John's wort has been found to interact with estrogen receptors, although the mechanisms are not fully understood. It is believed that the herb's constituents may mimic or modulate the effects of estrogen, which could contribute to the alleviation of menopausal symptoms.
10. **Immune System Support:** Hypericin and hyperforin have been shown to have immunomodulatory properties. These compounds may help regulate the immune response, enhancing the activity of immune cells such as T-cells and macrophages, which play a crucial role in identifying and neutralizing harmful pathogens.

While St. John's wort is generally considered safe to consume, there are several medical contradictions and important warnings to be aware of. This herb may interact with certain medications, particularly those metabolized by the liver enzymes CYP3A4 and CYP2C9, potentially reducing their effectiveness. Medications such as antidepressants (SSRIs and MAOIs), birth control pills, anticoagulants, immunosuppressants, HIV medications, and some anticonvulsants may experience altered efficacy when taken simultaneously with St. John's wort. Individuals with certain medical conditions, such as bipolar disorder, schizophrenia, or autoimmune diseases, should avoid using St. John's wort due to the risk of exacerbating symptoms. St. John's wort can cause photosensitivity, increasing the skin's sensitivity to sunlight, so it's essential to avoid excessive sun exposure during use. Allergy warnings include potential hypersensitivity reactions, which can manifest as skin rashes, itching, or respiratory symptoms in susceptible individuals. As St. John's wort belongs to the Hypericaceae family, other plants in the same family, like Hypericum elegans, also known as Graceful St. John's wort, may elicit similar allergic reactions. Safety during pregnancy and lactation is a critical consideration, as St. John's wort may have adverse effects on fetal development and pass into breast milk, potentially affecting nursing infants. Pregnant and breastfeeding women should avoid using St. John's wort.

SUMAC BERRIES

Sumac berries, scientifically known as Rhus coriaria, weave a captivating tale through the centuries, leaving an indelible mark on Middle Eastern and Mediterranean cultures. Originating from the resilient sumac shrub, indigenous to the arid landscapes of the Mediterranean, North America, and the Middle East, these vibrant red berries have been more than just culinary and medicinal assets. A century ago, in the sun-soaked villages of the Mediterranean and the culturally rich landscapes of the Middle East, sumac-ade emerged as a local marvel. Crafted by resourceful individuals within close-knit communities, this homemade drink offered a tart and refreshing alternative to commercially available beverages. The process involved soaking sumac berries in water, extracting their vibrant flavors, and skillfully sweetening the elixir to perfection. Throughout history, sumac berries have been used as a flavoring agent in dishes, imparting a tangy and slightly citrusy taste to food. They have also been employed in medicinal preparations.

Now, let's explore ten extensive health and longevity benefits associated with sumac berries:

1. **Immune System Support:** Sumac berries are packed with vitamin C, a potent antioxidant that strengthens the immune system and helps protect against age-related ailments. Vitamin C boosts the production of white blood cells, enhancing the body's defense against infections and supporting overall immune function.
2. **Digestive Health:** Sumac berries have traditionally been used to aid digestion by stimulating the production of digestive enzymes, promoting healthy gut function, and alleviating digestive discomfort. Active compounds like tannins and flavonoids in sumac berries contribute to these digestive benefits by supporting the breakdown of food and enhancing nutrient absorption.
3. **Anti-inflammatory Effects:** The antioxidants found in sumac berries, such as flavonoids and polyphenols, possess anti-inflammatory effects, supporting overall well-being and longevity. These compounds scavenge free radicals and inhibit inflammatory pathways, helping to reduce chronic inflammation, which is a key factor in many age-related diseases.
4. **Antimicrobial Effects:** Sumac berries contain natural compounds with antimicrobial properties, which may help combat harmful bacteria and support a healthy microbial balance in the body. One such compound is gallic acid, which exhibits antimicrobial activity against various bacteria and fungi.

5. **Cardiovascular Health:** The flavonoids present in sumac berries have been linked to improved heart health by reducing inflammation, lowering blood pressure, and promoting healthy blood vessel function. Quercetin and kaempferol are two flavonoids found in sumac berries that support cardiovascular health through their vasodilatory and anti-inflammatory effects.
6. **Skin Health:** Sumac berries offer skin-cleansing support primarily through their antimicrobial and astringent properties. The berries contain natural compounds with antimicrobial effects, which may help combat harmful bacteria and fungi on the skin's surface. These antimicrobial properties make sumac berries beneficial for cleansing the skin and maintaining its overall health.
7. **Antioxidant Powerhouse:** Sumac berries are rich in antioxidants, which help neutralize free radicals, protect cells from damage, and contribute to graceful aging. These antioxidants include quercetin, kaempferol, and gallic acid, all of which play a role in reducing oxidative stress and promoting cellular health.
8. **Anti-cancer Effects:** Certain compounds found in sumac berries, such as gallic acid and quercetin, may have anti-cancer properties, inhibiting the growth of cancer cells and reducing the risk of certain types of cancer. These compounds exert their effects by inducing apoptosis (programmed cell death) in cancer cells and inhibiting tumor growth.
9. **Wound Healing:** Sumac berries offer support for wound healing when applied topically due to their antimicrobial, astringent, and anti-inflammatory properties. These natural compounds found in sumac berries play a crucial role in promoting the healing process and protecting the wounded skin. The berries' antimicrobial properties help combat harmful bacteria and fungi on the wound's surface, creating a cleaner environment for healing and minimizing the risk of infections. Additionally, the astringent nature of sumac berries contributes to the tightening and toning of the skin, reducing bleeding from minor wounds and promoting clotting while creating a protective barrier over the wound. The presence of flavonoids and other anti-inflammatory compounds in sumac berries helps reduce excessive inflammation at the wound site, facilitating tissue repair and regeneration.

10. **Anti-allergic Effects:** Anti-allergic properties in sumac berries can be attributed to specific compounds found in the berries, such as quercetin and kaempferol. Quercetin, a flavonoid with potent antioxidant and anti-inflammatory properties, plays a crucial role in reducing allergic reactions. When the body is exposed to allergens, it releases histamine and other allergic mediators, leading to allergy symptoms. Quercetin inhibits the release of histamine and other inflammatory substances, thereby reducing the severity of allergic reactions and symptoms. Similarly, kaempferol, another flavonoid present in sumac berries, contributes to the anti-allergic effects. Kaempferol has been shown to suppress mast cell activation, which is responsible for the release of histamine and other allergic mediators. By inhibiting mast cell activation, kaempferol helps to prevent the release of histamine, providing relief from allergy symptoms and reducing the overall allergic response.

> While sumac berries are generally considered safe to consume, there are certain medical contradictions and warnings that should be considered. It is also important to note that sumac berries may interact with certain medications. For example, due to its high tannin content, sumac berries may interfere with the absorption of iron from iron supplements or medications, potentially reducing their effectiveness. Individuals taking warfarin or aspirin should consult with a healthcare professional before consuming sumac berries, as they may have mild anticoagulant properties and could potentially increase the risk of bleeding. Individuals with known allergies or sensitivities to sumac or related plants, such as mango or cashew, should avoid its consumption, as it may trigger allergic reactions. Pregnant or breastfeeding individuals should exercise caution and consult with their herbalist/practitioner before consuming sumac berries in large therapeutic quantities. Using small culinary amounts of sumac berries is generally safe to consume during these times.

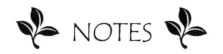

SWEETGUM BALLS

The sweetgum tree, scientifically known as the liquidambar styraciflua tree, is a fascinating and majestic deciduous tree native to the eastern United States and Mexico. It is highly regarded for its distinctive starshaped leaves, vibrant fall foliage, and unique fruiting structures called sweetgum balls. The sweetgum balls, also known as spiky seed pods, are formed when the tree's flowers mature and develop into round, woody capsules adorned with numerous prickly projections. These intriguing seed pods have a rich history of use and are known for their various health benefits. Now, let's explore ten extensive health and longevity benefits associated with sweet gum balls:

1. **Respiratory Health:** Sweetgum ball seeds contain shikimic acid, a compound known for its antiviral properties. Shikimic acid is used as a key ingredient in the production of antiviral medications, making sweetgum ball seeds potentially beneficial for supporting respiratory health.
2. **Immune System Support:** The presence of shikimic acid in sweetgum ball seeds also contributes to their immune-boosting properties. It supports the body's defense against pathogens and strengthens the immune system.
3. **Antioxidant Powerhouse:** Sweetgum ball seeds are rich in antioxidants, such as flavonoids and phenolic compounds. These antioxidants help neutralize harmful free radicals, protecting cells from oxidative damage and supporting overall health and healthy aging.
4. **Liver Health:** The antioxidants present in sweetgum ball seeds, along with their potential anti-inflammatory effects, can support liver health and promote detoxification processes, aiding in the elimination of toxins from the body.
5. **Anti-inflammatory Effects:** The compounds found in sweetgum ball seeds, including flavonoids and tannins, possess anti-inflammatory properties. These properties may help reduce inflammation throughout the body and alleviate related conditions.
6. **Skin Health:** The antioxidant properties of sweetgum ball seeds may help protect the skin from oxidative damage and promote a youthful appearance. These antioxidants may also support overall skin health and vitality.

7. **Cognitive Support:** Sweetgum ball seeds are a source of antioxidants, including flavonoids and phenolic compounds, which have been linked to cognitive benefits. These antioxidants help combat oxidative stress and inflammation in the brain, reducing damage caused by free radicals and promoting overall brain health. Oxidative stress is believed to play a role in age-related cognitive decline and certain neurodegenerative conditions. By neutralizing free radicals, the antioxidants in sweetgum ball seeds may help protect brain cells and maintain cognitive function. Certain flavonoids found in sweetgum ball seeds can cross the blood-brain barrier, further supporting their potential cognitive benefits. These flavonoids may have neuroprotective effects, preserving brain cells from damage and promoting synaptic plasticity, which is crucial for learning and memory.
8. **Adaptogenic Effects:** Sweetgum ball seeds may offer adrenal support through potential adaptogenic properties. Adaptogens are natural substances that are believed to help the body adapt and respond more effectively to stressors, as they have the potential to support the adrenal glands and promote a healthy stress response. The adrenal glands play a crucial role in the body's stress response by producing hormones such as cortisol and adrenaline. By supporting the adrenal glands and promoting a balanced stress response, sweetgum ball seeds, with their bioactive compounds like flavonoids and polyphenols known for antioxidant and anti-inflammatory properties, may help the body cope more effectively with stress.
9. **Cardiovascular Health:** The antioxidants and anti-inflammatory compounds in sweetgum ball seeds may contribute to cardiovascular health by reducing oxidative stress and inflammation, both of which are associated with heart disease.
10. **Antimicrobial Effects:** Sweetgum ball seeds exhibit antimicrobial effects, which can be attributed to the presence of bioactive compounds like tannins and polyphenols. These compounds have shown the ability to hinder the growth and proliferation of harmful microorganisms, including bacteria and fungi. The antimicrobial properties of sweetgum ball seeds make them effective in promoting a healthy microbial balance in the body. By combatting the growth of these pathogenic microorganisms, sweetgum ball seeds help prevent infections and maintain overall health.

While sweetgum ball seeds are generally considered safe to consume, it's important to be aware of certain medical contradictions and potential interactions. Individuals with bleeding disorders or those taking anticoagulant medications should exercise caution, as sweetgum ball seeds may have anticoagulant properties that can increase the risk of bleeding. Sweetgum ball seeds may also interact with certain medications, such as anticoagulants, antiplatelet drugs, and diabetes medications. Allergy warnings should be noted for individuals sensitive to plants in the Altingiaceae family, including sweetgum trees. As for pregnancy and lactation, it is advisable for pregnant and lactating women to consult with their herbalist/practitioner before using sweetgum ball seeds.

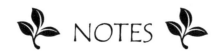

SWEET WOODRUFF

Sweet woodruff, also known as Galium odoratum, is a perennial herbaceous plant native to Europe, Asia, and North America. It has a rich history dating back centuries and has been widely used in traditional herbal medicine. Sweet woodruff is known for its delicate white flowers and distinct aroma, which has been described as sweet and hay-like. Historically, it was used as a strewing herb to add fragrance to homes and as a natural insect repellent. Sweet woodruff has also been used in culinary preparations, particularly in beverages and desserts, for its unique flavor. The herb is often associated with May Day celebrations and is considered a symbol of good luck and protection. Its popularity has endured through the years, and today, sweet woodruff continues to be appreciated for its medicinal properties and various health benefits. Now, let's explore ten extensive health and longevity benefits associated with sweet woodruff:

1. **Adrenal Support:** Sweet woodruff contains specific compounds such as asperuloside and coumarins, which have been suggested to support adrenal health and help maintain balanced cortisol levels. These compounds may have adaptogenic properties, meaning they can assist the body in adapting to stress and promote overall adrenal function.
2. **Brain Health:** The coumarins and flavonoids in sweet woodruff are known for their antioxidant properties, which help neutralize harmful free radicals in the brain. By doing so, these compounds protect brain cells from oxidative damage, reducing the risk of age-related cognitive decline and promoting overall brain health. The antioxidant action of these coumarins and flavonoids also aids in combating inflammation in the brain. These compounds also possess neuroprotective qualities, shielding neurons from damage and supporting their proper functioning.
3. **Cardiovascular Health:** Sweet woodruff contains flavonoids and polyphenols that may help maintain cardiovascular health by supporting healthy blood pressure levels, improving blood circulation, and reducing oxidative stress.
4. **Skin Health:** The antioxidant compounds in sweet woodruff, such as phenolic acids and flavonoids, help protect the skin from oxidative damage, promoting a healthy complexion and youthful-looking skin.

5. **Liver Health:** Asperuloside possesses hepatoprotective properties, which means it plays a vital role in safeguarding the liver from damage and promoting its overall well-being. Asperuloside is known to help shield liver cells from harmful toxins and substances, effectively reducing the risk of liver injury. This compound has been found to support the liver's natural detoxification processes, enhancing its ability to metabolize and eliminate harmful substances from the body. By supporting the liver's detoxification pathways, asperuloside assists in maintaining a healthy liver function, which is essential for overall health and vitality. As the liver is a central organ responsible for filtering and processing toxins in the body, the hepatoprotective properties of asperuloside are crucial for promoting optimal liver health.
6. **Digestive Health:** The coumarins and tannins in sweet woodruff contribute to its ability to support digestive health. Coumarins have been found to have antispasmodic properties, helping to relax the smooth muscles of the digestive tract and alleviate gastrointestinal discomfort, such as cramps and spasms. Tannins have astringent properties that may help reduce inflammation and irritation in the digestive system, providing relief from symptoms like bloating and indigestion.
7. **Anti-inflammatory Effects:** Coumarins like Daphnetin, Umbelliferone, and Scopoletin, known for their diverse bioactive properties, contribute to anti-inflammatory actions. These coumarins help to neutralize harmful free radicals, reducing inflammatory molecules, and modulating immune responses. In addition to coumarins, sweet woodruff also contains flavonoids, including quercetin and rutin, which further contribute to its anti-inflammatory effects by modulating immune responses and suppressing inflammatory markers. Together, these compounds work synergistically to support the body's natural inflammatory response, promoting a balanced and healthy immune system.
8. **Sleep Support:** Sweet woodruff offers relaxation and sleep aid properties attributed to its bioactive compounds that interact with the nervous system to induce calming effects. Coumarins like Daphnetin, Umbelliferone, and Scopoletin have been associated with sedative effects and the modulation of neurotransmitters. These compounds interact with receptors in the brain, such as GABA receptors, known to promote relaxation and reduce anxiety.

9. **Antimicrobial Effects:** Daphnetin, Umbelliferone, and Scopoletin, inhibit the growth of certain bacteria and fungi, combatting pathogens on the skin and mucous membranes. Flavonoids such as quercetin and rutin also inhibit microbial growth, supporting a healthy microbial balance and bolstering the immune system. Additionally, phenolic acids like chlorogenic acid and caffeic acid have antimicrobial effects, further promoting a healthy immune system and overall well-being. Together, these compounds make sweet woodruff a natural defense against harmful microorganisms and support optimal immune function.
10. **Detoxification:** Coumarins and phenolic acids support the body's natural detoxification processes. Asperuloside has been found to enhance liver function and aid the detoxifying process. Phenolic acids, such as chlorogenic acid and caffeic acid, exhibit antioxidant properties that help neutralize free radicals and protect cells from oxidative damage during the detoxification process.

> While sweet woodruff is generally considered safe to consume, there are some medical contradictions and potential drug interactions that should be noted. Individuals with liver conditions or taking medications that affect the liver should exercise caution when using sweet woodruff. Sweet woodruff may interact with anticoagulant medications, potentially enhancing their effects and increasing the risk of bleeding. Sweet woodruff belongs to the Rubiaceae family. Therefore, individuals with known allergies to any members of this family should exercise caution when handling sweet woodruff. Sweet woodruff should not be used in large quantities or taken for prolonged periods. It's recommended to consult with your herbalist/practitioner prior to using sweet woodruff, especially for those who are pregnant or lactating.

NOTES

TANSY

Tansy, a fascinating flowering herb with a rich and storied history, boasts origins that can be traced back to both Europe and Asia, where it has flourished for centuries. The plant's remarkable beauty lies in its vibrant yellow flowers, which have captivated the imagination of people throughout the ages. Beyond its appearance, tansy's distinct aroma has made it an intriguing addition to various cultural practices and traditions. Delving into its historical significance, tansy has served multifaceted roles in human societies. Its use as a medicinal herb can be dated back to ancient times when it was highly valued for its potential health benefits and even rumored age-reversal properties. Ancient civilizations explored its therapeutic potential, and through generations, it continued to be a staple in traditional medicine and folk remedies. The intriguing part of tansy's journey lies in its symbolic and spiritual associations. Often, this herb found its way into various rituals and ceremonies, believed to bring luck, protection, and blessings to those who incorporated it into their lives.
Now, let's explore ten extensive health and longevity benefits associated with tansy:

1. **Digestive Health:** Tansy's ability to support digestion and alleviate gastrointestinal discomfort, such as bloating and gas, can be attributed to several active compounds present in the herb. One of these compounds is thujone, which is believed to stimulate the secretion of digestive juices, promoting better digestion. Additionally, tansy contains flavonoids like quercetin and myricetin, which have been shown to have antispasmodic properties that help relax the smooth muscles of the gastrointestinal tract, easing cramps and discomfort.
2. **Menstrual Support:** The regulation of menstrual cycles and easing of menstrual cramps by tansy can be linked to its active compounds, including camphor and isopinocamphone. These compounds have been suggested to have hormone-regulating effects, potentially aiding in menstrual cycle regularity. Tansy's antispasmodic properties, attributed to compounds like camphor and borneol, may help relieve the intensity of menstrual cramps, promoting overall menstrual health.
3. **Fever Reduction:** Tansy's historical use in reducing fever can be attributed to camphor and borneol. These compounds possess antipyretic properties, which may help lower body temperature and provide relief from fever.

4. **Respiratory Health:** Tansy's role in addressing respiratory issues, such as coughs and congestion, can be associated with its active compounds like camphor and 1,8-cineole. These compounds have expectorant properties, facilitating the removal of mucus and phlegm from the airways, thus promoting easier breathing. Tansy's antimicrobial properties, attributed to compounds like thujone and camphor, may help combat respiratory infections that contribute to congestion.
5. **Skin Health:** Tansy's potential antimicrobial effects, attributed to compounds like camphor and thujone, contribute to its support of skin health. These compounds may help combat bacteria and fungi that may cause minor skin irritations, contributing to a clearer complexion. Additionally, the presence of flavonoids and sesquiterpenes like chamazulene may also play a role in reducing skin inflammation and redness.
6. **Insect Repellent:** Tansy's historical use as a natural insect repellent can be linked to the presence of compounds like thujone and camphor, which have insecticidal properties. These compounds help deter mosquitoes, flies, and other bothersome insects, making tansy an effective natural solution for insect control.
7. **Anti-parasitic Effects:** Tansy's potential to combat certain digestive parasites may be associated with the presence of thujone and other essential oils like camphor. These compounds are believed to possess anthelmintic properties, which may help eliminate intestinal worms and parasites. However, it's crucial to emphasize that using tansy for this purpose requires professional guidance to ensure safe and appropriate dosage.
8. **Appetite Stimulant:** Tansy's ability to stimulate the appetite is thought to be linked to its active compounds, including camphor and thujone. These compounds can influence the secretion of digestive enzymes, potentially enhancing hunger signals and promoting a healthy appetite.
9. **Anti-inflammatory Effects:** The active compound parthenolide, found in tansy, plays a significant role in its anti-inflammatory effects. Parthenolide is a sesquiterpene lactone that has been shown to inhibit the activity of pro-inflammatory enzymes, such as COX-2 and 5-LOX, responsible for producing inflammatory mediators. Chamazulene has also been suggested to inhibit the production of pro-inflammatory molecules like cytokines and prostaglandins, further reducing inflammation and related symptoms.

10. **Sleep Support:** Tansy's potential calming properties, promoting relaxation and aiding in sleep, can be associated with compounds like camphor and myrcene. These compounds have been suggested to have sedative effects, contributing to the herb's ability to support relaxation and improve sleep quality.

> While tansy is generally considered safe to consume, there are several medical contradictions and drug interactions that should be taken into account. Tansy may interact with medications metabolized by the liver, such as CYP450 substrates, and it is essential to consult a healthcare professional before using it alongside such drugs to avoid adverse interactions. Tansy should be avoided or used with caution in individuals with liver disorders. Tansy contains thujone, and large doses taken for prolonged periods may exacerbate liver conditions. Individuals with epilepsy or a history of seizures should use caution and consult with a health care provider prior to using tansy. Tansy belongs to the Asteraceae family, and individuals with known allergies to plants in this family, such as ragweed, marigold, and chamomile, should exercise caution or avoid tansy to prevent allergic reactions. Regarding pregnancy and lactation, tansy is not recommended for use during these times, as it may stimulate uterine contractions and potentially lead to complications. It can also pass into breast milk and may be harmful to nursing infants.

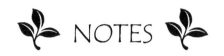

NOTES

THUJA

Thuja, scientifically known as Thuja occidentalis or arborvitae, is a fascinating evergreen tree with a rich history and origin. This majestic tree is native to North America and has played a crucial role in the medicinal practices of various indigenous cultures for centuries. The very name "thuja" finds its roots in the Greek word "thuo," meaning "to sacrifice" or "to fumigate," highlighting its historical use in ceremonial rituals and as an incense. Beyond its practical applications, thuja held significant symbolic value and was often planted near homes as a protective charm, embodying a sense of sacredness and spiritual significance. However, it's important to exercise caution when using thuja. Internal use of the herb is not recommended unless done so under the expert guidance of a knowledgeable herbalist. This underlines the need for responsible and informed utilization of the plant's potential benefits while being aware of any potential risks or side effects.

Now, let's explore ten extensive health and longevity benefits associated with thuja:

1. **Skin Soothing:** Thuja has soothing properties attributed to its active compounds, including thujone and camphor. These compounds possess anti-inflammatory effects, which help calm irritated or inflamed skin. This makes it highly beneficial for conditions like eczema, psoriasis, and dermatitis when used in topical preparations.
2. **Wound Healing:** Thuja contains compounds such as thujic acid and flavonoids, which promote wound healing by supporting tissue regeneration and reducing the risk of infection. These compounds stimulate the body's natural healing processes when applied topically to minor cuts, scrapes, and burns.
3. **Antimicrobial Effects:** The essential oil of thuja, contains thujone and other terpenoids such as sabinene, myrcene, and thujopsene that exhibit antimicrobial properties. These compounds help inhibit the growth of bacteria and fungi on the skin, making it useful for topically treating fungal infections like athlete's foot or nail fungus.
4. **Skin Tags and Warts:** Thuja's potential antiviral properties come from its active compounds, including thujone and thujopsene. When applied topically as oil or extract, it may help stimulate the immune response against skin tags and warts, aiding in their removal.

5. **Acne Support:** Thuja's antimicrobial and anti-inflammatory properties are attributed to compounds like thujone, sabinene, myrcene, and thujopsene, which make it effective for managing acne when applied topically. It helps reduce acne-causing bacteria, soothes inflammation, and supports clearer skin.
6. **Respiratory Health:** Thuja contains eucalyptol, thujone, and camphor, which may act as bronchial dilators and expectorants. When prepared as a steam inhalation, thuja helps to loosen mucus in the respiratory tract, promoting its expulsion. The anti-inflammatory effects of these compounds reduce airway inflammation, facilitating easier breathing and providing relief from respiratory distress.
7. **Scalp Health:** Thujone, myrcene, and alpha-pinene are the constituents which possess anti-inflammatory properties. When carefully applied topically to the scalp in specialized preparations by your herbalist, these compounds can effectively soothe inflammation and irritation, addressing factors that may contribute to hair loss and scalp issues. Thuja contains camphor, which, when applied to the scalp, stimulates blood circulation. This boost in blood flow facilitates the delivery of vital nutrients and oxygen to hair follicles, fostering an environment conducive to healthy hair growth.
8. **Joint and Muscle Pain Relief:** The soothing effect of thuja-based topical preparations in specialized preparations by their herbalist, likely attributed to thujone, eucalyptol, a-pinene, and limonene, may offer relief from joint and muscle discomfort when applied to the affected areas.
9. **Insect Repellent:** Thuja's aromatic nature makes it a natural insect repellent when used externally. The active compound thujone, along with sabinene, eucalyptol, and limonene, with its strong odor and insecticidal activity, acts as a natural repellent against mosquitoes and other insects, providing protection from bites.
10. **Minor Burn Support:** Thujone and sabinene, active compounds found in thuja, offer potential support for minor burns. These compounds possess anti-inflammatory properties, reducing swelling and redness, providing relief, and promoting a comfortable healing process. Their antimicrobial action helps prevent or minimize infection risks in compromised burn sites. Applying thuja-based topical preparations with thujone and sabinene can soothe the affected area, alleviate pain, and potentially stimulate skin cell regeneration for the growth of new, healthy tissue. Patch tests should be performed on the skin prior to broader application.

> While topical applications of thuja in carefully prepared formulations by a qualified herbalist are generally considered safe for external use, internal ingestion of this herb can be toxic and is not recommended unless otherwise stipulated by your herbalist/practitioner. Thuja may interact with certain medications, particularly those affecting the immune system, such as immunosuppressants and corticosteroids, potentially altering their effectiveness. It is advised to exercise caution and seek medical advice before using thuja if you have bleeding disorders, as it may increase the risk of bleeding. Allergy-wise, individuals sensitive to plants in the Cupressaceae family, including cypress, cedar, and juniper, may also have allergic reactions to thuja. Pregnant and breastfeeding women should avoid using thuja to prevent potential adverse effects on the developing fetus or nursing infant.

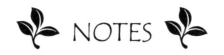
NOTES

THYME

Thyme, a fragrant herb with a rich history, has its origins deeply rooted in the Mediterranean region, where it has flourished for centuries. This perennial herb, known for its small aromatic leaves and delicate flowers, holds a special place in ancient cultures, where it was cultivated and cherished for both culinary and medicinal purposes. The ancient Egyptians, Greeks, and Romans revered thyme for its diverse uses and considered it a symbol of courage and strength. Its distinct flavor, warm aroma, and captivating fragrance have made thyme a staple ingredient in various cuisines around the world. Thyme boasts a long history of medicinal applications. Ancient healers and herbalists recognized its therapeutic properties, utilizing it to treat ailments ranging from respiratory issues to digestive complaints. In medieval Europe, thyme was associated with courage, and knights often carried sprigs of thyme into battle to boost their spirits and protect themselves from harm.

Now, let's explore ten extensive health and longevity benefits associated with thyme:

1. **Cardiovascular Support:** Thyme's antioxidant properties, along with its potential to reduce inflammation, lower blood pressure, and modulate cholesterol levels, contribute to its heart-protective effects, promoting cardiovascular health. The active constituents responsible for these benefits include thymol, carvacrol, flavonoids like luteolin and apigenin, rosmarinic acid, and phytosterols, making thyme a valuable herb for maintaining a healthy heart.
2. **Anti-inflammatory Effects:** Thyme's notable anti-inflammatory benefits can be attributed to its diverse array of flavonoids, such as luteolin and apigenin, which serve as powerful phytochemical compounds with significant anti-inflammatory and antioxidant properties. Luteolin and apigenin act as potent antioxidants, neutralizing harmful free radicals that contribute to oxidative stress and inflammation. By scavenging these free radicals, these flavonoids help protect the body's cells and tissues from damage, reducing the inflammatory response. Luteolin and apigenin exert anti-inflammatory effects by inhibiting the production of pro-inflammatory molecules, such as cytokines and enzymes, which are involved in the inflammatory process. By modulating the immune response and down-regulating these inflammatory mediators, luteolin and apigenin help to mitigate inflammation and promote a more balanced and harmonious immune system.

3. **Stress Relief:** The delightful aroma of thyme has been linked to relaxation and stress relief through its interaction with the olfactory system. Thyme contains various phytochemical compounds responsible for these effects. The primary constituents contributing to stress relief are thymol and carvacrol, both of which are essential oils found in thyme. These compounds have been shown to possess anxiolytic properties, meaning they can reduce anxiety and promote a sense of calm. When the aroma of thyme is inhaled, these volatile compounds stimulate the olfactory receptors, which send signals to the brain's limbic system, the area responsible for emotions and memory. As a result, thymol and carvacrol can modulate neurotransmitter activity, such as increasing the release of serotonin, a neurotransmitter associated with mood regulation and well-being. The calming effect of thyme's aroma may help soothe the mind, alleviate stress, and promote emotional well-being and mental clarity, making it a valuable natural option for managing stress and anxiety.
4. **Digestive Health:** Thymol acts as a natural antispasmodic and relaxant for the gastrointestinal muscles, easing cramps and promoting smoother digestion. Thymol has been shown to stimulate the secretion of digestive enzymes, such as bile, which aids in the breakdown of fats and enhances overall digestion. Thyme is a source of flavonoids, including luteolin and apigenin, which possess anti-inflammatory properties. These flavonoids help reduce inflammation in the digestive tract, soothing discomfort and promoting a healthier gut environment. The presence of volatile oils, such as p-cymene and terpinene, in thyme, contributes to its carminative effects. These compounds help expel gas from the digestive system, alleviating bloating and reducing discomfort.
5. **Antioxidant Powerhouse:** Thymol and carvacrol are powerful phenolic compounds that exhibit strong antioxidant properties. These compounds neutralize harmful free radicals that can damage cells and contribute to aging and various diseases. Thyme contains flavonoids, such as luteolin and apigenin, which also act as antioxidants, further enhancing its ability to combat oxidative stress. The presence of terpenes like limonene and alpha-pinene in thyme contributes to its antioxidant power. These phytochemical compounds work in synergy, providing comprehensive cellular protection, promoting cellular health, and potentially extending longevity.

6. **Skin Health:** Thyme's extraordinary benefits for skin health can be attributed to its rich array of phytochemical compounds, specifically thymol, carvacrol, linalool, and terpinene-4-ol, which confer potent antimicrobial and anti-inflammatory properties. These compounds work synergistically to combat harmful bacteria and fungi that may contribute to acne and other skin conditions, effectively reducing inflammation and redness associated with skin irritations. Thymol and carvacrol act as natural antimicrobial agents, inhibiting the growth of acne-causing bacteria and supporting the treatment of skin infections. Thyme's anti-inflammatory properties, mainly attributed to linalool and terpinene-4-ol, help soothe skin inflammation, providing relief for conditions like eczema and dermatitis. By reducing inflammation and combating microbial growth, thyme supports the healing process of various skin issues, promoting a healthier and more radiant complexion.
7. **Oral Health:** Thymol has been extensively studied for its effectiveness against a wide range of bacteria, including both Gram-positive and Gram-negative strains. Thymol disrupts the cell membranes of bacteria, leading to their death or inhibition of growth, making it a valuable natural agent in combating oral infections and maintaining a healthy oral microbiome. Like thymol, carvacrol is a phenolic compound with remarkable antimicrobial properties. It works synergistically with thymol to enhance thyme's overall antimicrobial activity. Together, these two compounds create a formidable defense against harmful microorganisms that may reside in the mouth, contributing to the prevention of oral infections and supporting oral hygiene. Thyme contains other bioactive compounds, such as caryophyllene, p-cymene, and borneol, which also contribute to its antimicrobial effects. These compounds exhibit broad-spectrum antimicrobial activity and play a role in maintaining the balance of beneficial bacteria in the oral cavity.
8. **Respiratory Health:** Thymol is one of the main bioactive compounds in thyme. It possesses antispasmodic and expectorant properties, which may help relax the smooth muscles of the respiratory tract and promote the clearance of mucus. Carvacrol is another significant compound in thyme. It has been studied for its potential anti-inflammatory effects and its ability to relax the bronchial muscles, providing relief from coughing and bronchial discomfort.

9. **Cognitive Support:** Thyme possesses a diverse array of compounds associated with supporting cognitive function and enhancing memory and concentration. One key compound found in thyme is rosmarinic acid, which exhibits antioxidant properties, safeguarding brain cells from oxidative stress and promoting optimal cognitive health. Thyme contains essential oils like thymol and carvacrol, known for their neuroprotective effects and ability to enhance neurotransmitter activity in the brain. By increasing the availability of acetylcholine, a neurotransmitter crucial for learning and memory processes, these essential oils may contribute to improved memory and concentration. Flavonoids like luteolin and apigenin also play a crucial role in thyme's neuroprotective effects and cognitive benefits. These flavonoids possess antioxidant and anti-inflammatory properties, combatting oxidative stress and reducing inflammation in the brain, thereby protecting brain cells from damage and degeneration.
10. **Immune System Support:** Thymol has been extensively studied for its antimicrobial effects, helping to fend off harmful pathogens and infections that could compromise the body's defenses. Carvacrol, another vital phenolic compound in thyme, complements thymol's immune-boosting actions by further enhancing the body's ability to combat infections. Thyme also contains flavonoids, such as luteolin and apigenin, which exhibit antioxidant and anti-inflammatory properties. These flavonoids aid in reducing oxidative stress and inflammation, supporting the immune system's response to threats and promoting overall well-being.

While thyme is generally considered safe to consume, there are certain medical contradictions and warnings that should be considered. Thyme may have an impact on blood clotting due to its coumarin content, and individuals with bleeding disorders or those taking anticoagulant or antiplatelet medications, such as warfarin or aspirin, should consult with a healthcare professional before consuming thyme, as it may increase the risk of bleeding. Individuals with a known allergy or hypersensitivity to thyme or other plants in the Lamiaceae family, such as basil, mint, or oregano, should avoid its consumption, as it may trigger allergic reactions. Thyme is safe to use in culinary amounts during pregnancy and lactation, but concentrated thyme supplements should be avoided unless otherwise stipulated by your herbalist/practitioner.

TURKEY TAIL MUSHROOM

Turkey tail, scientifically known as Trametes versicolor, is a fascinating medicinal mushroom with a rich and storied history and origin. Widely distributed across the globe, this mushroom thrives in diverse ecosystems, often found flourishing on decaying trees, fallen logs, and forest floors. Its presence in nature has caught the attention of ancient civilizations and indigenous communities, leading to its integration into traditional healing practices. Throughout history, turkey tail has held a prominent place in traditional Chinese medicine and various indigenous healing systems, where it has been highly regarded for its therapeutic properties and potential health benefits. The mushroom's extensive use spans back centuries, with records of its inclusion in remedies and therapies aimed at supporting overall health and well-being. In ancient times, indigenous cultures recognized and respected turkey tail's healing potential, incorporating it into their traditional remedies to address various health conditions. The vibrant and intricate colors of turkey tail's fruiting bodies have also sparked artistic inspiration, and the mushroom's beauty has been immortalized in historical artworks and cultural symbolism. Today, modern research continues to unveil the potential health-promoting compounds found within turkey tail, further affirming its significance in both traditional and contemporary health practices.

Now, let's explore ten extensive health and longevity benefits associated with turkey tail:

1. **Immune System Support:** Turkey tail contains a variety of bioactive compounds, including polysaccharopeptides, polysaccharides, and beta-glucans, which have immunomodulating effects. These compounds enhance the activity of immune cells and support immune response.
2. **Antiviral Effects:** Turkey tail contains a variety of bioactive compounds, including polysaccharides (such as PSK and PSP), beta-glucans, and other active compounds like ergosterol, lanosterol, and mycophenolic acid. Together, these compounds exhibit potent antiviral activity, making turkey tail a valuable natural ally in combating viral infections. Research has shown that these active compounds can effectively inhibit the growth of various viruses, including influenza, herpes, and human papillomavirus (HPV). With its multifaceted antiviral potential, turkey tail mushroom offers promising support in defending against viral pathogens and promoting overall immune health.

3. **Antioxidant Powerhouse:** Turkey tail is rich in antioxidants, such as phenols and flavonoids, which help protect cells from oxidative damage caused by free radicals. These antioxidants scavenge harmful molecules and contribute to cellular health, promoting healthy aging and reducing the risk of chronic diseases.
4. **Digestive Health:** The prebiotic properties of turkey tail's polysaccharides support the growth of beneficial gut bacteria, such as Bifidobacterium and Lactobacillus. A healthy gut microbiome is essential for digestion, nutrient absorption, and overall immune function.
5. **Anti-inflammatory Effects:** Turkey tail contains compounds like polysaccharides and triterpenoids that possess anti-inflammatory properties. These compounds help reduce inflammation in the body, which is associated with various chronic diseases and age-related conditions.
6. **Anti-cancer Effects:** Turkey tail has been the subject of several studies that demonstrate its potential anti-cancer effects. Its active compounds, including polysaccharides (such as PSK and PSP), triterpenoids, and phenolic compounds, have shown the ability to inhibit the growth and spread of cancer cells. These bioactive components stimulate the immune system's response against cancer, enhancing the body's natural defense mechanisms. The combination of these properties makes turkey tail mushroom a promising candidate for supporting cancer management and overall health.
7. **Liver Health:** Turkey tail contains triterpenoids, such as ergosterol and lanosterol, that contribute to its liver-protective effects. These bioactive compounds exhibit antioxidant activity, scavenging harmful free radicals and reducing oxidative stress in the liver. The polysaccharides present in turkey tail also support the liver's natural detoxification processes by enhancing the activity of enzymes involved in detoxification pathways.
8. **Cognitive Support:** The polysaccharides in turkey tail have been shown to support brain health by enhancing neuroplasticity, promoting the growth and survival of brain cells, and improving communication between neurons. These effects may help reduce mental fatigue and enhance cognitive performance, including memory, attention, and focus.

9. **Respiratory Health:** Turkey tail's exceptional immune-stimulating properties, attributed to compounds like polysaccharides (PSK and PSP) and triterpenoids, make it a valuable supporter of respiratory health. These bioactive constituents bolster the immune system, enabling the body to defend against respiratory infections and reducing their occurrence and severity. Turkey tail's antiviral activity, driven by its polysaccharides and other active compounds, targets respiratory viruses, making it beneficial in managing conditions such as the flu. The mushroom's anti-inflammatory effects, linked to polysaccharides and triterpenoids, may further alleviate symptoms of respiratory conditions by reducing inflammation in the airways and enhancing overall breathing.
10. **Skin Health:** Turkey tail's abundant bioactive compounds, such as phenols, flavonoids, polysaccharides (including beta-glucans), and triterpenoids, play crucial roles in supporting skin health. The mushroom's antioxidants combat oxidative stress, safeguarding skin cells from free radical damage. Its anti-inflammatory properties soothe skin, promoting a calmer complexion. Turkey tail's polysaccharides, including beta-glucans, contribute to collagen synthesis, improving skin elasticity. Additionally, these polysaccharides aid in skin cell regeneration, enhancing overall skin tone and texture.

While turkey tail mushroom is generally considered safe for consumption, there are certain medical contradictions and precautions to be aware of. Individuals undergoing organ transplantation or taking immunosuppressant medications should avoid turkey tail due to its potential immune-enhancing effects. It is important to note that turkey tail may interact with certain medications, such as anticoagulants or antiplatelet drugs, due to its potential blood-thinning properties. It is advisable to consult with a healthcare professional before using turkey tail alongside these medications. Allergy warnings should be noted for individuals sensitive to mushrooms or other fungi, as an allergic reaction may occur. Turkey tail belongs to the Polyporaceae family, which includes other medicinal mushrooms such as reishi (Ganoderma lucidum) and Chaga (Inonotus obliquus). Those who are pregnant or lactating should consult with their herbalist/practitioner before using turkey tail in high therapeutic quantities.

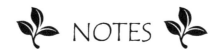

TURMERIC

Turmeric, scientifically known as Curcuma longa, is a vibrant golden spice widely used in culinary traditions around the world. It boasts a rich and fascinating history with a captivating origin. Native to Southeast Asia, specifically India and Indonesia, turmeric has been an integral part of the region's culture for millennia. Its journey as a medicinal and culinary gem dates back thousands of years, taking center stage in traditional Ayurvedic medicine, revered for its potent healing properties. The spice is derived from the rhizomes of the Curcuma longa plant, a member of the ginger family known for its striking orange-yellow hue and distinctive aroma. Throughout history, turmeric has been cherished not only for its delightful flavor in dishes but also for its remarkable medicinal benefits. Its active compound, curcumin, is a powerful antioxidant and anti-inflammatory agent, contributing to its pro-aging and health-boosting qualities. In addition to its therapeutic uses, turmeric holds intriguing cultural significance. It has been used as a dye for textiles and even played a part in religious ceremonies in some regions. In ancient times, traders carried turmeric along the famous Silk Road, facilitating its spread to different parts of the world and solidifying its global presence.

Now, let's explore ten extensive health and longevity benefits associated with turmeric:

1. **Anti-inflammatory Effects:** Turmeric's reputation for its potent anti-inflammatory effects can be attributed to its active compound, curcumin, as well as its other components, like demethoxycurcumin and bisdemethoxycurcumin. These compounds work synergistically to suppress inflammatory pathways, thus alleviating chronic inflammation, which is a contributing factor to various age-related conditions.
2. **Joint and Muscle Support:** The anti-inflammatory action of turmeric, primarily facilitated by curcumin, demethoxycurcumin, and bisdemethoxycurcumin, plays a crucial role in relieving joint pain and stiffness. By modulating inflammatory responses, turmeric supports overall musculoskeletal health and promotes flexibility.
3. **Antioxidant Powerhouse:** Curcumin, along with other constituents like turmerone, atlantone, and turmerin found in turmeric, acts as a powerful scavenger of free radicals. These compounds neutralize harmful oxidative species, protecting cells from damage and supporting cellular health.

4. **Cognitive Function:** Turmeric's positive impact on cognitive function and its potential to reduce age-related cognitive decline can be attributed to curcumin's neuroprotective effects. Curcumin's ability to cross the blood-brain barrier allows it to combat oxidative stress and inflammation in the brain, supporting brain health and potentially contributing to graceful aging.
5. **Digestive Health:** Turmeric aids digestion through its stimulation of bile production, which aids in the breakdown of fats. Curcumin's anti-inflammatory properties may also soothe digestive discomfort, contributing to a healthy gut environment.
6. **Cardiovascular Health:** Turmeric's role in promoting heart health is influenced by curcumin's ability to improve cholesterol levels and reduce the risk of blood clot formation. These effects, along with the support of other components like turmerone, atlantone, and turmerin, contribute to overall cardiovascular function.
7. **Detoxification:** Turmeric enhances liver detoxification by increasing the production of enzymes responsible for eliminating toxins from the body. Curcumin, along with other compounds like turmerone, supports the liver's detoxification processes, promoting healthy liver function.
8. **Blood Sugar Balance:** Turmeric's potential to aid in blood sugar regulation is driven by curcumin's ability to enhance insulin sensitivity. This compound, along with turmerone, atlantone, and turmerin, helps the body effectively utilize and regulate blood sugar levels. The presence of essential vitamins and minerals, such as vitamin B6, magnesium, and manganese in turmeric, further contributes to better carbohydrate metabolism and insulin function, ultimately promoting better blood sugar control.
9. **Immune System Support:** Turmeric's immune-boosting properties are attributed to curcumin and a range of other beneficial compounds, such as turmerone, atlantone, and turmerin. Together, these compounds modulate immune responses, promote a balanced immune system, and help defend against pathogens. Curcumin's anti-inflammatory action reduces chronic inflammation, while the antioxidants found in turmeric, including curcumin, neutralize free radicals, supporting immune cell function. Additionally, turmeric's antiviral and antibacterial effects, driven by curcumin, further aid in the body's defense. Curcumin supports gut health by promoting beneficial gut bacteria. These combined benefits contribute to a robust immune response, enhancing overall well-being and potential protection against infections.

10. **Skin Health:** The antioxidant and anti-inflammatory properties of turmeric, particularly curcumin, help improve skin health by neutralizing free radicals and reducing inflammation. This can result in a youthful appearance, reduction of acne, and overall support for graceful aging.

> While turmeric is generally considered safe to consume, there are several medical contradictions and drug interactions to be aware of. Turmeric may interact with blood-thinning medications like warfarin, increasing the risk of bleeding. People with gallbladder issues should exercise caution and consult with their healthcare provider before using high-dose supplemental turmeric. Turmeric may lower blood sugar levels, potentially affecting those with diabetes or hypoglycemia, and should be used with caution in combination with diabetes medications. Turmeric may interact with medications that slow blood clotting, increasing the risk of bruising or bleeding. Allergy-wise, individuals with a sensitivity to plants in the Zingiberaceae family, which includes ginger and cardamom, may experience allergic reactions to turmeric. Pregnant and breastfeeding individuals should consult with their herbalist/practitioner before consuming turmeric in high quantities for prolonged periods during these times. Consuming culinary amounts of turmeric during pregnancy and lactation is generally considered safe.

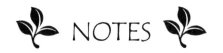

NOTES

UVA URSI

Uva ursi, scientifically known as Arctostaphylos uva-ursi, and also known as bearberry, is a small shrub with a rich history and origin, spanning across North America, Europe, and Asia. Throughout the ages, this remarkable plant has been highly regarded for its diverse medicinal properties and has played a significant role in the traditional practices of various cultures. Among those who esteemed uva ursi, Native American tribes stand out, valuing its therapeutic benefits for generations. The very name "uva ursi" is derived from Latin, translating to "bear's grape," a whimsical reference to the bears' fondness for its fruit. This endearing connection with bears adds a touch of charm to the plant's lore. Uva ursi's journey as a medicinal herb stretches back centuries, with documented usage by herbalists and healers throughout history.

Now, let's explore ten extensive health and longevity benefits associated with uva ursi:

1. **Urinary Tract Health:** Uva ursi has a long history of traditional use in supporting urinary tract health and promoting proper kidney function. This remarkable herb contains a compound called arbutin, which undergoes conversion into hydroquinone, specifically within the urinary tract. Hydroquinone, known for its potent antimicrobial properties, acts to inhibit the growth of bacteria in the urinary tract, contributing to the herb's effectiveness in promoting urinary health.
2. **Anti-inflammatory Effects:** Uva ursi's anti-inflammatory effects are attributed to ursolic acid and tannins, reducing inflammation caused by injury, infection, rheumatoid arthritis, and inflammatory bowel disease. Ursolic acid inhibits inflammatory mediators and relieves associated pain and swelling, while tannins soothe irritated tissues, reducing redness and swelling.
3. **Oral Health:** One of the key active compounds responsible for its antibacterial effects is arbutin. Arbutin is a glycoside that is metabolized in the body to release hydroquinone, a potent antibacterial agent. Hydroquinone acts against bacteria that contribute to oral health issues, including tooth decay and gum disease. Uva ursi contains tannins, such as gallic acid and ellagitannins, which also possess antimicrobial properties. These tannins help create an unfavorable environment for bacteria in the oral cavity, contributing to combat bad breath and supporting overall oral health.

4. **Diuretic Effects:** Uva ursi possesses diuretic properties primarily attributed to its active compounds, including arbutin and hydroquinone. Arbutin, when metabolized in the body, converts to hydroquinone, which has been recognized for its ability to increase urine production. This diuretic effect can help flush out excess water and toxins from the body, potentially alleviating bloating and supporting detoxification.
5. **Antioxidant Powerhouse:** Uva ursi boasts a wealth of powerful antioxidants, including flavonoids and phenolic compounds. These potent antioxidants play a vital role in neutralizing harmful free radicals, safeguarding the body against oxidative stress, and helping to maintain overall health. By combating oxidative damage, uva ursi's antioxidant activity supports the body's resilience and contributes to graceful aging.
6. **Digestive Health:** Uva ursi contains specific tannins, such as gallic acid, ellagitannins, and catechins, alongside flavonoids like quercetin and myricetin. These compounds contribute to the herb's digestive properties by soothing irritated tissues in the digestive tract and supporting smooth digestive functioning. Gallic acid and ellagitannins offer potent antioxidant and anti-inflammatory effects, while catechins, quercetin, and myricetin provide additional antioxidant activity and potential anti-inflammatory benefits. Uva ursi's combination of tannins and flavonoids makes it a valuable herbal remedy for promoting digestive health and offering relief from digestive discomfort.
7. **Antiviral Effects:** Uva Ursi demonstrates antiviral activity through its key constituents. Arbutin, found in uva ursi, undergoes a conversion into hydroquinone within the body. Hydroquinone exhibits potent antiviral properties and is effective against viruses like the herpes simplex virus. In addition to arbutin, uva ursi contains quercetin, a flavonoid that contributes to its antiviral effects. Quercetin works by inhibiting viral replication and interfering with virus-host cell interactions. Together, these combined constituents make Uva Ursi a potential herbal remedy for managing viral infections, particularly those caused by the herpes simplex virus.
8. **Antifungal Effects:** Uva ursi possesses various compounds that enhance its antifungal properties, playing a role in sustaining a healthy microbial balance. A key component, arbutin, transforms into hydroquinone within the body, showcasing robust antifungal activity by disrupting fungal cell membranes and impeding their growth. Additionally, the presence of tannins, quercetin, and gallic acid in uva ursi further strengthens its antimicrobial potential, creating an inhospitable environment for fungal growth.

9. **Skin Health:** Arbutin, a naturally occurring compound, undergoes metabolism in the body, releasing hydroquinone known for its remarkable skin-lightening properties. This effectively diminishes the visibility of dark spots and hyperpigmentation, promoting a more even and radiant complexion. Additionally, uva ursi is rich in antioxidants, including quercetin and gallic acid, which actively combat free radicals and safeguard the skin from oxidative stress, thereby supporting a youthful and radiant complexion. This herb's anti-inflammatory properties, attributed to compounds like ursolic acid and tannins, play a crucial role in soothing irritated skin, reducing redness, and promoting overall skin health.
10. **Astringent Effects:** The astringent properties of uva ursi can be attributed to its rich content of tannins, specifically gallic acid and ellagitannins. When applied topically, uva ursi acts as a natural astringent, helping to tighten and tone the skin. Tannins work by constricting the skin's tissues and blood vessels, which can lead to a temporary reduction in pore size and oiliness. This effect provides a smoother appearance to the skin and may help in managing conditions like acne and oily skin. The astringent action of uva ursi can be particularly beneficial in reducing puffiness and swelling in the under-eye area, making it a popular choice in some skincare products targeting these concerns.

While uva ursi is generally considered safe to consume, there are important medical contradictions to be aware of. Uva ursi should be avoided by those with bleeding disorders or taking anticoagulant medications, as uva ursi can increase the risk of bleeding. This herb may interact with medications like diuretics, lithium, and antacids, affecting their effectiveness or potentially leading to adverse effects. Allergy-wise, individuals sensitive to plants in the Ericaceae family, which includes blueberries, cranberries, and rhododendrons, may be at higher risk of allergic reactions to uva ursi. Those who are pregnant or breastfeeding should avoid uva ursi during these periods unless otherwise stipulated by their herbalist/practitioner.

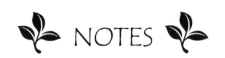

VALERIAN ROOT

Valerian root, derived from the Valeriana officinalis plant, boasts a fascinating and rich history that dates back to ancient civilizations. Native to Europe and Asia, this herb has been a treasured natural remedy for centuries. Its origin can be traced to the renowned Greek physician Hippocrates, often hailed as the father of modern medicine, who documented its therapeutic properties and recognized its potential to address various ailments. Valerian root's use has endured throughout history, gaining prominence for its remarkable calming and relaxing effects on both the body and mind. Interestingly, its name, "Valeriana," is said to have been derived from the Latin word "valere," which means "to be strong" or "to be healthy," a testament to the herbal remedy's esteemed reputation. Notably, valerian root was used during World War II to help alleviate the stress and anxiety experienced by civilians during air raids, underscoring its enduring value as a natural aid for promoting tranquility. Ancient civilizations, including the Greeks and Romans, esteemed valerian for its medicinal attributes, using it to address sleep disturbances, nervous tension, and overall well-being.

Now, let's explore ten extensive health and longevity benefits associated with valerian root:

1. **Sleep Support:** Valerian root's ability to improve sleep quality and alleviate insomnia is attributed to its active compounds, including valerenic acid and valerenol. These compounds act as mild sedatives, interacting with GABA receptors in the brain to reduce nerve excitability, leading to a calming effect. This helps individuals fall asleep faster and enjoy a deeper, more restful sleep.
2. **Menopausal Relief:** Valerian root's benefits for menopausal symptoms can be attributed to its ability to interact with estrogen receptors. The active compounds in valerian root, such as isovaleric acid and valepotriates, may help regulate hormonal imbalances and reduce discomforts like hot flashes and mood swings during menopause.
3. **Cognitive Support:** Studies suggest that valerian root may improve cognitive function through its active compounds, including valerenic acid and linarin. These compounds are thought to enhance blood flow to the brain and may support memory and concentration, making it beneficial for individuals experiencing mental fatigue or difficulty focusing.

4. **Anxiety and Stress Relief:** Valerian root's anxiolytic properties are mainly due to valerenic acid and its interaction with GABA receptors. By increasing GABA levels in the brain, valerian root helps calm the nervous system and reduce anxiety and stress. This can promote a sense of relaxation and ease tension.
5. **Mood Support:** Valerian root's mood-enhancing effects are attributed to alkaloids like valerine, which interact with neurotransmitters in the brain, including serotonin and norepinephrine. By inhibiting the breakdown of serotonin, valerine may increase its availability in the brain, leading to improved emotional well-being and potentially alleviating symptoms of depression. Valerine's impact on norepinephrine reuptake may contribute to increased alertness and focus, further supporting a positive mood.
6. **Muscle Pain Support:** Valerian root's antispasmodic properties, attributed to valtrates and isovaltrates, help ease muscle pain and cramps by relaxing muscle contractions. This makes it useful for relieving conditions like menstrual cramps and tension headaches.
7. **Digestive Health:** Valerian root's soothing effect on the gastrointestinal tract is due to its volatile oils, including borneol and bornyl acetate. These compounds help reduce inflammation and calm digestive discomfort, such as bloating, gas, and indigestion.
8. **Cardiovascular Health:** Valerian root's anti-inflammatory effects may help reduce the risk of cardiovascular issues. Linarin, an active compound in valerian root, has been studied for its ability to relax blood vessels and promote healthy blood pressure levels.
9. **Immune System Support:** Valerian root's immune-boosting properties are linked to its antioxidants, such as flavonoids and terpenes. These compounds help neutralize free radicals, reducing oxidative stress and supporting overall immune system health, which may lower the risk of infections.
10. **Graceful-aging Effects:** The antioxidants present in valerian root help combat free radicals and protect cells from damage, potentially contributing to a more youthful appearance and slowing down the aging process. By reducing oxidative stress, valerian root may support graceful aging and skin health.

While valerian root is generally considered safe to consume, there are some medical contradictions and drug interactions to be aware of. Valerian root may interact with medications that depress the central nervous system, such as sedatives, tranquilizers, and anti-anxiety drugs, potentially enhancing their effects and leading to excessive drowsiness or sedation. Individuals with liver disorders should exercise caution, as valerian root can affect liver enzymes and may exacerbate liver conditions. Avoid using valerian root with other substances that cause drowsiness, including alcohol, as it may increase the risk of excessive sedation. Allergy-wise, those with known sensitivities to plants in the Valerianaceae family may experience allergic reactions to valerian root. Women who are pregnant or lactating should consult with their herbalist/practitioner prior to using this herb.

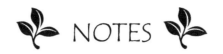

NOTES

WAKAME

Wakame, scientifically known as Undaria pinnatifida, is a fascinating and culturally significant edible seaweed with a rich history that traces its origins to the coastal waters of Japan, China, and Korea. For centuries, wakame has played a pivotal role in Asian cuisine, where it was revered as a culinary delight and an essential ingredient in various traditional dishes. The history of wakame stretches back to ancient times when coastal communities of fishermen skillfully harvested this marine algae from the sea. The harvesting and preparation of wakame were passed down through generations, becoming a cherished part of local traditions and culinary heritage. Beyond its gastronomic appeal, wakame held great importance for its nutritional richness and therapeutic properties. Throughout history, it has been believed to confer numerous health benefits, promoting overall well-being and vitality. Wakame's cultural significance also extended beyond the culinary realm, as it was often incorporated into various rituals and ceremonies, symbolizing prosperity, longevity, and a deep connection to the sea.

Now, let's explore ten extensive health and longevity benefits associated with wakame:

1. **Thyroid Health:** Wakame is a natural source of iodine, an essential mineral that plays a crucial role in the synthesis of thyroid hormones. The thyroid gland utilizes iodine to produce thyroxine (T4) and triiodothyronine (T3), hormones that are involved in regulating metabolic processes in the body, such as energy production and utilization of nutrients. Adequate iodine intake from sources like wakame ensures the thyroid gland has the necessary building blocks to produce thyroid hormones effectively.
2. **Cardiovascular Health:** Wakame is rich in omega-3 fatty acids, specifically eicosapentaenoic acid (EPA), which supports cardiovascular health. EPA helps reduce inflammation, lower blood pressure, and improve overall heart function.
3. **Brain Health:** The presence of essential omega-3 fatty acids in wakame contributes to brain health and cognitive function. These fatty acids support the development and maintenance of brain cells, improving memory, focus, and overall brain performance.
4. **Bone Health:** Wakame is a good source of calcium, magnesium, and vitamin K, essential nutrients for maintaining strong and healthy bones. These nutrients promote bone density and help prevent conditions like osteoporosis.

5. **Immune System Support:** Wakame contains antioxidants, such as fucoxanthin and vitamin C, which help strengthen the immune system and protect the body against harmful pathogens. These antioxidants work by neutralizing free radicals, reducing oxidative stress, and allowing the immune system to function more efficiently in identifying and fighting off viruses, bacteria, and other microorganisms. Additionally, the antioxidants in wakame directly protect against harmful pathogens, inhibiting their growth and activity to prevent infections.
6. **Anti-inflammatory Effects:** The active compounds in fucoidan work by modulating the body's inflammatory response, leading to a reduction in inflammation throughout the body. This anti-inflammatory effect can provide relief from various inflammatory conditions, such as arthritis, allergies, and skin irritations.
7. **Digestive Health:** Fucoidan has been shown to have prebiotic properties, which means it promotes the growth of beneficial bacteria in the gut. These bacteria play a vital role in maintaining a healthy digestive system by aiding in the breakdown and absorption of nutrients, supporting immune function, and preventing the growth of harmful bacteria.
8. **Skin Support:** The skin rejuvenation benefits of wakame are attributed to the presence of fucoxanthin and vitamin C. These antioxidants play a crucial role in protecting the skin from oxidative damage caused by free radicals, which can lead to premature aging and skin deterioration. Fucoxanthin and vitamin C work together to neutralize free radicals, reducing their harmful effects on the skin's structure and function. As a result, the antioxidants help promote healthy aging, preserving the skin's elasticity and firmness.
9. **Detoxification:** Fucoxanthin has been shown to have antioxidant and anti-inflammatory properties, which contribute to its detoxification benefits. It helps protect the liver from oxidative stress and supports the liver's ability to break down and eliminate toxins and harmful substances from the body. Wakame is also rich in essential minerals like magnesium and potassium, which are important for maintaining proper liver function and aiding in the detoxification process.

10. **Anti-cancer Effects:** Fucoidan and fucoxanthin have shown the ability to inhibit the growth and proliferation of cancer cells, impeding their spread and metastasis. These compounds have demonstrated their potential to induce apoptosis, a natural process of programmed cell death, in cancer cells, which helps eliminate malignant cells from the body. Additionally, fucoidan and fucoxanthin's anti-cancer properties have been associated with their capacity to modulate certain signaling pathways involved in cancer development.

> While wakame is generally considered safe to consume, there are certain medical contradictions and precautions to be aware of. Wakame may interact with certain medications, such as anticoagulants or blood thinners, due to its potential blood-thinning properties. It is important to consult with a healthcare professional before incorporating wakame into your diet if you have any underlying medical conditions or are taking medications that may interact with it. Allergy warnings should be noted for individuals sensitive to seaweeds or other members of the family Alariaceae, which includes kelp, kombu, and arame. It is also crucial to source wakame from the Atlantic Ocean to avoid higher levels of contamination from pollutants in the Pacific Ocean. As for safety during pregnancy and lactation, it is advisable to consult with your herbalist/practitioner before consuming wakame to ensure it is safe and appropriate for your specific situation.

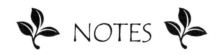

NOTES

WHITE OAK BARK

White oak bark, scientifically known as Quercus alba, holds its origins in the ancient bark of the white oak tree, a magnificent and resilient hardwood native to the vast woodlands of North America. This bark boasts a truly rich and storied history, deeply intertwined with the traditions and wisdom of indigenous cultures that inhabited these lands for centuries. The historical significance of white oak bark extends beyond its medicinal applications; it also found various practical uses in the daily lives of indigenous peoples. For instance, the strong and durable wood of the white oak tree was employed in constructing essential tools, crafting vessels for storing food, and even fashioning canoes for navigation across waterways. Additionally, its bark's tannin-rich nature contributed to its application in the tanning of animal hides, an indispensable process for transforming raw materials into leather. Through generations, white oak bark has remained an enduring symbol of resilience, strength, and resourcefulness, embodying the deep-rooted connection between humans and the bountiful gifts of nature.

Now, let's explore ten extensive health and longevity benefits associated with white oak bark:

1. **Skin Health:** The presence of tannins in white oak bark serves as a potent astringent, reducing skin irritation and redness while providing a soothing effect. These tannins also contribute to minimizing itchiness, making it particularly effective for relieving discomfort associated with various skin conditions. The bark contains flavonoids like quercetin and kaempferol, known for their antioxidant and anti-inflammatory effects. These compounds help combat free radicals, reducing oxidative stress and inflammation, which can improve the appearance of acne and eczema.
2. **Digestive Health:** White oak bark consumption can effectively soothe digestive discomfort, including diarrhea, indigestion, and gastric ulcers, thanks to its rich content of beneficial compounds. The presence of tannins in white oak bark acts as an astringent, helping to tone and constrict tissues, which can reduce diarrhea symptoms and promote firmer stools. This bark's potent anti-inflammatory properties, attributed to compounds like quercetin and kaempferol, assist in calming inflammation in the digestive tract, thereby providing relief from indigestion and gastric ulcer discomfort.

3. **Oral Health:** White oak bark's astringent properties make it an effective natural remedy for various oral health issues, including gum disease, toothache, and canker sores. The presence of tannins, such as quercitannic acid and pedunculagin, contributes to its astringent action, which helps tighten and tone tissues in the mouth. This tightening effect can provide relief from gum inflammation and discomfort associated with conditions like gingivitis. The astringent nature of white oak bark may help alleviate toothache by reducing swelling and inflammation around the affected tooth. Its antimicrobial properties may aid in combatting bacteria that contribute to oral infections and canker sores, promoting a healthier oral environment.
4. **Cardiovascular Health:** White oak bark offers support for cardiovascular health by promoting healthy blood pressure levels and improving blood circulation. Tannins, a prominent compound in the bark, possess astringent properties that help constrict blood vessels, aiding in the regulation of blood pressure. Flavonoids like quercetin, kaempferol, and myricetin found in white oak bark have antioxidant properties, reducing oxidative stress and inflammation in the cardiovascular system. These flavonoids also strengthen blood vessels and enhance their flexibility, thereby improving blood circulation. Ellagitannins, particularly pedunculagin and castalagin, further enhance cardiovascular benefits by promoting healthy cholesterol levels.
5. **Antimicrobial Effects:** White oak bark's antimicrobial properties are attributed to the presence of specific compounds, including tannins and ellagic acid. Tannins act as natural astringents, disrupting the growth and survival of certain bacteria and fungi. These compounds bind to proteins in the microbial cell walls, causing structural damage and hindering their ability to thrive. Ellagic acid found in white oak bark contributes to its antimicrobial effects by interfering with microbial enzymes and inhibiting their replication. The combined action of these compounds makes white oak bark a potential natural remedy for infections and skin conditions caused by microbial agents, offering a botanical solution for promoting overall skin health and combating microbial-related issues.

6. **Wound Healing:** White oak bark's wound healing capabilities are attributed to its high tannin content, specifically gallic acid tannins and ellagitannins. These tannins exhibit astringent properties that help constrict blood vessels, reduce inflammation, and promote blood clotting at the wound site. By applying a poultice or using products containing white oak bark extract, these tannins accelerate the healing process of minor wounds, cuts, and skin irritations. The astringent action also aids in forming a protective barrier over the wound, preventing infection and promoting tissue repair. The presence of antioxidants in white oak bark helps neutralize harmful free radicals, further supporting the body's natural healing response and contributing to the overall effectiveness of the wound healing process.
7. **Urinary Tract Health:** White oak bark's diuretic properties, attributed to the presence of compounds like quercitrin, myricitrin, and ellagic acid, promote healthy urinary function and aid in relieving urinary tract infections, kidney stones, and bladder-related issues. These active compounds enhance kidney filtration, increasing urine production and facilitating the elimination of toxins and waste products from the body. The diuretic action helps to flush out harmful bacteria, preventing their proliferation and reducing the risk of urinary tract infections. The increased urine flow may assist in breaking down kidney stones and easing their passage through the urinary system. White oak bark's anti-inflammatory properties contribute to alleviating inflammation and discomfort associated with bladder-related problems, providing comprehensive support for urinary health.
8. **Antioxidant Powerhouse:** White oak bark's remarkable antioxidant capacity is attributed to specific compounds, including ellagitannins, with a notable presence of pedunculagin. This compound has gained recognition for its exceptional ability to scavenge free radicals, the harmful molecules responsible for oxidative stress and cellular damage. White oak bark contains myricetin, kaempferol, and quercetin, each contributing to its antioxidant prowess and providing further support to the body. These compounds work synergistically to counteract the detrimental effects of free radicals, forming a protective shield that safeguards the body from oxidative harm, thereby promoting overall cellular health.

9. **Respiratory Health:** The presence of tannins in white oak bark acts as an astringent, tightening and toning the tissues in the respiratory tract, which may help soothe coughs and reduce irritation. This bark contains mucilage, a gel-like substance that helps in promoting the expulsion of mucus from the respiratory passages, providing relief from chest congestion. The expectorant properties of white oak bark are due to compounds like quercetin and other flavonoids, which facilitate the clearance of phlegm from the airways, making it beneficial in alleviating symptoms of bronchitis and asthma.
10. **Anti-inflammatory Effects:** White oak bark boasts potent anti-inflammatory properties, primarily attributed to its active compounds such as tannins, quercetin, and myricetin. These compounds work synergistically to provide relief from a range of inflammatory conditions, including arthritis, joint pain, and rheumatism. Tannins act as powerful astringents, helping to constrict blood vessels and reduce inflammation, while quercetin and myricetin function as antioxidants, quenching free radicals and suppressing inflammation at the cellular level. By addressing the inflammatory response, white oak bark serves as a natural remedy, soothing discomfort and supporting joint and musculoskeletal health.

While white oak bark is generally considered safe to consume, there are important medical contradictions and warnings to consider. Individuals taking anticoagulant or antiplatelet medications like warfarin or aspirin should consult with a healthcare professional before using white oak bark, as it may have mild anticoagulant properties and could increase the risk of bleeding. White oak bark may also interact with certain medications, including antibiotics and drugs for blood pressure or diabetes management. Individuals with known allergies or sensitivities to oak trees or other members of the Fagaceae family, which includes beech and chestnut, should avoid the use of white oak bark, as it may trigger allergic reactions. Women who are pregnant or lactating should consult with their herbalist/practitioner prior to using this herb.

WHITE PINE BARK

White pine (Pinus strobus) bark has a rich history and fascinating origin that dates back centuries. Native to eastern North America, the white pine tree holds significant cultural and historical importance among various indigenous tribes. Known for its majestic appearance and valuable resources, the white pine has been cherished by early settlers and Native Americans alike. Among the Native American tribes, white pine bark was highly revered for its versatile uses. It played a central role in their traditional medicine, where it was utilized for its medicinal properties. The inner bark of the white pine tree, often referred to as "quills," was carefully harvested and used to create poultices, teas, and tinctures. The Iroquois regarded the white pine as the "Tree of Peace," using it in peace ceremonies and even crafting the symbolic Peace Pipe from its wood. During colonial times, the white pine became a vital resource for early European settlers. Its tall and straight trunks were favored for shipbuilding, making it crucial in maritime history. Apart from its practical applications, white pine also holds a place in folklore and legend. Native American tribes had their own myths and stories about the white pine, attributing spiritual significance and supernatural qualities to this magnificent tree. The white pine was often considered a symbol of strength, resilience, and connection to the divine.

Now, let's explore ten extensive health and longevity benefits associated with white pine bark:

1. **Respiratory Health:** White pine bark offers valuable support for respiratory health due to its rich content of beneficial compounds such as pinosylvin and various polyphenols. These active constituents work synergistically to combat respiratory inflammation and provide soothing relief for bothersome coughs. By reducing inflammation in the respiratory tract, white pine bark may help ease breathing difficulties and promote overall respiratory wellness. Its properties may assist in calming cough reflexes, making it beneficial for individuals dealing with respiratory discomfort.
2. **Detoxification:** White pine bark contains bioactive compounds, including proanthocyanidins and polyphenols, which have been found to support the body's natural detoxification processes. These compounds help enhance liver function, the primary organ responsible for detoxification, by promoting the production of detoxifying enzymes and supporting antioxidant activity.

3. **Immune System Support:** White pine bark boasts a wealth of immune-supportive compounds beyond its vitamin C content. It contains proanthocyanidins, potent antioxidants that fortify the immune system by combating free radicals and reducing oxidative stress. Additionally, the bark harbors catechins, flavonoids, and phenolic acids, which work in synergy to bolster the body's defenses and promote overall health and vitality. These active constituents contribute to a strengthened immune response, helping the body ward off infections and maintain optimal immune function.
4. **Cognitive Support:** White pine bark is enriched with flavonoids and phenolic compounds, such as pinosylvin and other polyphenols, that play a pivotal role in supporting brain health and enhancing cognitive function. These bioactive constituents contribute to improved memory retention, mental clarity, and overall cognitive performance. The flavonoids found in white pine bark have been linked to increased blood flow to the brain, aiding in delivering essential nutrients and oxygen to brain cells, supporting their optimal functioning. The presence of phenolic compounds in white pine bark provides potent antioxidant support to brain cells, guarding them against oxidative stress and potential damage caused by free radicals.
5. **Cardiovascular Health:** White pine bark's active compounds, particularly proanthocyanidins and catechins, play a crucial role in promoting cardiovascular health through their beneficial effects on blood pressure and blood vessel function. Proanthocyanidins are potent antioxidants that scavenge free radicals, reduce oxidative stress, and protect blood vessels from damage. They help enhance the flexibility and strength of blood vessel walls, promoting healthy circulation and reducing the risk of hypertension. Catechins in white pine bark have been shown to improve endothelial function, which is essential for the proper dilation and constriction of blood vessels. This supports healthy blood flow, helps maintain normal blood pressure levels, and contributes to overall cardiovascular well-being.
6. **Digestive Health:** White pine bark contains tannins, which are a type of polyphenolic compound known for their astringent properties. These tannins have been found to support digestive health by promoting healthy digestion and alleviating digestive discomfort. They may help tone and tighten the tissues of the gastrointestinal tract, improving the overall function of the digestive system.

7. **Antioxidant Powerhouse:** White pine bark is rich in powerful antioxidants, specifically catechins, that play a crucial role in combating oxidative stress and safeguarding cells from damage caused by harmful free radicals. These catechins work by neutralizing free radicals, highly reactive molecules that can cause cellular damage and contribute to aging and various health issues. By effectively neutralizing these free radicals, white pine bark's antioxidants help promote healthy aging, supporting overall well-being and longevity. The catechins in white pine bark work within the body's antioxidant defense system, preventing oxidative damage and maintaining cellular integrity.
8. **Joint and Muscle Pain Relief:** White pine bark's ability to provide relief for joint and muscle discomfort can be attributed to its potent anti-inflammatory properties, primarily associated with its active compounds like proanthocyanidins and polyphenols. These constituents act as powerful antioxidants that help quench free radicals and reduce oxidative stress in the body. These compounds are believed to modulate the inflammatory response, inhibiting the production of pro-inflammatory molecules and enzymes. As a result, white pine bark can effectively reduce inflammation in the joints and muscles, leading to a noticeable alleviation of discomfort and supporting improved joint flexibility and mobility.
9. **Antimicrobial Effects:** Phenolic acids, flavonoids, and tannins work synergistically to contribute to its potent antimicrobial properties. Studies have demonstrated that these constituents possess inhibitory effects against harmful bacteria and fungi, making white pine bark an effective natural agent to help maintain a healthy microbial balance within the body. Phenolic acids, such as ferulic acid and gallic acid, have been found to interfere with the growth and replication of pathogenic microorganisms, while flavonoids like quercetin and kaempferol exert strong antimicrobial actions against various bacterial strains. The tannins present in white pine bark have astringent properties that help inhibit microbial growth and contribute to its overall antimicrobial effect. These collective actions of phenolic acids, flavonoids, and tannins enable white pine bark to act as a formidable defense against harmful pathogens, making it a valuable natural remedy to support the body's immune system and promote overall well-being.

10. **Skin Health:** By neutralizing harmful free radicals, proanthocyanidins help preserve the skin's collagen and elastin fibers, promoting skin elasticity and reducing the appearance of wrinkles. The antioxidants present in white pine bark contribute to the skin's overall health by preventing cellular damage caused by environmental pollutants and UV radiation. These antioxidants also aid in promoting a youthful complexion by supporting a smoother and more radiant skin tone.

While white pine bark is generally considered safe to consume, there are some medical contradictions and potential drug interactions to be aware of. White pine bark should be used with caution in individuals with bleeding disorders, as it may increase the risk of bleeding. It may also interact with certain medications, including anticoagulants and antiplatelet drugs, potentially affecting their effectiveness. Allergy-wise, individuals with known hypersensitivity to plants in the Pinaceae family, which includes other pine species like cedar and spruce, may also experience allergic reactions to white pine bark. Women who are pregnant or lactating should consult with their herbalist/practitioner prior to using white pine bark.

WHITE WILLOW BARK

White willow bark, scientifically known as Salix alba, has a fascinating and rich history that dates back thousands of years. Its medicinal use can be traced to ancient civilizations such as Egypt, China, and Mesopotamia, where it was employed to alleviate pain and reduce inflammation. Even renowned physician Hippocrates prescribed willow bark tea for pain relief and fever. In the 18th century, the naturalist Edmund Stone's discovery of its pain-relieving properties piqued interest in the medical community. Later, in the 19th century, the active compound "salicin" was isolated from white willow bark, leading to the development of modern-day aspirin. Mythologically, it held significance as a symbol of renewal and wisdom in Greek and Celtic folklore. The name "Salix alba" itself has historical roots, with "Salix" being Latin for "willow" and "alba" signifying "white." This enduring botanical's history showcases its vital role in shaping herbal medicine and its profound connection to human healthcare throughout the ages.

Now, let's explore ten extensive health and longevity benefits associated with white willow bark:

1. **Pain Relief:** White willow bark contains salicin, a compound that provides natural pain relief by inhibiting the production of pain-inducing chemicals in the body. It supports the management of various types of pain, including headaches, muscle aches, and joint discomfort.
2. **Anti-inflammatory Effects:** The salicin in white willow bark possesses anti-inflammatory properties, which may help reduce inflammation in the body. This can benefit conditions such as arthritis, tendonitis, and other inflammatory disorders.
3. **Mood Support:** These effects are attributed to the presence of certain constituents that support the body's natural production of neurotransmitters, such as serotonin and dopamine. The active compounds salicin, and flavonoids found in white willow bark play a crucial role in this process. Salicin, for instance, is a precursor to salicylic acid, which has been associated with mood enhancement and potential antidepressant effects. Flavonoids present in the bark can exert neuroprotective effects and modulate neurotransmitter levels. By supporting the production of serotonin and dopamine, two key neurotransmitters that influence mood regulation and emotional balance, white willow bark may help promote a sense of calm and relaxation.

4. **Fever Reduction:** Salicin is a natural compound that exhibits antipyretic effects, helping to lower body temperature during fever. In the body, salicin is converted into salicylic acid, which acts as a fever-reducing agent. By promoting perspiration and enhancing the body's natural cooling mechanisms, white willow bark helps to alleviate fever and support the body's response to infections or inflammatory conditions.
5. **Digestive Health:** White willow bark contains active constituents such as salicin, flavonoids, tannins, and catechins that contribute to its ability to soothe digestive discomfort. One of the key components, salicin, possesses anti-inflammatory properties that aid in reducing inflammation in the gastrointestinal tract. This can be particularly beneficial for alleviating stomachaches and indigestion, as the reduction in inflammation may help ease discomfort and promote digestive well-being. The presence of polyphenols, flavonoids, and tannins further supports the bark's therapeutic effects, as these compounds may help soothe irritated tissues and provide a gentle, natural remedy for digestive issues.
6. **Cardiovascular Health:** White willow bark offers significant benefits for cardiovascular health, primarily attributed to its rich content of antioxidants. Among these antioxidants are flavonoids and phenolic compounds, such as salicin and catechins, which play a crucial role in its cardioprotective properties. These antioxidants work to combat oxidative stress within the cardiovascular system, neutralizing harmful free radicals that can lead to cell damage and inflammation. By reducing oxidative stress, white willow bark supports the health of blood vessels, helping to maintain their flexibility and integrity. The flavonoids present in white willow bark have been shown to promote healthy blood flow, which can aid in maintaining optimal circulation and lowering the risk of cardiovascular complications. The phenolic compounds found in this herbal remedy may help regulate blood pressure levels and reduce the risk of blood clot formation.
7. **Respiratory Health:** White willow bark contains specific compounds, including salicin, quercetin, and polyphenols, which contribute to its respiratory health benefits. Salicin possesses expectorant properties that help promote the clearance of mucus from the respiratory tract. The anti-inflammatory properties of white willow bark, attributed to its flavonoids and polyphenols, help reduce inflammation in the respiratory system, alleviating symptoms of bronchitis and supporting overall respiratory function.

8. **Skin Health:** White willow bark can be used both topically and internally to promote skin health. Its anti-inflammatory properties, attributed to compounds such as salicin and flavonoids like quercetin, help reduce inflammation in the skin, providing relief from conditions like acne, eczema, and psoriasis. White willow bark's antimicrobial properties help combat bacteria on the skin's surface, supporting a healthier skin microbiome. When applied topically, it can soothe inflammation, reduce redness, and promote the healing of skin irritations. Consuming white willow bark may also provide systemic benefits for skin health due to its anti-inflammatory and antioxidant properties.
9. **Urinary Tract Health:** Salicin promotes increased urine production, helping the body flush out toxins and waste products more efficiently. By enhancing the frequency of urination, white willow bark aids in maintaining a healthy urinary system and preventing urinary stagnation. This diuretic action can also be beneficial for individuals dealing with conditions like edema, where excess fluid accumulates in the body's tissues. The presence of other active compounds, such as flavonoids and polyphenols in white willow bark, may contribute to its overall urinary health benefits, as these compounds possess antioxidant and anti-inflammatory properties, which may help reduce oxidative stress and inflammation in the urinary tract.
10. **Oral Health:** White willow bark offers valuable benefits for oral health due to its rich content of essential compounds, such as salicin and polyphenols. These constituents play a crucial role in promoting dental well-being by exhibiting potent antimicrobial properties. The presence of salicin in white willow bark provides it with natural anti-inflammatory and analgesic effects, which may help alleviate toothaches and oral discomfort. The polyphenols found in the bark contribute to its strong antimicrobial activity. These properties make white willow bark particularly effective in combating oral bacteria, including the notorious Streptococcus mutans, a bacterium closely associated with tooth decay and gum disease. By targeting and reducing harmful bacteria in the mouth, white willow bark can aid in preventing the formation of plaque and tartar, thereby supporting overall dental health and contributing to a healthier, cleaner mouth.

While white willow bark is generally considered safe to consume, there are some medical contradictions and precautions to be aware of. This herb may interact with certain medications, including nonsteroidal anti-inflammatory drugs (NSAIDs), such as ibuprofen, and medications that affect blood clotting. Individuals with bleeding disorders or those taking blood-thinning medications, such as warfarin, should exercise caution when using white willow bark due to its potential anticoagulant effects. It is not recommended for individuals with known allergies to aspirin or salicylates, as white willow bark contains salicin, which is metabolized into salicylic acid in the body. Pregnant and breastfeeding women should avoid white willow bark unless otherwise stipulated by their herbalist/practitioner.

WILD CHERRY BARK

Wild cherry bark, scientifically known as Prunus serotina, has a fascinating and rich history that dates back centuries. Native to North America, this deciduous tree has played a significant role in various indigenous cultures and early civilizations. Native American tribes had a deep reverence for the wild cherry tree, not only for its medicinal properties but also for its cultural significance. The bark of the wild cherry tree was used in traditional ceremonies and rituals, symbolizing renewal, growth, and the cycle of life. Beyond its ceremonial importance, the wood of the wild cherry tree was highly valued for crafting beautiful and durable tools, weapons, and ceremonial objects. Early European settlers later recognized its usefulness and incorporated it into their own folk medicine practices. The Cherokee people, in particular, utilized wild cherry bark for various medicinal purposes, including its potential as an expectorant and cough suppressant. Its name, "serotina," is derived from Latin, meaning "late," referring to the tree's characteristic of blooming later in the season than most other cherry trees. Throughout history, wild cherry bark's captivating aroma and taste led to its use as a flavoring agent in candies, syrups, and liqueurs.

Now, let's explore ten extensive health and longevity benefits associated with wild cherry bark:

1. **Respiratory Health:** Wild cherry bark's effectiveness in soothing and relieving respiratory issues such as coughs, bronchitis, and congestion can be attributed to its natural expectorant properties. Active compounds such as prunasin, quercetin, and kaempferol contribute to the herb's expectorant action. These compounds help to loosen and expel mucus from the respiratory tract, providing relief from respiratory discomfort and facilitating easier breathing.
2. **Pain Relief:** Wild cherry bark's analgesic properties, supported by compounds like prunasin and caffeic acid, make it effective in alleviating pain. Traditionally used for managing headaches, muscle aches, and joint pain, this herb's natural pain-relieving properties have been valued for centuries.
3. **Digestive Health:** Wild cherry bark's bitter components, including quercetin and kaempferol, stimulate digestion by increasing the production of digestive enzymes and promoting bile flow. These compounds help relieve indigestion, bloating, and other digestive complaints, supporting overall digestive health.

4. **Anti-inflammatory Effects:** The potent anti-inflammatory compounds found in wild cherry bark, including quercetin, kaempferol, caffeic acid, and p-coumaric acid, contribute to its ability to reduce inflammation throughout the body. By targeting and inhibiting inflammatory pathways, this herb may offer relief from symptoms associated with arthritis, gout, and other inflammatory conditions.
5. **Anxiety and Stress Relief:** Wild cherry bark is known for its mild sedative properties, which may help calm the nervous system and promote relaxation. These effects are attributed to specific compounds found in the bark, such as prunasin, which is a glycoside. When ingested in appropriate amounts, prunasin is safely metabolized by the body and does not pose any risks of cyanide release. Instead, it contributes to the herb's calming benefits. Wild cherry bark contains quercetin, a flavonoid with antioxidant properties that may help modulate neurotransmitter activity in the brain, promoting a sense of calm and tranquility. When used in herbal preparations or ingested in safe doses, wild cherry bark's constituents interact with the body's neurochemical pathways, inhibiting excessive nerve impulses that may lead to anxiety and nervous tension. This calming effect extends to the musculoskeletal system, easing tension and supporting overall relaxation. As a result, wild cherry bark may aid in reducing symptoms of anxiety, nervousness, and restlessness, making it a valuable herbal option for individuals seeking natural remedies to unwind and improve sleep quality.
6. **Skin Health:** Wild cherry bark, rich in antioxidants like quercetin, kaempferol, and caffeic acid, plays a crucial role in supporting skin health by protecting against free radical damage. These antioxidants neutralize harmful free radicals, safeguarding the skin from premature aging and environmental damage. Quercetin reduces inflammation and redness, making it effective for skin conditions like eczema and rosacea. Kaempferol supports the skin's defense against UV radiation, protecting it from sun-induced damage and maintaining a youthful appearance. Caffeic acid, on the other hand, offers anti-inflammatory and antimicrobial benefits, reducing acne breakouts and promoting collagen production for improved skin elasticity and texture. Wild cherry bark's astringent properties, attributed to tannins and catechins, contribute to better skin tone and reduced oiliness by tightening the skin and minimizing pore size.

7. **Immune System Support:** Wild cherry bark's immune-strengthening properties can be attributed to various compounds and nutrients. Prunasin, a cyanogenic glycoside, exhibits antioxidant and anti-inflammatory effects, helping to scavenge harmful free radicals and promote a healthy immune response. Flavonoids like quercetin and kaempferol enhance immune cell activity and reduce inflammation, bolstering the body's defenses against pathogens. Phenolic acids such as caffeic acid and p-coumaric acid further contribute to the bark's immune-supporting effects.
8. **Antimicrobial Effects:** One of this herb's key constituents is prunasin, a cyanogenic glycoside, which acts as a natural defense mechanism for the tree against pathogens. When used in humans, prunasin helps inhibit the growth of harmful microorganisms, including bacteria and fungi, making it an essential ally in supporting overall well-being. Wild cherry bark contains quercetin and kaempferol, both of which are flavonoids with strong antimicrobial properties. These compounds work by disrupting the integrity of microbial cell membranes and inhibiting key enzymes necessary for their survival and reproduction. As a result, the growth and proliferation of bacteria and fungi are inhibited, helping to alleviate infections and promote a healthier microbial balance in the body.
9. **Cardiovascular Health:** This herb's remarkable effects on the cardiovascular system can be attributed to its rich array of active compounds, including quercetin, kaempferol, and prunasin, among others. Quercetin, a potent flavonoid antioxidant found in wild cherry bark, plays a crucial role in reducing oxidative stress and inflammation within blood vessels, promoting better vascular function, and helping to regulate blood pressure. Kaempferol, another flavonoid present in the herb, has been linked to lowering LDL (bad) cholesterol levels, thus contributing to maintaining a healthy lipid profile. Prunasin, a compound unique to wild cherry bark, has shown potential cardioprotective properties by supporting smooth muscle relaxation within blood vessels, leading to improved blood flow and reduced strain on the heart. The combined actions of these active constituents in wild cherry bark work synergistically to enhance overall heart function, maintain cardiovascular well-being, and potentially reduce the risk of heart-related issues.

10. **Sore Throat Support:** Wild cherry bark has long been revered for its remarkable anti-inflammatory and analgesic properties, making it a reliable remedy for providing relief from sore throat symptoms, particularly pain and inflammation. These soothing effects are attributed to the presence of several key constituents in wild cherry bark, such as prunasin and caffeic acid. Prunasin, a glycoside found in the bark, acts as an anti-inflammatory agent, working to reduce swelling and discomfort in the throat. Caffeic acid, on the other hand, exhibits analgesic properties, serving as a natural pain reliever to ease the discomfort associated with a sore throat.

> While wild cherry bark is generally considered safe to consume, there are certain medical contradictions and precautions to be aware of. Individuals taking blood pressure-lowering drugs, anticoagulants, or antiplatelet medications, should exercise caution as wild cherry bark may potentiate their effects, leading to adverse reactions. Caution is advised for individuals taking medications metabolized by the liver, as wild cherry bark may interfere with the liver's enzymatic processes. Individuals with known allergies to plants in the Rosaceae family, such as cherries, plums, peaches, or almonds, may also experience allergic reactions to wild cherry bark. Pregnant or lactating women should consult with their herbalist/practitioner before using wild cherry bark.

WILD YAM

Wild yam, scientifically known as Dioscorea villosa, boasts a rich history and origin that spans centuries and continents. Native to North and Central America, this perennial vine has been an integral part of the traditional medicine practices of various indigenous cultures. The indigenous peoples of these regions utilized wild yam for its numerous potential medicinal properties and attributed it to a host of folkloric beliefs. Interestingly, despite its name, wild yam is not closely related to true yams (genus Dioscorea) commonly found in tropical regions but belongs to the Dioscoreaceae family, making it a distant botanical cousin. Historically, wild yam has been revered for its purported ability to support women's health, particularly during menopause, earning it the nickname "colic root" due to its traditional use in easing menstrual discomfort. It was once believed that the twisted shape of the wild yam tubers resembled the human figure, leading to the belief that its consumption would bestow a person with strength and vitality.

Now, let's explore ten extensive health and longevity benefits associated with wild yam:

1. **Liver Health:** Diosgenin is thought to interact with certain liver enzymes responsible for metabolizing toxins, which may help enhance the liver's detoxification capabilities. By promoting these enzymatic processes, wild yam could facilitate the efficient removal of harmful substances from the body, reducing the burden on the liver and supporting its overall health and function.
2. **Menopausal Relief:** The potential of wild yam to alleviate menopausal symptoms, such as hot flashes and night sweats, stems from its diosgenin content. While it does not directly convert into hormones in the human body, it has been the subject of scientific interest due to its structural similarity to human hormones like progesterone and estrogen. This resemblance has led researchers to explore whether diosgenin could interact with hormone receptors in a way that may provide relief from menopausal discomfort. While more research is needed to fully understand the mechanisms at play, preliminary studies have indicated that diosgenin might have mild estrogenic effects, meaning it could exert some activity similar to estrogen, though not as potent.

3. **Anti-inflammatory Effects:** Wild yam has been recognized for its potential to exhibit anti-inflammatory effects, primarily attributed to its bioactive compounds like diosgenin, saponins, and alkaloids. Diosgenin, in particular, has been extensively studied for its anti-inflammatory properties, as it is structurally similar to certain corticosteroids, suggesting potential modulation of inflammation-related pathways. Wild yam also contains saponins, natural plant chemicals that may inhibit pro-inflammatory mediators and enzymes, complementing diosgenin's effects. The presence of alkaloids in wild yam further contributes to its anti-inflammatory potential.
4. **Antioxidant Powerhouse:** Within this herb, various bioactive compounds, including flavonoids, polyphenols, and saponins, contribute to its antioxidant properties and act as potent free radical scavengers, neutralizing harmful oxidative species and reducing oxidative stress on cells and tissues. Polyphenols, including tannins, further enhance the antioxidant defense by inhibiting the formation of free radicals. These compounds play a vital role in protecting cellular structures and genetic material from oxidative damage, thereby potentially mitigating the risk of chronic diseases and premature aging.
5. **Digestive Health:** Diosgenin in wild yam enhances the secretion of digestive enzymes, which are essential for breaking down food into smaller, more absorbable components. This process facilitates efficient nutrient extraction and assimilation by the body, leading to improved digestion and reducing the likelihood of digestive discomfort and bloating. Diosgenin's positive impact on digestion extends to its ability to enhance nutrient absorption. It has been shown to improve the absorption of various nutrients, including vitamins, minerals, and essential nutrients, from the digestive tract into the bloodstream. This enhanced nutrient absorption ensures that the body can effectively utilize these essential building blocks for various bodily functions, contributing to overall wellness and vitality.
6. **Immune System Support:** Dioscin, a compound present in wild yam, may interact with immune cells and signaling pathways, resulting in beneficial effects on immune function. Additionally, saponins found in wild yam have been associated with immune-modulating effects. These saponins may assist in stimulating the activity of specific immune cells, including macrophages and lymphocytes. These immune cells play crucial roles in identifying and eliminating harmful pathogens within the body.

7. **Skin Health:** Diosgenin is believed to exert positive effects on skin health through alternative mechanisms. One such mechanism involves its influence on collagen production. Collagen is a crucial protein responsible for maintaining skin's firmness, elasticity, and overall youthfulness. As we age, collagen production naturally declines, leading to the formation of fine lines, wrinkles, and a loss of skin elasticity. However, diosgenin's presence in wild yam may help stimulate collagen synthesis, potentially contributing to improved skin texture and firmness.
8. **Anti-cancer Effects:** Diosgenin has shown cytotoxic effects, meaning it can induce cell death in specific cancer cells. These effects are particularly notable in breast, ovarian, and prostate cancer cell lines. The mechanism behind diosgenin's anti-cancer activity is believed to involve multiple pathways that inhibit cancer cell growth and promote apoptosis (programmed cell death) in cancer cells. Diosgenin may exert anti-angiogenic effects, meaning it could impede the formation of new blood vessels that support tumor growth, thus further inhibiting cancer progression.
9. **Hormone Health:** Wild yam is known for its diosgenin content, a compound that bears a structural similarity to human hormones (only relatively mild compared to actual hormones). This distinctive characteristic has led to the belief that wild yam could potentially support hormonal balance in the body. However, it is crucial to clarify that diosgenin itself does not transform into hormones. This conversion can only happen in a laboratory with specific processing. Diosgenin itself is believed to interact with hormone receptors in the body, although its effects are considered relatively mild compared to our actual hormones. Wild yam also contains saponins, along with various other phytochemicals. These saponins are natural plant chemicals known for their diverse biological activities, including potential interactions with hormone receptors in the body. While the precise mechanisms of action are not fully understood, it is believed that saponins may also influence hormone activity through their ability to bind to hormone receptors and modulate their responses. By interacting with hormone receptors, many of these phytochemicals could potentially exert mild estrogenic or progesterone-like effects, though not to the same extent as our actual hormones. Therefore, while wild yam may not provide direct hormonal benefits, its unique bioactive compounds offer potential supportive effects on women's hormonal health.

10. **Antimicrobial Effects:** Dioscorin and dioscin, present in wild yam demonstrates antimicrobial properties, potentially inhibiting the growth of harmful microorganisms. Dioscorin, a protein found in wild yam, acts as a natural defense mechanism for the plant against potential pathogens. Similarly, dioscin, a steroidal saponin in wild yam, has shown antimicrobial activity by disrupting the integrity of microbial cell walls or membranes.

> While wild yam is generally considered safe to consume, there are certain medical contradictions and drug interactions to be aware of. Individuals with a history of hormone-sensitive conditions such as breast, ovarian, or uterine cancer should exercise caution when using wild yam due to its potential hormonal effects. Wild yam may also interact with medications that affect hormones, such as hormone replacement therapy, birth control pills, or certain blood-thinning medications. As for allergies, individuals with known sensitivities to plants in the Dioscoreaceae family, such as yams, sweet potatoes, or other Dioscorea species, may also be at risk of allergic reactions to wild yam. During pregnancy and lactation, it is advisable to avoid using wild yam unless otherwise stipulated by your herbalist/practitioner.

WINTERGREEN LEAF

Wintergreen, scientifically known as Gaultheria procumbens, an intriguing herb with a rich history, has been cherished for centuries by various indigenous tribes of North America. The name "wintergreen" originates from its evergreen leaves, which retain their vibrant green hue throughout the winter season, providing a delightful contrast against the snow-covered landscape. The scientific name Gaultheria procumbens pays homage to Dr. Jean-François Gaultier, an 18th-century French physician who first identified and documented the herb's use by Native Americans. Wintergreen holds a significant place in cultural practices, with its leaves used in teas, poultices, and balms for various purposes. Its captivating minty aroma has also been employed in spiritual ceremonies and rituals. Beyond its cultural significance, wintergreen found its way into the world of confections, serving as a flavoring agent in candies, chewing gums, and beverages, thanks to its pleasant taste and aromatic profile. Throughout history, wintergreen has fascinated botanists and explorers, drawing attention to its distinctive appearance and aroma. In modern times, wintergreen continues to hold its place in herbalism and aromatherapy, with its essential oil extracted for various applications.

Now, let's explore ten extensive health and longevity benefits associated with wintergreen leaf:

1. **Headache Relief:** Methyl salicylate is a natural analgesic that acts as a counterirritant, producing a cooling effect when applied topically to the skin. When wintergreen leaf extract is used, the methyl salicylate is absorbed through the skin and works to reduce pain sensations associated with headaches and migraines. Headaches often result from tension and constriction of blood vessels in the head and neck region. Methyl salicylate, with its cooling effect, helps to relax tense muscles in the area, promoting increased blood flow and relieving the constriction of blood vessels. This increased blood flow can alleviate the pressure and tension that contribute to headache symptoms, leading to relief.
2. **Pain Relief:** Wintergreen leaf contains methyl salicylate, a natural analgesic that provides relief from pain and inflammation. Methyl salicylate acts as a counterirritant, producing a cooling effect on the skin and reducing pain sensations, making it beneficial for conditions such as arthritis, muscle aches, and headaches.

3. **Anti-inflammatory Effects:** The presence of methyl salicylate in wintergreen leaf also offers potent anti-inflammatory properties. It inhibits the production of inflammatory mediators, helping reduce inflammation in the body and providing relief from conditions like rheumatoid arthritis and inflammatory bowel disease.
4. **Acne Support:** Methyl salicylate acts as an anti-inflammatory and antimicrobial agent. Its anti-inflammatory properties help soothe skin irritation and redness, making it beneficial for individuals dealing with acne or other inflammatory skin conditions. Its antimicrobial activity helps inhibit the growth of acne-causing bacteria, contributing to a reduction in acne breakouts.
5. **Respiratory Health:** Methyl salicylate acts as an expectorant, meaning it helps promote the clearance of mucus from the respiratory passages. When individuals experience respiratory issues like coughs, congestion, or bronchitis, excess mucus can accumulate in the airways, leading to discomfort and difficulty breathing. Methyl salicylate works by thinning the mucus, making it easier to expel from the lungs, and facilitating a more productive cough. Wintergreen leaf contains other supportive constituents that contribute to its respiratory benefits. For instance, the herb contains essential oils like alpha-pinene and eucalyptol, which are known for their respiratory benefits. Alpha-pinene has been shown to have bronchodilator properties, which help relax and widen the airways, facilitating easier breathing. Eucalyptol, on the other hand, has mucolytic properties, meaning it can break down and dissolve mucus, aiding in its expulsion.
6. **Digestive Health:** Methyl salicylate acts as a carminative by relaxing the smooth muscles in the digestive tract, allowing trapped gas to be released more easily. This can provide relief from symptoms such as bloating, indigestion, and cramps. In addition to methyl salicylate, wintergreen leaf contains other supportive constituents such as alpha-pinene, beta-pinene, and limonene, which also possess mild carminative and anti-inflammatory properties. These compounds can further aid in soothing the gastrointestinal tract and easing digestive discomfort.
7. **Joint Pain Relief:** Wintergreen leaf's combination of anti-inflammatory and analgesic properties, primarily due to methyl salicylate, contributes to its benefits for arthritis. It helps reduce joint pain, swelling, and stiffness associated with various forms of arthritis.

8. **Antimicrobial Effects:** Methyl salicylate exhibits broad-spectrum antimicrobial properties, acting against various bacteria and fungi. Its antibacterial effects help inhibit the growth of harmful bacteria, including strains associated with infections such as Staphylococcus aureus and Escherichia coli.
9. **Cognitive Support:** When individuals inhale the aromatic compounds present in wintergreen leaf, such as methyl salicylate, these compounds interact with the olfactory system. The olfactory system is closely linked to the brain's limbic system, which plays a crucial role in regulating emotions, memory, and cognitive functions. The refreshing and invigorating scent of wintergreen leaf, thanks to methyl salicylate, can activate the limbic system, leading to increased alertness and mental clarity. This may help improve focus and concentration, making it beneficial for tasks that require sustained attention and mental acuity.
10. **Astringent Effects:** When applied to the skin, methyl salicylate causes vasoconstriction, which is the narrowing of blood vessels. This narrowing reduces blood flow to the skin's surface, leading to a temporary tightening of the skin and pores. The astringent properties of wintergreen can be particularly beneficial for individuals with oily or acne-prone skin. By tightening the pores, it helps to regulate excess sebum production and minimizes the appearance of pores, giving the skin a smoother and more refined look. The astringent action may help reduce redness and inflammation associated with certain skin conditions. Apart from methyl salicylate, wintergreen also contains other supportive constituents that contribute to its astringent properties. These include tannins, which are natural plant compounds known for their astringent effects. Tannins can further enhance the skin-tightening and toning effects of wintergreen when applied topically.

While wintergreen leaf is generally considered safe to consume, there are important medical contradictions and drug interactions to be aware of. Wintergreen contains methyl salicylate, which is chemically similar to aspirin, and excessive use or ingestion of wintergreen products could lead to salicylate toxicity, especially in individuals with a history of aspirin sensitivity, bleeding disorders, or those taking blood-thinning medications like warfarin. Wintergreen should be avoided by individuals with known allergies to salicylates or aspirin, as it may trigger allergic reactions. Wintergreen belongs to the Ericaceae family, which includes other plants like cranberry, blueberry, and rhododendron; individuals with known allergies to these plants should also exercise caution when using wintergreen. Pregnant and lactating individuals should avoid large quantities of wintergreen as methyl salicylate can cross the placenta and may be excreted in breast milk, potentially posing risks to the developing fetus or nursing baby. Women who are pregnant or lactating should consult with their herbalist/practitioner prior to using this herb to ensure safe quantities are being used.

WITCH HAZEL BARK

Witch hazel bark, scientifically known as Hamamelis virginiana, boasts a rich history and fascinating origin. Native to North America, this remarkable herb has held a prominent place in the medicinal practices of various indigenous cultures for centuries. The Native American tribes, particularly the Algonquian people, utilized witch hazel bark as a traditional remedy to address a diverse range of ailments. The name "witch hazel" itself is said to have originated from the Old English word "wych" or "wyche," meaning "bendable," which refers to the plant's flexible branches. The unique characteristic of witch hazel lies in its peculiar flowering time. Unlike most plants that bloom during spring or summer, witch hazel flowers grace the autumn landscape, blooming from late September to November, even after their leaves have fallen. This phenomenon has earned it the moniker "the last flower of fall." The herb's distinctive ability to produce bright yellow flowers during this season has enchanted many nature enthusiasts. In addition to its medicinal use, witch hazel bark was also embraced for its astringent properties and applied topically for various skincare purposes, making it a staple in the world of natural beauty.

Now, let's explore ten extensive health and longevity benefits associated with witch hazel bark:

1. **Astringent Effects:** The beneficial effects of witch hazel bark when applied to the skin topically are attributed to its rich composition of tannins such as hamamelitannin and proanthocyanidins, which act as natural astringents by constricting the skin's tissues and reducing excess oil production.
2. **Anti-inflammatory Effects:** The topical anti-inflammatory action of witch hazel bark, attributed to its gallic acid and proanthocyanidins content, plays a vital role in alleviating skin irritation, reducing redness, and soothing conditions such as eczema, psoriasis, and dermatitis. Gallic acid, known for its potent anti-inflammatory properties, helps to calm and soothe inflamed skin when applied topically. Similarly, proanthocyanidins contribute to this effect by providing additional antioxidant support, reducing oxidative stress on the skin, and promoting overall skin health. Together, these constituents in witch hazel bark offer a holistic approach to skincare, making it a valuable natural remedy for various inflammatory skin conditions.

3. **Wound Healing:** When topically applied, the constituents present in witch hazel bark, including tannins, act as astringents, causing the tightening of blood vessels around the wound, reducing bleeding, and promoting the formation of a protective barrier. This aids in clot formation and minimizes the risk of infection. Witch hazel bark's anti-inflammatory properties help soothe the wounded area, reducing redness and swelling, which is vital for the healing process. The bark's antioxidant effects are attributed to its flavonoids and gallic acid content, contributing to cell repair and regeneration and accelerating the formation of new skin tissue.
4. **Antimicrobial Effects:** The bark contains compounds such as tannins, gallic acid, and proanthocyanidins, which contribute to its antimicrobial properties. As a topical preparation, these compounds work synergistically to combat bacteria and fungi on the skin, making witch hazel bark effective in treating minor cuts, scrapes, and other skin infections. The antimicrobial action helps inhibit the growth of harmful microorganisms, reducing the risk of infection and promoting the natural healing process for various skin issues.
5. **Hemorrhoid Relief:** Witch hazel bark contains tannins that play a significant role in providing topical relief from hemorrhoidal discomfort. These tannins have astringent properties that help constrict blood vessels and reduce swelling, thereby alleviating the symptoms associated with hemorrhoids. Witch hazel bark contains flavonoids, which exhibit anti-inflammatory effects, further aiding in the reduction of inflammation and soothing the affected area. Additionally, the presence of gallic acid in witch hazel bark contributes to tissue healing and repair due to its antioxidant properties.
6. **Scalp Health:** Witch hazel bark, when incorporated into hair care products, can play a pivotal role in maintaining a healthy scalp. This is due to its ability to balance the scalp's oil production, alleviate itchiness, and promote a more favorable scalp environment. Witch hazel bark contains several constituents that support these claims, including tannins, which contribute to its astringent properties and help regulate oil production on the scalp. This aids in managing excess oiliness or dryness, promoting a balanced scalp. The bark contains gallic acid and proanthocyanidins, which possess anti-inflammatory and antioxidant effects, providing relief from itchiness and creating a soothing environment for the scalp.

7. **Antioxidant Powerhouse:** Witch hazel contains several polyphenols, including hamamelitannin and tannins, which act as antioxidants for the skin when used topically. These compounds play a crucial role in protecting skin cells from oxidative damage caused by free radicals, which can contribute to premature aging and skin damage. By neutralizing free radicals, the antioxidant properties of witch hazel help maintain the skin's health and vitality, supporting a more youthful and radiant complexion.
8. **Soothing Sunburns:** Applying witch hazel bark topically may help soothe sunburns, providing relief from pain, reducing inflammation, and promoting the healing of damaged skin. Witch hazel bark contains tannins as one of its major constituents, which contribute to its astringent properties. The astringent action of tannins helps to constrict and tighten the skin, reducing inflammation and relieving pain associated with sunburns. Witch hazel bark contains gallic acid, which possesses anti-inflammatory properties that further aid in calming the skin and reducing redness caused by sunburns. The presence of gallic acid and other antioxidants in witch hazel bark helps protect the skin from oxidative stress, promoting the healing process of damaged skin cells.
9. **Varicose Veins Support:** This herb's astringent properties, attributed to tannins and gallic acid, help tighten blood vessels when used as a topical application. This topical application can help reduce blood vessel dilation and minimize the appearance of varicose veins over time (providing the liver is in a healthy, well-functioning state). The anti-inflammatory effects of gallic acid help to reduce swelling in the affected areas. By toning and constricting blood vessels while reducing inflammation, witch hazel bark may aid in improving the appearance of varicose veins.
10. **Acne Support:** Witch hazel bark's antimicrobial properties, attributed to its tannins, gallic acid, and proanthocyanidins content, make it effective in treating acne when applied topically. These compounds work synergistically to combat acne-causing bacteria and reduce inflammation in the skin. The astringent action of tannins helps tighten skin tissues, reducing excess oil production and minimizing pore size. Gallic acid's anti-inflammatory effects further soothe redness and irritation associated with acne.

Witch hazel bark is generally considered safe for external use, such as in topical skin care products and as an astringent for various skin conditions. However, it is not typically consumed as a dietary supplement or herbal remedy in the form of an oral preparation. Consuming witch hazel bark orally is not recommended, as it may contain certain compounds that can be toxic or irritating when ingested. Witch hazel products intended for external use are specially formulated and often contain a distilled extract of the plant, which is designed to be applied to the skin.

WOOD BETONY

Wood betony, scientifically known as Stachys officinalis, has a rich history and origin dating back centuries. This perennial herb is native to Europe and western Asia, where it has been revered for its various uses and intriguing folklore. In ancient times, wood betony held a reputation as a potent healing herb and was highly regarded by herbalists and traditional healers. Its historical prominence is evidenced by the inclusion of "officinalis" in its botanical name, signifying its recognized medicinal value. Wood betony was traditionally employed for various purposes and prepared in different forms to harness its unique properties. Beyond its uses, wood betony was considered a protective herb, believed to ward off evil spirits and negative energies. Its mystical associations made it an essential ingredient in various rituals and incantations.

Now, let's explore ten extensive health and longevity benefits associated with wood betony:

1. **Digestive Health:** Wood betony contains several active compounds that contribute to its digestive benefits. Its carminative properties are attributed to constituents like pinene, limonene, and cineole, which help soothe the digestive system, reduce gas, and alleviate bloating. The presence of tannins and bitter principles, such as stachydrine, supports healthy digestion by stimulating the secretion of digestive juices and enzymes, aiding in the breakdown of food and easing indigestion.
2. **Headache and Migraine Support:** The analgesic and sedative effects of wood betony can be attributed to compounds like betonicine and betaine. These constituents are believed to have calming properties that may help reduce the intensity and frequency of headaches and migraines. By promoting relaxation and reducing tension, wood betony offers potential relief from these painful conditions.
3. **Menstrual Support:** Wood betony possesses antispasmodic properties attributed to compounds like betonicine, which may aid in relaxing uterine muscles and reducing menstrual cramps. Through its ability to ease muscular tension and promote smooth muscle relaxation, wood betony offers potential relief from menstrual discomfort. This herbal remedy has been traditionally used to support women during their menstrual cycles by alleviating the intensity and duration of menstrual cramps.

4. **Cognitive Support:** Wood betony's cognitive-enhancing properties are thought to be related to its alkaloids, such as stachydrine and betaine, which have been linked to improved memory and mental clarity. This herb's flavonoids, including apigenin and luteolin, possess antioxidant properties that protect brain cells from oxidative stress, supporting overall brain health and cognitive function.
5. **Respiratory Health:** Wood betony's expectorant properties are linked to compounds like saponins and tannins. These constituents help loosen mucus and facilitate its expulsion, making it beneficial for respiratory conditions like bronchitis and coughs. Its anti-inflammatory effects, attributed to flavonoids like quercetin, may alleviate airway inflammation and improve respiratory function.
6. **Immune System Support:** Wood betony's immune-supportive effects are associated with compounds like tannins, flavonoids, and alkaloids. These constituents help enhance the body's immune response by stimulating the production and activity of immune cells, making it more effective in defending against infections and illnesses.
7. **Cardiovascular Health:** Wood betony's vasodilatory effects are attributed to flavonoids, particularly apigenin and luteolin, which help relax blood vessels, improve blood flow, and lower blood pressure. The presence of minerals like potassium and magnesium further supports cardiovascular health by regulating fluid balance and promoting proper muscle function within blood vessel walls.
8. **Liver Health:** Wood betony's hepatoprotective properties are attributed to its constituents, namely flavonoids and tannins, that are thought to aid in detoxifying the liver and improving its function. Flavonoids are known for their antioxidant effects, helping to neutralize harmful free radicals that may damage liver cells. Tannins, on the other hand, possess astringent properties that aid in tightening and strengthening liver tissues.
9. **Sleep Support:** Wood betony's ability to improve sleep quality is attributed to its sedative and calming effects, primarily influenced by the presence of compounds such as betaine and betonicine. These constituents work synergistically to induce relaxation and tranquility, making wood betony a potential natural sleep aid. Betaine and betonicine act on the central nervous system, promoting a sense of calmness and reducing anxiety.

10. **Anxiety and Stress Relief:** Wood betony's anxiolytic effects can be attributed to its bioactive compounds, such as aucubin and betaine, which may help reduce anxiety and nervousness. By promoting a sense of calm and relaxation, wood betony can be a natural remedy for alleviating stress and tension.

> While wood betony is generally considered safe to consume, there are certain medical contradictions and warnings that should be considered. Wood betony may interact with certain medications, including anticoagulants or antiplatelet drugs, such as warfarin or aspirin, due to its potential to possess mild anticoagulant properties. Individuals with low blood pressure or those taking medications for hypertension should avoid wood betony, as it may have hypotensive effects and potentially lower blood pressure further. Individuals with known allergies or sensitivities to plants in the Lamiaceae family, such as mint, basil, and oregano, should exercise caution when consuming wood betony. Women who are pregnant or lactating should consult with their herbalist/practitioner prior to using this herb.

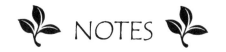

NOTES

WORMWOOD

Wormwood, scientifically known as Artemisia absinthium, boasts a rich history and intriguing origin that spans centuries. This perennial herb has deep-rooted historical significance, dating back to ancient civilizations. Wormwood's name is believed to have originated from its use in ancient times to expel intestinal worms, highlighting one of its traditional medicinal applications. The herb is famously associated with the production of the infamous spirit "absinthe," a highly alcoholic beverage known for its potent green color and alleged hallucinogenic effects. In the 19th and early 20th centuries, absinthe gained notoriety among artists, writers, and bohemian circles, leading to its eventual ban in several countries due to concerns about its safety and potential for addiction. Wormwood's association with absinthe also gave rise to the nickname "Green Fairy." Beyond its connections to absinthe, wormwood has been valued for its aromatic and culinary uses in various cultures. It was used as a flavoring agent in ancient Greek wines and is still occasionally employed today in some traditional cuisines for its distinct bitter taste. Throughout history, wormwood has also been recognized for its purported medicinal properties, finding applications in traditional medicine for digestive issues and other ailments.

Now, let's explore ten extensive health and longevity benefits associated with wormwood:

1. **Digestive Health:** Wormwood stimulates digestion by promoting the production of digestive juices and enzymes. The constituents responsible for these effects include bitter compounds such as absinthin and sesquiterpene lactones. These bitter constituents effectively promote the release of essential gastric juices, including hydrochloric acid, which is crucial for proper digestion and appetite stimulation. By encouraging the production of digestive enzymes and gastric juices, wormwood supports the breakdown of food and facilitates nutrient absorption, contributing to improved digestive efficiency and overall digestive health.
2. **Anxiety and Stress Relief:** Wormwood contains constituents, thujone and chamazulene. Thujone acts as a mild sedative, helping to alleviate feelings of restlessness and nervous tension. Chamazulene, with its anti-inflammatory properties, may contribute to reducing stress-related inflammation in the body, promoting a sense of tranquility.

3. **Bile Flow Stimulation:** This herb contains active constituents such as sesquiterpene lactones, flavonoids, and essential oils, which contribute to its bile-stimulating effects. The sesquiterpene lactones, especially absinthin, is believed to be the primary compound responsible for promoting bile secretion. When wormwood is ingested or prepared as an herbal remedy, these constituents work together to support the liver's function, enhance bile production, and facilitate the breakdown of fats and detoxification processes in the body.
4. **Fever Support:** The active constituents in wormwood responsible for these effects include cineole, camphor, and borneol. These compounds help to loosen and expel mucus from the respiratory passages, making it easier to breathe and relieving congestion. Wormwood's anti-inflammatory properties may help reduce inflammation in the airways, further contributing to respiratory relief.
5. **Respiratory Health:** The active constituents in wormwood responsible for these effects include cineole, camphor, and borneol. These compounds help to loosen and expel mucus from the respiratory passages, making it easier to breathe and relieving congestion. Wormwood's anti-inflammatory properties may help reduce inflammation in the airways, further contributing to respiratory relief.
6. **Menstrual Support:** Sesquiterpene lactones, flavonoids, and essential oils found in wormwood are thought to play a role in its therapeutic effects on menstrual health. Sesquiterpene lactones are believed to have anti-inflammatory properties that may help reduce uterine muscle contractions and ease menstrual pain. Flavonoids found in wormwood, such as quercetin, are known for their antioxidant and hormone-modulating effects, which could contribute to hormonal balance.
7. **Skin Health:** Topical application of wormwood extracts may provide benefits for skin health due to the presence of sesquiterpene lactones, flavonoids, and essential oils. The sesquiterpene lactones, including artemisinin, exhibit anti-inflammatory properties, which may help soothe skin irritations and reduce redness. Flavonoids, such as quercetin, possess antioxidant activity, supporting the skin's defense against free radicals and promoting a healthier complexion. Additionally, wormwood's essential oils offer antiseptic properties that aid in wound healing by protecting against infections.

8. **Anti-inflammatory Effects:** Sesquiterpene lactones, flavonoids, and coumarins are bioactive compounds that work together to inhibit inflammatory pathways and modulate the body's immune response, thereby helping to alleviate inflammation-related symptoms and improve overall well-being.
9. **Immune System Support:** Sesquiterpene lactones such as artemisinin, and flavonoids, along with essential oils in wormwood are believed to possess immune-stimulating properties. These constituents may enhance the body's natural defense mechanisms, supporting overall immune system health. Artemisinin, in particular, has gained attention for its potential immunomodulatory effects.
10. **Antimicrobial Effects:** Thujone has been shown to exhibit antibacterial and antifungal effects against various pathogens, including Escherichia coli, Staphylococcus aureus, and Aspergillus species. Wormwood contains other bioactive compounds, such as artemisinin, flavonoids, and phenolic acids, which contribute to its antimicrobial activity. Artemisinin, in particular, has been extensively studied for its potent antiparasitic and antimalarial effects.

> While wormwood is generally considered safe to consume when used in mindful amounts, there are several medical contradictions and drug interactions that need to be taken into account. Wormwood should be avoided by individuals with epilepsy or seizure disorders due to its potential to trigger seizures. It may also interact with anticoagulant medications, such as warfarin, leading to an increased risk of bleeding. Additionally, people with liver diseases should exercise caution and consult with their healthcare provider before using wormwood. Allergy-wise, individuals with allergies to plants in the Asteraceae family, such as ragweed, daisies, or marigolds, may also be sensitive to wormwood and should avoid its use. It is important to note that wormwood contains thujone, a compound that can be toxic in high doses over prolonged periods. As for pregnancy and lactation, wormwood is not recommended, as it may cause uterine contractions and potentially harm the developing fetus.

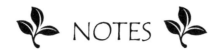
NOTES

YARROW

Yarrow, scientifically known as Achillea millefolium, boasts a rich history and fascinating origin that spans millennia. This herb holds deep cultural significance and has been revered by various civilizations throughout history. Yarrow's history can be traced back to ancient times when it was a revered plant by the ancient Greeks, Egyptians, and Chinese. The name "Achillea" is attributed to the legendary Greek hero Achilles, who, according to mythology, used yarrow to heal the wounds of his soldiers on the battlefield. The species name "millefolium" comes from the Latin words "mille" (thousand) and "folium" (leaf), referencing the herb's finely divided feathery leaves, a distinctive characteristic of the plant. Yarrow has been regarded as a sacred herb by some Native American tribes, who used it in various ceremonial rituals. This hardy and versatile herb is native to regions of Asia, Europe, and North America, where it thrives in meadows, pastures, and along roadsides. Yarrow's unique and fun characteristic is its traditional use in divination practices; the ancient Chinese I Ching oracle system employed yarrow stalks to provide insight and guidance.

Now, let's explore ten extensive health and longevity benefits associated with yarrow:

1. **Digestive Health:** Yarrow's bitter constituents, including sesquiterpene lactones like achillin and lactucopicrin, stimulate digestive juices and enhance appetite. Yarrow also contains flavonoids like apigenin and luteolin, which possess anti-inflammatory properties, soothing inflamed tissues in the digestive tract and alleviating issues such as indigestion, bloating, and cramps. Yarrow's essential oils, such as chamazulene and borneol, help increase bile production, aiding in the breakdown of fats and the absorption of nutrients, thus promoting proper nutrient absorption and bowel regularity.
2. **Cardiovascular Health:** Yarrow's potential benefits for cardiovascular health are attributed to compounds like flavonoids, particularly rutin, which may help improve blood circulation and reduce blood pressure. Yarrow contains alkaloids like achilleine, which may have vasodilatory effects, potentially supporting cardiovascular function. The presence of antioxidants in yarrow, such as caffeic acid and quercetin, may contribute to reducing oxidative stress and aiding in maintaining healthy blood vessels and cholesterol levels.

3. **Immune System Support:** Yarrow's immune-boosting properties can be attributed to its active compounds, which include flavonoids, such as quercetin and rutin, and antioxidants, like caffeic acid and coumarins. These compounds have been shown to have antimicrobial, antiviral, and anti-inflammatory effects, supporting the immune system's ability to fight off infections and reduce inflammation, thereby enhancing overall immune function.
4. **Respiratory Health:** Active compounds like cineole and camphor found in yarrow essential oil help loosen mucus, facilitating its expulsion and providing relief from coughs and congestion. This herb's anti-inflammatory effects, attributed to compounds like sesquiterpenes and flavonoids, further contribute to respiratory comfort and clearer breathing.
5. **Wound Healing:** Yarrow contains essential oils like chamazulene and thujone, which provide antiseptic benefits, helping cleanse wounds and prevent infections. Yarrow's tannins, flavonoids, and phenolic acids, including salicylic acid and gallic acid, contribute to its astringent properties, promoting blood clotting and facilitating the healing process of wounds.
6. **Anti-inflammatory Effects:** Yarrow's anti-inflammatory properties may provide relief from various inflammatory conditions such as arthritis, rheumatism, and inflammatory bowel disease. This herb's flavonoids, including apigenin and luteolin and sesquiterpene lactones like achillin, exhibit anti-inflammatory effects, reducing pain, swelling, and inflammation associated with these conditions, thereby improving overall comfort and mobility.
7. **Skin Health:** Yarrow's antimicrobial and anti-inflammatory properties make it beneficial for maintaining healthy skin. The presence of compounds like camphor and borneol in its essential oils contributes to its antimicrobial effects, helping to alleviate skin conditions like acne and soothe irritation. Flavonoids, such as apigenin and luteolin, along with tannins, provide anti-inflammatory relief, promoting skin rejuvenation and overall skin health.
8. **Mood Support:** Yarrow has calming and relaxant properties attributed to compounds like sesquiterpene lactones and flavonoids, which may help relieve anxiety, stress, and tension. These compounds contribute to promoting relaxation, improving sleep quality, and reducing symptoms of mood disorders, potentially enhancing mental well-being.

9. **Menstrual Support:** Yarrow contains flavonoids, including apigenin and luteolin, which possess antispasmodic properties. These compounds help relax the uterine muscles and ease the intensity of menstrual cramps by inhibiting the release of certain chemicals that trigger muscle contractions. Yarrow's tannins, such as catechins, contribute to its astringent properties, aiding in regulating menstrual flow by constricting blood vessels and reducing excessive bleeding. Sesquiterpene lactones, such as achillin, also support this effect by providing anti-inflammatory relief during menstruation.
10. **Urinary Tract Health:** Yarrow's diuretic properties are attributed to compounds such as flavonoids, phenolic acids, and essential oils. These constituents help increase urine production and promote the flushing out of toxins, potentially reducing the risk of urinary tract infections and supporting overall urinary tract health.

While yarrow is generally considered safe to consume, there are a few important warnings and contradictions to consider. It is important to note that yarrow can interact with certain medications, particularly blood-thinning medications like warfarin and may increase the risk of bleeding. Therefore, individuals taking such medications should exercise caution and consult with their healthcare provider before incorporating yarrow into their regimen. People with kidney disorders should use caution when using yarrow, as its diuretic properties may increase urine output and could potentially impact kidney function. Individuals with known allergies to plants in the Asteraceae family, such as ragweed or daisies, may also be sensitive to yarrow and should avoid its use. As for pregnancy and lactation, yarrow is not recommended for use during these periods, as it may stimulate uterine contractions and potentially lead to miscarriage. Nursing mothers should avoid yarrow unless otherwise specified by their herbalist/practitioner.

NOTES

YELLOW DOCK

Yellow dock, scientifically known as Rumex crispus, boasts a fascinating history and origin deeply rooted in ancient civilizations. This herb has a rich historical background that spans continents, with its origins believed to lie in Europe, North Africa, and parts of Asia. Its use dates back thousands of years, and it holds cultural significance among Native American tribes and early European settlers. Yellow dock has a distinctive appearance with its long, lance-shaped leaves and tall flower spikes, which can grow up to four feet in height. Interestingly, the leaves are known to taste sour and slightly astringent, leading some to refer to the herb as "sour dock." Native Americans used yellow dock for various purposes, including as a food source due to its nutritious leaves and as a traditional medicinal herb for its potential health benefits. Early European settlers brought yellow dock to North America, where it became naturalized and continued to be embraced for its herbal properties.

Now, let's explore ten extensive health and longevity benefits associated with yellow dock:

1. **Bile Stimulation:** Yellow dock stimulates bile production, promoting digestive health. It contains anthraquinone glycosides, including emodin and chrysophanol, known for their digestive benefits. These compounds enhance the breakdown of fats and aid in digestion by promoting bile production and flow, supporting overall digestive well-being.
2. **Blood Cleansing:** The herb exhibits blood-purifying properties, assisting in the elimination of toxins and impurities from the bloodstream. It contains anthraquinones, such as emodin and rhein, which may support healthy blood circulation and help cleanse the blood of toxins.
3. **Hair and Scalp Health:** Yellow dock offers benefits for both internal and topical applications when it comes to hair and scalp health. Internally, its antioxidant properties help protect hair follicles from oxidative damage, contributing to stronger and healthier hair growth. By reducing oxidative stress within the body, yellow dock supports the overall vitality of hair. Topically, yellow dock can be applied to the scalp to soothe and nourish it, potentially alleviating scalp conditions like itching and irritation. The anti-inflammatory effects of yellow dock can provide relief for those experiencing discomfort on the scalp, promoting an environment conducive to healthy hair growth.

4. **Skin Health:** Yellow dock has a long history of traditional use in addressing various skin conditions, such as eczema, psoriasis, and acne, dating back centuries. Its therapeutic effects are attributed to its anti-inflammatory and antioxidant properties, which contribute to its potential in reducing skin inflammation, itchiness, and redness. The constituents that support these claims include anthraquinone glycosides (such as emodin and chrysophanol), tannins, and flavonoids. Anthraquinone glycosides exhibit anti-inflammatory properties that may help soothe irritated skin and alleviate symptoms of skin conditions. Tannins, on the other hand, provide astringent effects, which can tighten and protect the skin. Flavonoids act as antioxidants, scavenging free radicals and protecting the skin from oxidative stress.
5. **Iron Absorption:** This plant supports the body's ability to absorb and utilize iron effectively. Among its constituents, yellow dock contains iron, calcium, vitamin C, emodin, and chrysophanol. Iron is essential for the production of hemoglobin, which carries oxygen in the blood. Calcium is known to enhance iron absorption, and vitamin C aids in converting non-heme iron (the form found in plant-based foods) into a more absorbable form. Additionally, emodin and chrysophanol, two bioactive compounds found in yellow dock, have been shown to influence iron metabolism positively. By providing this combination of beneficial constituents, yellow dock can contribute to improved iron absorption and overall iron status in the body, making it a potentially effective and natural option for individuals seeking ways to address iron deficiency anemia.
6. **Joint Health:** This herb's anti-inflammatory properties may help reduce swelling and discomfort, ultimately promoting improved joint mobility and flexibility. The anthraquinone glycosides act as anti-inflammatory agents, helping to mitigate inflammation in the joints and surrounding tissues. Tannins also contribute to the herb's anti-inflammatory effects, while flavonoids exhibit antioxidant activity, protecting the joints from oxidative stress and potential damage.
7. **Liver Health:** Yellow dock is rich in anthraquinone glycosides, particularly emodin and chrysophanol, which are known for their hepatoprotective properties. These compounds aid in detoxification processes by supporting the liver's ability to metabolize and eliminate toxins from the body, promoting overall liver health.

8. **Respiratory Health:** Yellow dock possesses expectorant properties that may help alleviate respiratory congestion and promote healthy lung function. It may provide relief from coughs, bronchitis, and other respiratory conditions. The primary constituent responsible for these effects is a compound called emodin, which acts as an expectorant, helping to loosen and expel mucus from the respiratory tract. Yellow dock contains anthraquinone glycosides, flavonoids, and tannins which contribute to its overall therapeutic properties for respiratory health. The expectorant action of emodin, combined with the antioxidant and anti-inflammatory effects of the other constituents, supports respiratory comfort and aids in clearing the airways, making yellow dock a valuable herb for respiratory well-being.
9. **Antioxidant Powerhouse:** Yellow dock contains antioxidants, such as flavonoids like quercetin and kaempferol, which work synergistically to neutralize harmful free radicals and prevent cellular damage. Additionally, yellow dock contains anthraquinone compounds, including emodin and chrysophanol, which exhibit antioxidant activity. These compounds help scavenge free radicals and reduce oxidative stress, leading to improved cellular function, reduced inflammation, and enhanced overall health. The combination of flavonoids and anthraquinones contributes to yellow dock's potent antioxidant properties, which play a crucial role in protecting cells and tissues from oxidative damage and supporting general well-being.
10. **Immune System Support:** Yellow dock is rich in various phytochemicals, including anthraquinone glycosides, tannins, and flavonoids, which could potentially play a role in supporting immune function. These compounds might stimulate the immune response, aiding the body in combating infections and illnesses more effectively. By bolstering the body's natural defense mechanisms, yellow dock may help strengthen the immune system.

While yellow dock is generally considered safe to consume, there are some medical contradictions and drug interactions to be aware of. The herb may interact with certain medications, including blood thinners like warfarin, as yellow dock contains vitamin K, which could interfere with the anticoagulant effects. People taking diuretic medications should also be cautious, as yellow dock has natural diuretic properties and could potentially lead to excessive fluid loss. Yellow dock's potential effects on blood clotting and platelet function may pose risks during and after surgical procedures. It is recommended to discontinue yellow dock use at least two weeks before any scheduled surgery. Allergy-wise, individuals sensitive to plants in the Polygonaceae family, such as buckwheat or rhubarb, may also be at risk of developing an allergic reaction to yellow dock. Pregnant and breastfeeding individuals should avoid yellow dock unless otherwise stipulated by their herbalist/ practitioner.

WHY NO INDEX?

In this herbal textbook, you will notice the absence of an index, and that is intentional. This book is *not* intended to serve as a diagnostic tool; it's not a protocol book nor a guide for treating specific symptoms or medical conditions. Instead, its purpose is to provide comprehensive, educational, and insightful information about all the plant medicine I have in my herbal pantry. In this textbook, the goal is to empower you, the reader, by presenting you with my botanical longevity tools, their properties, historical uses, and potential health benefits. Through these insights, you'll gain a deeper understanding of the medicinal herbs I have in my longevity toolkit, and become familiar with various plant constituents and their supportive roles in the human body. This herbal textbook encourages curiosity and exploration, fostering a respectful and responsible approach to herbalism. As you delve into the pages, you'll find a wealth of knowledge to enrich your understanding of these medicinal herbs, supporting your journey toward greater herbal literacy and appreciation. Remember, always seek the guidance of your trusted herbalist or practitioner for personalized treatment plans and the safe use of herbal preparations and remedies for specific health concerns.

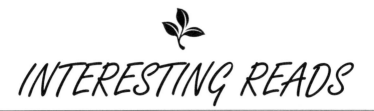

INTERESTING READS

Advanced Herbal Pharmacy: The Practitioner's Guide to Preparation, Formulation and Compounding, 2020
Scripta Rustica

American Herbal Pharmacopoeia: Botanical Pharmacognosy - Microscopic Characterization of Botanical Medicines, 2016
Roy Upton, Alison Graff, Georgina Jolliffe, Reinhard Länger, Elizabeth Williamson

American Herbal Products Association: Botanical Safety Handbook, 2013
Zoë Gardner, Michael McGuffin

Ayurvedic Herbs: A Clinical Guide to the Healing Plants of Traditional Indian Medicine, 2012
M.S Premila

Botanical Medicine Manual, 2019
Dr. Marisa Marciano, Dr. Nikita Vizniak

Encyclopedia of Herbal Medicine: 550 Herbs and Remedies for Common Ailments, 2016
Andrew Chevallier

Essentials of Botanical Extraction: Principles and Applications, 2015
Subhash C. Mandal, Vivekananda Mandal, Anup Kumar Das

Health from God's Garden: Herbal Remedies for Glowing Health and Well-Being, 1987
Maria Treben

Health Through God's Pharmacy: Advice and Proven Cures with Medicinal Herbs, 2017
Maria Treben

Healing Adaptogens: The Definitive Guide to Using Super Herbs and Mushrooms for Your Body's Restoration, Defense, and Performance, 2022
Tero Isokauppila, Danielle Ryan Broida

Healing Plants of the Celtic Druids: Ancient Celts in Britain and their Druid Healers Used Plant Medicine to Treat the Mind, Body and Soul, 2018
Angela Paine

Herbal Antibiotics, 2nd Edition: Natural Alternatives for Treating Drug-resistant Bacteria, 2012
Stephen Harrod Buhner

Herbal Antibiotics: What BIG Pharma Doesn't Want You to Know - How to Pick and Use the 45 Most Powerful Herbal Antibiotics for Overcoming Any Ailment, 2017
Mary Jones

Herbal Antivirals, 2nd Edition: Natural Remedies for Emerging & Resistant Viral Infections, 2021
Stephen Harrod Buhner

Herbal Constituents, 2nd Edition: Foundations of Phytochemistry, 2021
Lisa Ganora

Herbal Contradictions and Drug Interactions: Plus Herbal Adjuncts with Medicines, 4th Edition, 2010
Francis Brinker

Herbal Formularies for Health Professionals, Volume 5: Immunology, Orthopedics, and Otolaryngology, including Allergies, the Immune System, the Musculoskeletal System, and the Eyes, Ears, Nose, Mouth, and Throat, 2021
Dr. Jill Stansbury

Medical Herbalism: The Science Principles and Practices of Herbal Medicine, 2003
David Hoffmann

Native American Herbalism for Beginners of Natural Remedies:
A 7 Simple Chapter Herbal Medicine Book
With 100 Native American Herbs, 2022
Kit Nick Herb

Native Americtheir herbalist's Bible - 14 Books in 1: 500+ Ancient
Herbal Remedies to Improve Your Wellness Naturally.
Create Your Own Herbal Dispensatory and Unleash
the Secret Power of Plants, 2022
Amayeta Acothley

Native Americtheir herbalist's Bible: 10 Books in 1 -
The Encyclopedia to Build Your Home-Based Herb Lab
& Increase Your Longevity & Quality of Life with Ancient Practices
& Natural Herbal Preparations, 2022
Vanessa Grant

Natural Healing and Medical Research:
Learn the Secrets of Natural Medicine, 2022
Evexiandros

The Encyclopedia of Medicinal Plants, 1996
Andrew Chevallier

The Green Pharmacy: The Ultimate Compendium
of Natural Remedies from the World's Foremost Authority
on Healing Herbs, 1998
James A. Duke Ph.D.

Phytochemistry and Pharmacy for Practitioners
of Botanical Medicine, 2003
Eric Yarnell

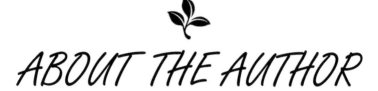

ABOUT THE AUTHOR

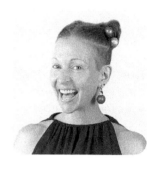

The Smile Enthusiast, affectionately known as Smile, embodies the essence of a modern-day medicine woman who, through her own will and determination, reversed all of her chronic symptoms and conditions using plant-forward, grassroots healing practices. Smile's journey to wellness was not driven by supplement-heavy healing protocols.

Smile, a woman who dances to the beat of her own drum, believes in genuine enlightenment through continuous learning and personal growth, independent of formal institutions. With a decade of herbalism studies and practical experience, Smile's commitment to continuous learning empowers her to exercise discernment in making choices and decisions that she believes will optimize her health, vitality, and commitment to graceful aging throughout her journey.

As an author and advocate for longevity through the utilization of Mother Nature's resources, she passionately shares her knowledge, wisdom, and the unique lifestyle she has cultivated for herself across various social media platforms. Her authenticity and transparency have captivated the attention of women worldwide who seek to enhance their quality of life and attain better health. With her invaluable insights, she serves as a beacon of knowledge and empowerment, inspiring others to embark on transformative journeys and forge paths toward a higher quality of life.

Discover Smile's remarkable journey as she challenges conventional wisdom and explores the limits of longevity. With determination and humility, Smile has set herself a goal - to make history by becoming a Guinness World Record holder for longevity. This ambitious aspiration requires a lifelong commitment, leading to a momentous celebration on November 13, 2097, when she aims to surpass the current record holder for the oldest person ever (Jeanne Louise Calment, at the time of this book's publication). Smile's fearless pursuit exemplifies her courage, determination, and unwavering dedication to her vision. She serves as an inspiring role model, unafraid to break norms and pave her own unique path towards living her best, longest life.

At the core of her philosophy lies a powerful mantra: "I'm all about making choices and decisions today that my future self will thank me for."

Connect with me on Instagram:
@The_Smile_Enthusiast

Printed in the USA
CPSIA information can be obtained
at www.ICGtesting.com
LVHW020200190724
785891LV00002B/27